Principles of
Electronics
in
Medical Research

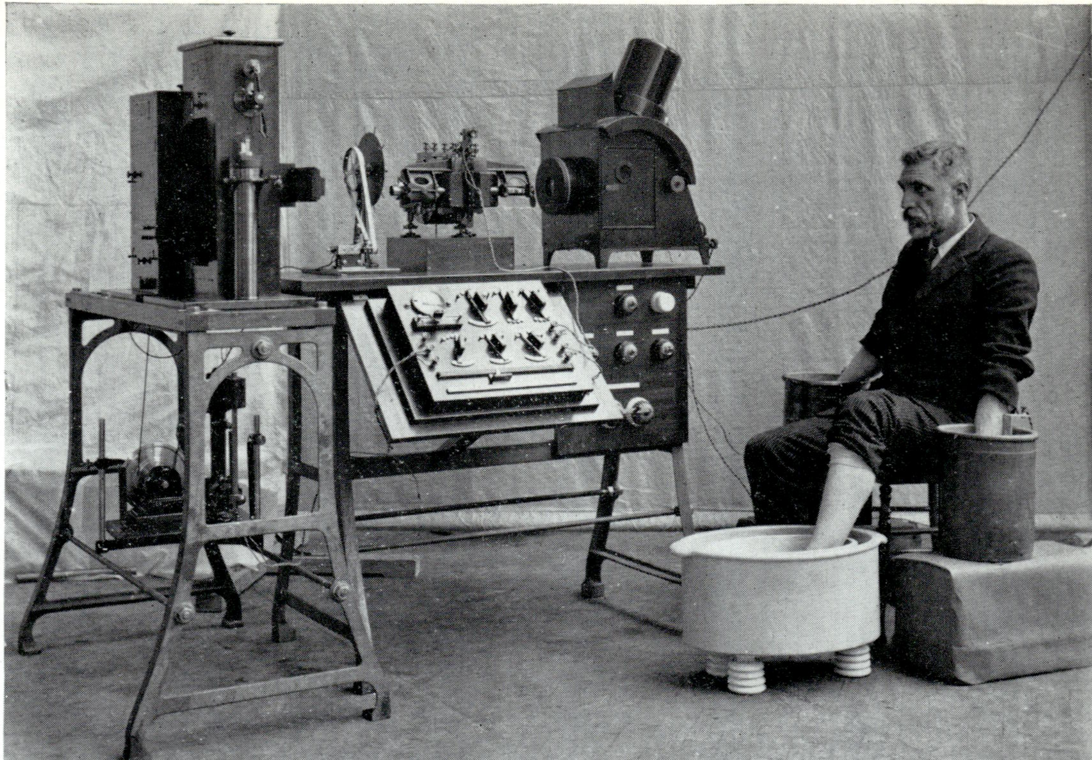

An early electrocardiograph

(By courtesy of Cambridge Instrument Co. Ltd.)

Principles of Electronics in Medical Research

D. W. HILL

M.Sc., Ph.D., F.Inst.P., F.I.E.E.

Reader in Medical Physics,
Royal College of Surgeons of England

Second Edition

LONDON
BUTTERWORTHS

ENGLAND:	BUTTERWORTH & CO. (PUBLISHERS) LTD. LONDON: 88 Kingsway, WC2B 6AB
AUSTRALIA:	BUTTERWORTHS PTY. LTD. SYDNEY: 586 Pacific Highway, 2067 MELBOURNE: 343 Little Collins Street, 3000 BRISBANE: 240 Queen Street, 4000
CANADA:	BUTTERWORTH & CO. (CANADA) LTD. TORONTO: 14 Curity Avenue, 374
NEW ZEALAND:	BUTTERWORTHS OF NEW ZEALAND LTD. WELLINGTON: 26–28 Waring Taylor Street, 1
SOUTH AFRICA:	BUTTERWORTH & CO. (SOUTH AFRICA) (PTY) LTD. DURBAN: 152–154 Gale Street

1st Edition..............1965

2nd Edition..............1973

Suggested U.D.C. Number 621·38:61

Suggested Additional Number 537:61

ISBN 0 407 36401 3

Made and printed in Great Britain at the
St Ann's Press, Park Road, Altrincham, Cheshire WA14 5QQ

Contents

Preface to the Second Edition

Since the publication of the first edition of this book seven years ago, the most important changes have been the almost complete change-over from thermionic valves to semiconductor devices and the striking impact on both analogue and digital circuitry of integrated circuits. On the one hand, this has led to an increasing awareness in medical electronics of the potential available from an association with digital computers. On the other hand, the reduction in size of equipments made possible by the use of integrated circuits has proved beneficial for apparatus associated with patients. The thin film circuitry of cardiac pacemakers can be hermetically sealed and offers a greater reliability than has been obtainable with conventional encapsulation in the past. Progress with the circuitry focuses attention on the need for reliable, longer life power supplies for implanted circuits and is leading to developments such as the lithium cell and radioactive power supplies. As new measuring and monitoring techniques are introduced, so the amount of apparatus which can be connected to a patient during a comprehensive investigation increases. This leads to an increasing possibility of the patient receiving an electric shock. As a result, the input circuitry of apparatus connected to patients is designed to be as well isolated from the mains supply and other potentially dangerous voltages as possible. It must also be able to withstand the application of a defibrillator to the patient.

The aim of this book continues to be, as in the first edition, to provide an introduction to the subject for workers in medicine and biology and to encourage them to read further and take expert advice in the particular field in which they are interested.

D.W.H.

Preface to the First Edition

The contents of this book are based on the series, 'Some Fundamentals of Medical Electronics', which appeared in the *British Journal of Anaesthesia*, and experience gained over several years of teaching scientists and doctors on the 'Laboratory Course in Medical Electronics', held at the Royal College of Surgeons of England.

Increasing instrumentation is being used in medical and biological laboratories, but many of the staff lack a basic grounding in the fundamentals of electronic engineering. When doctors are responsible for electronics staff, and for ordering equipment and spares, it is desirable that they have some knowledge of what is involved, and what the various technical terms mean, if only in outline. This applies also to technicians responsible for operating equipment in medical departments, in order to obtain the most effective functioning of the apparatus.

The basic devices and circuits are dealt with in a descriptive fashion, since a knowledge of detailed design is best left to the electronic engineer. In a single volume, it is not possible to give details of all the applications of electronic techniques in medicine. Wherever possible, references have been given for further reading, so that workers in a particular specialty can find information on techniques which will be of use to them. Counting techniques for use with radioisotopes have been deliberately excluded, since these are well covered elsewhere.

It is a pleasure to acknowledge the encouragement of the editorial staff of the *British Journal of Anaesthesia*, and of my colleagues on the staff, and many students, at the Royal College of Surgeons. Without their patient co-operation, I would not have been able to gain an appreciation of the power of modern instrumental techniques in medical research.

D.W.H.

Chapter 1

Magnetism and Electromagnetism

PERMANENT MAGNETS

The fact that an iron needle, when rubbed with a lodestone and freely suspended, acts as a compass and aligns itself in a North–South direction has been known from early times. A piece of lodestone (leading stone) can also be used as a compass, hence the name. Needham (1962) mentions a Chinese text describing the use of a magnetic needle compass as early as A.D. 1080, about a century before its first European use. The magnetic attraction of lodestone to iron was mentioned in the late third century B.C. An interesting connection between magnetism and electricity is provided by William Gilbert (1546–1603), Personal Physician to Queen Elizabeth I, who published his work *On the Magnet and on Magnetic Bodies, and concerning that great magnet the Earth, a new physiology*.

The availability of compact, powerful permanent magnets has made possible the construction of a wide range of recorders and scientific instruments. Permanent magnets are found in moving-coil galvanometers, moving-coil meters, loudspeakers, magnetic stirrers, paramagnetic oxygen analysers and mass spectrometers. In the case of recorders, whether the method of writing is ink on paper, a heated stylus, an ink jet or a light beam on photographic paper, a powerful magnet is needed. It is interesting to recall that in order to obtain a high degree of sensitivity for his experiments on animal electricity, Emil Du Bois Reymond had to wind 3·17 miles of wire on to his galvanometer coils (Bence Jones, 1852). This was before the availability of powerful magnets.

THE MAGNETIC FIELD

In the space surrounding every magnet there exists what is called a magnetic field. If a strip of magnetic material (a bar magnet) is dipped in iron filings, then the filings will be attracted to each end of the magnet. These preferred regions of attraction are called Magnetic Poles. If the magnet is freely suspended, it will take up a North–South position. The end pointing towards North is called the 'N' or north-seeking pole. The other end is the 'S' or south-seeking pole. Like magnetic poles repel and unlike poles attract each other. Two similar poles of unit strength placed one centimetre apart in a vacuum will repel each other with a force of one dyne (10^{-5} Newtons).

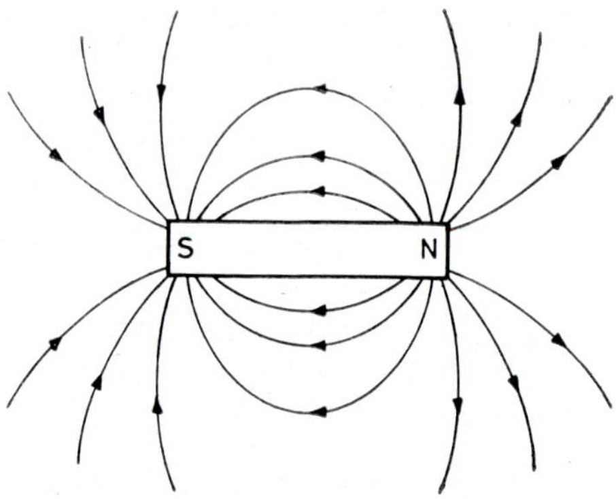

Figure 1.1. The magnetic field due to a bar magnet

If a small compass is placed at some point near the North pole of a straight bar magnet and then moved always in the direction that the compass is pointing, the centre of the compass needle will trace out a magnetic line of force. By starting at different points, many such lines may be plotted as shown in *Figure 1.1.* These magnetic lines of force do not really exist. They are simply useful devices for describing magnetic phenomena. Where the magnet exerts its strongest attraction close to the poles, the field is greatest, and the lines are closest together.

The magnets used in fast response pen recorders are shaped as in *Figure 1.2.* The magnetic field is concentrated in the gap between the pole pieces (*Figure 1.3*). In order to obtain a radial field for the coil to move in, a cylindrical iron core is placed between the poles, but this has been omitted from *Figure 1.3.* On the c.g.s. (centimetre-gramme-second) system, the strength of a magnetic field is numerically equal to the force in dynes acting on a unit pole placed at the point considered. The unit is the oersted. In a field of 5,000 oersteds, a force of 5,000 dynes would act on a unit pole placed there.

It is not often that the magnets have to be removed from the magnet block of, for example, a multi-channel pen recorder. When this happens they should be treated with respect. Dropping

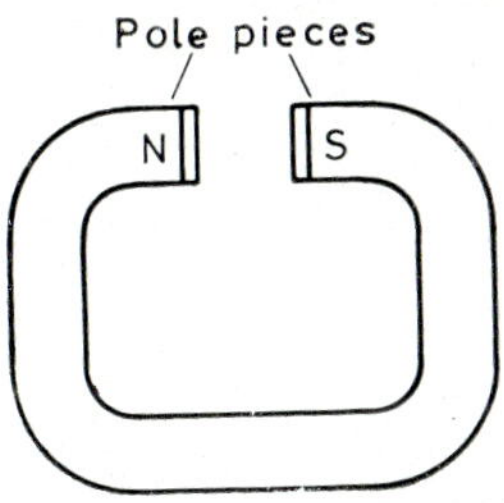

Figure 1.2. A galvanometer magnet

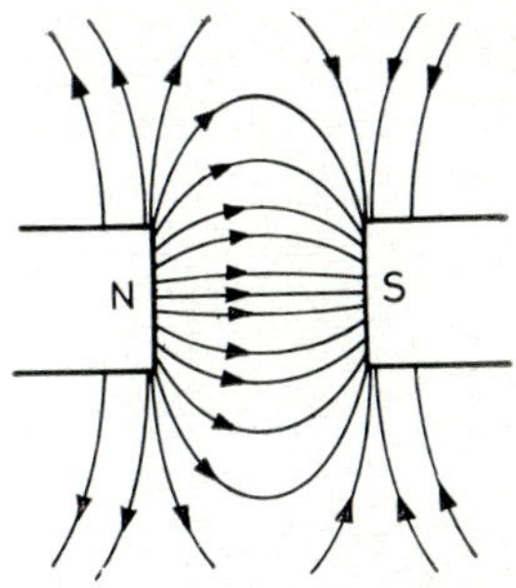

Figure 1.3. Field in the gap of a galvanometer magnet without any core present

them can reduce their strength and they can seriously upset the working of a watch that is brought too close. The use of a steel 'keeper' bar will prevent self-demagnetization which occurs when magnets are stored.

TYPES OF MAGNETISM

All materials have some magnetic property, but it is only the ferromagnetic substances such as iron, nickel and cobalt which have strong effects. Substances can be categorized as paramagnetic or diamagnetic. Paramagnetic materials will, when suspended in a magnetic field in the form of a needle-shaped specimen, align themselves along the lines of force and move to the strongest part of the field. On the other hand, diamagnetic materials under similar conditions will take up a position at right angles to the lines of force and move to the weakest part of the field. Ferromagnetic materials exhibit paramagnetism to a marked degree.

PROPERTIES OF MAGNETIC MATERIALS

Intensity of Magnetization (J)

The Magnetic Moment (M) of a magnet is given by M=Pole strength$\times$Magnetic length where the magnetic length is the distance separating the poles. If the length is measured in centimetres, then the pole strength is expressed in c.g.s. units. The

Intensity of Magnetization (J) of the material is defined as the magnetic moment per unit volume. If the cross-sectional area of the magnet is constant, the intensity of magnetization is equal to the 'pole' strength per unit area.

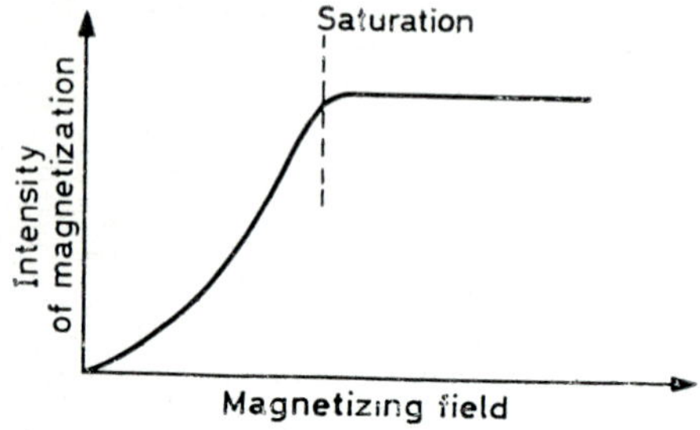

Figure 1.4. The onset of saturation in a high magnetizing field

When a magnetic material is magnetized by placing it in an increasing magnetic field, it is found that the intensity of magnetization increases to a maximum when the material becomes saturated (*Figure 1.4*).

Susceptibility (κ)

The susceptibility (κ) of a material is defined by $\kappa = J/H$ where J is the resulting intensity of magnetization when a magnetizing field H is applied. For any given field, if J is low the susceptibility is low, and if J is high the susceptibility is high.

Magnetic Induction (B)

In choosing a permanent magnet material, attention will be paid in particular to the intensity of magnetization which can be produced. For a transformer core material, the flux density (lines of

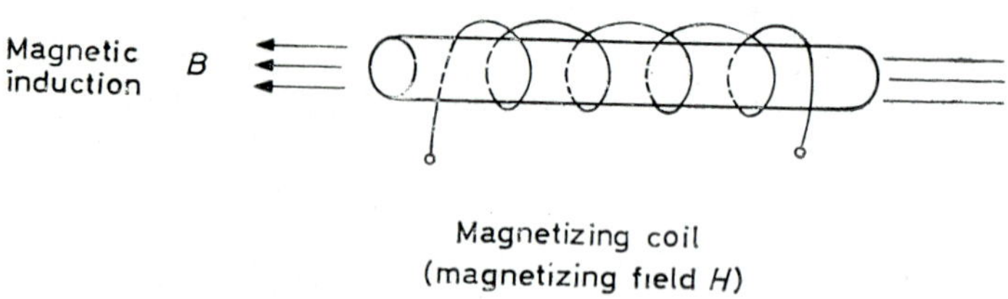

Figure 1.5. The production of an induced magnetic field by a magnetizing coil

force per unit area) that can be produced in it is important. This follows, since it is the total number of the lines that intersect a given coil which governs the e.m.f. induced in the coil. The permeability of the material is given by $\mu = B/H$ where H is the magnetizing field and B is the flux density developed in the material (*Figure 1.5*). B is in gauss on the c.g.s. system.

B–H Loop Hysteresis

On the application of a magnetizing field to a piece of unmagnetized steel, the magnetic induction increases by following the path OA in *Figure 1.6a*. When the field is reduced, the path AO is not retraced, but rather the path AD. As a result, the induction B lags behind the field H. This phenomenon is called Hysteresis. When the field is reversed, the path DEF is followed. The complete cycle is ADEFPQA. As the microscopic magnetic particles turn to follow the direction of the changing field, they encounter resistance and heat is generated. If the area enclosed by the loop is large, the hysteresis loss of energy is large. The loss is proportional to the area of the loop. The loop for a low-loss core material is compared with that for ordinary steel in *Figure 1.6b*.

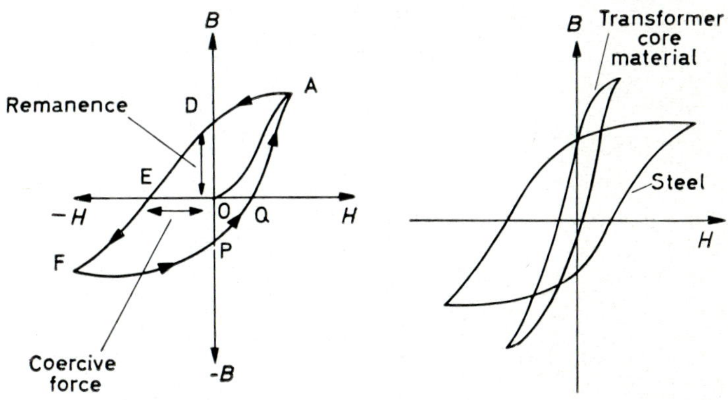

(*a*) (*b*)

Figure 1.6. (a) A typical B–H loop. (b) The B–H curves for soft iron and steel

Remanence and Coercive Force

After taking a specimen through a magnetizing cycle and removing the magnetizing field, the flux density remaining in the material is called the Remanence. The magnitude of the additional field which has to be applied in order to remove the remanence is called the coercive force. These facts are illustrated in *Figure 1.6b*. The limiting value of the coercive force is the coercivity which is the reverse field required to reduce the remanence to zero.

SOFT AND HARD MAGNETIC MATERIALS

'Soft' magnetic materials have small coercive forces and 'hard' magnetic materials have large coercive forces. Soft magnetic materials also have small loop areas and correspondingly small energy losses when they are magnetized by a cyclic procedure (*Figure 1.6b*). The commonest soft magnetic materials are soft iron and silicon–iron containing up to 4 per cent of silicon. Silicon–irons are widely used in transformer cores and the stators of electric motors. The high permeability of mumetal makes it suitable for the laminations of audio frequency transformers and for magnetic shielding. However, it is relatively expensive and requires heat treatment and careful handling. Hard magnetic materials have a large loop area and high energy losses per cycle of magnetization. Since their remanence is high and difficult to remove (high coercivity), they form good permanent magnets.

Table 1.1
Properties of Some Magnetic Materials

Material	*Maximum permeability*	*Saturation induction (gauss)*	*Coercivity (oersteds)*
Soft			
4 per cent Silicon–iron	8,000	19,500	0·6
Mumetal	80,000	8,500	0·1
Hard			
Alnico (52 per cent Fe, 12 per cent Co, 20 per cent Ni, 6 per cent Cu, 10 per cent Al)	12,000	7,000	500
Alcomax (55 per cent Fe, 8 per cent Al, 11 per cent Ni, 22 per cent Co, 4 per cent Cu)	16,000	12,500	550
Hycomax (50 per cent Fe, 9 per cent Al, 21 per cent Ni, 20 per cent Co)	14,000	9,000	850

PROPERTIES OF TRANSFORMER CORES, PERMANENT MAGNETS AND ELECTROMAGNETS

Transformer Cores

Subjected to the changing fluxes from the alternating currents in the primary winding, transformer cores are taken through many magnetizing cycles per second. Hence the core material must possess a low hysteresis loss, a high permeability (to produce a high flux density) and a high resistivity (to reduce eddy currents). Suitable alloys for the laminations are Permalloy (78 per cent Ni, 20 per cent Fe plus traces of Co and Mn) and Mumetal (78 per cent Ni, 17 per cent Fe, 5 per cent Cu plus small amounts of Cr, Si and Mn). Silicon–iron is used in the larger power frequency transformers.

Permanent Magnets

Materials for these should have a high remanence (so that a high intensity of magnetization remains on removing the magnetizing field), a high coercive force (difficult to demagnetize) and a high susceptibility (magnetized strongly by a small magnetizing field). Typical magnet alloys are Alnico (52 per cent Fe, 12 per cent Co, 6 per cent Cu, 10 per cent Al) and Ticonal (51 per cent Fe, 8 per cent Al, 13·5 per cent Ni, 24 per cent Co, 3 per cent Cu plus a trace of titanium).

Electromagnets

The core of electromagnets should have a high susceptibility at a low magnetic field intensity (so that a small magnetizing current produces a strong magnetization), a low coercive force (easy to demagnetize) and a low remanence (little magnetism left on removing the energizing field). Swedish iron makes a good electromagnet core material.

Pot Cores

Employing the techniques of powder metallurgy, it is possible to mould from ferrite material efficient core shapes for inductors and transformers for use at audio and radio frequencies. The core may be of a cylindrical shape containing an internal annular groove to hold the windings, slots being provided for the connection leads. The core is split into an upper and a lower half, which allows the winding to be inserted and the halves then clamped together. As an example, the type SA 500L ferrite material made by I.T.T. Ltd. is a low loss, low hysteresis material for use in inductors up to

300 kHz. The type SA 601 is a high stability low loss manganese–zinc ferrite for use in pulse and wideband transformer cores up to 5–10 MHz. It has a maximum permeability of 5,800, a saturation flux density of 4,200 gauss, a remanence of 900 gauss and a coercivity of 0·12 oersteds. Watkins (1971) discusses in detail the characteristics of ferrite materials.

THE BEHAVIOUR OF MAGNETIC SHIELDING

The effect of placing a piece of soft iron in a uniform magnetic field is shown in *Figure 1.7.* The soft iron is seen to have the effect of concentrating the magnetic lines of force so that they pass through the soft iron in preference to passing through the air. An alloy such as

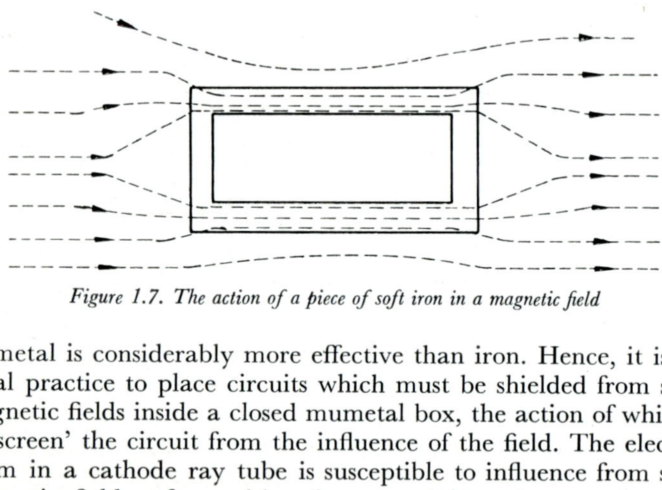

Figure 1.7. The action of a piece of soft iron in a magnetic field

mumetal is considerably more effective than iron. Hence, it is the usual practice to place circuits which must be shielded from stray magnetic fields inside a closed mumetal box, the action of which is to 'screen' the circuit from the influence of the field. The electron beam in a cathode ray tube is susceptible to influence from stray magnetic fields, often arising from a neighbouring power transformer. For this reason, the cathode ray tube gun is usually mounted inside a mumetal shield. Field (1970) gives an account of magnetic screening.

ELECTROMAGNETISM

The first discovery of any connection between electricity and magnetism was made by Hans Oersted in 1820. Oersted was born the son of an apothecary, graduated in medicine in Copenhagen, and subsequently became Professor of Physics there. He placed a current-carrying wire parallel to a magnetic compass needle and found that the needle was deflected. Soon after, Ampère found that a loop or coil of wire acted as a magnet when an electric current was passed through it. The magnetic field available was greatly increased if the coil was wound upon a soft iron core (*Figure 1.8*).

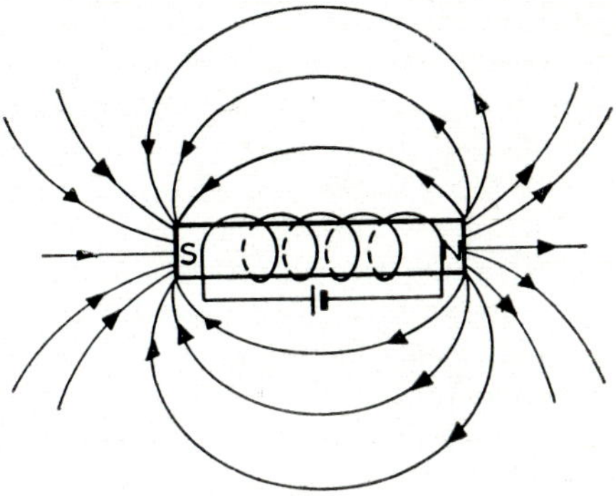

Figure 1.8. The magnetic field due to a simple electromagnet

The magnetic field intensity produced at a distance of d centimetres from a long straight wire carrying a current of I amperes is given by $H_{oersteds}=I/10\times 2/d$. On the SI system of units, $H=I/2\pi d$ where I is in amperes and D is in metres and H is now expressed in ampere-turns per metre.

In the case of a long cylindrical air-cored solenoid coil, having n turns per centimetre and carrying a current of I amperes, the magnetic field intensity well inside the coil has a value of $H=4\pi nI/10$ oersteds where I is in amperes. On the SI system this becomes $H=nI$ where n is the number of turns per metre and H is in ampere-turns per metre. The flux density inside the coil in SI units is given by $B=\mu_0 nI$ where μ_0, the permeability of free space (air for practical purposes), is $4\pi\times 10^{-7}H/n$ when H is in ampere-turns per metre and n is the number of turns per metre, and the flux density is expressed in Teslas. One Tesla=one Weber per square metre. The SI unit of magnetic flux is the Weber.

SOLENOIDS AND RELAYS

Electromagnets are commonly encountered in the form of 'solenoids' used to produce a mechanical movement in response to the passage of an electric current. The magnetic field developed when current is switched through the solenoid coil attracts an iron armature which is free to move and is attached to the object to be moved. Solenoid-operated valves are of great use in gas sampling arrangements and in control systems. Hill and Stone (1963) describe a solenoid-operated gas sampling pump which can be used to sample potentially explosive anaesthetic mixtures. D.C. solenoids operating from supplies in the range 6–50 V are commonly used in electronic apparatus. Solenoids are also available for operating from mains frequency a.c. supplies. Copper 'shading' rings are fitted to the core to produce a reasonably steady pull with a.c. energization. A.C. solenoids are useful when considerable power is required as the need for a heavy current d.c. supply is eliminated, but the unsteadiness (chatter) of the pull can be troublesome in some applications, and a.c. solenoids are likely to make more noise.

Another wide application of electromagnetism occurs in electromagnetic relays. The relay coil is wound on an iron core. The pull of this electromagnet attracts a pivoted iron armature. The movement of the armature is caused to open or close pairs of electrical contacts as required. For general purpose applications, Post Office type relays (Atkinson, 1947) are used. Special purpose high speed relays with low noise precious metal contacts are used in some 'chopper' type d.c. amplifiers, particularly in millivolt potentiometric recorders. Gayford (1969) provides a good account of the construction of relays and their testing, whilst Machin (1958) gives a concise account of relays for use in biological applications.

The closure or release of the relay contacts can be delayed by the mounting of the appropriate copper bands or 'slugs' on the iron core of the relay coil. Consider the case of a slow release relay. When the coil current is switched off, the collapsing magnetic field induces an eddy current in the low resistance slug. This gives rise to a temporary field which holds the relay armature attracted for a period of perhaps 100 ms before it releases. For normal relays, releasing times would be of the order of 30–40 ms. Slow release relays were used by Hill and Hook (1958) to switch the solenoids of a solenoid-operated inspiratory–expiratory valve. The slow release action ensures that when switching occurs, the valve that is shut stays shut until the other valve closes, whereupon the first valve opens. At no instant are both valves moving, as would occur with a simple change-over action. Thus leakage past the valves is prevented.

Compact reed relays are commonly used in association with transistorized circuitry, for example, when high voltages have to be switched. A typical reed relay insert placed inside its solenoid operating coil is shown in *Figure 1.9*. The ferromagnetic cantilever reed spring contacts are sealed into opposite ends of a special glass tube with their ends slightly overlapping, but spaced apart by a specified distance (Gayford, 1969). A solenoid or a permanent magnet is used to cause the reeds to be attracted to each other and make contacts at their ends. The reeds are usually constructed from nickel–iron and the contact area may be of diffused gold, platinum–cobalt or palladium. The glass envelope is filled with an inert gas such as nitrogen to which a small trace of hydrogen may be added.

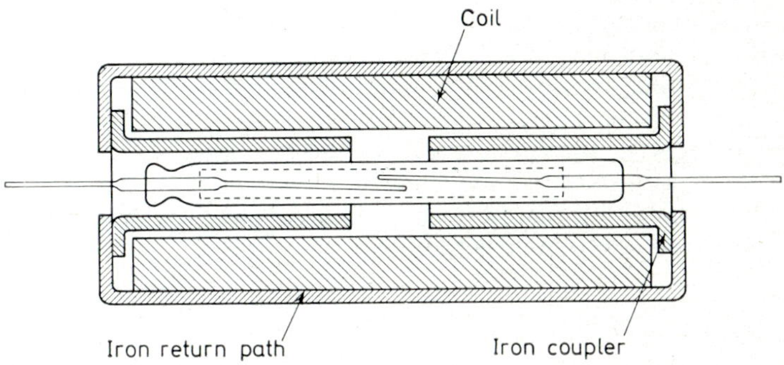

Figure 1.9. A double-ended glass-sealed dry reed switch unit fitted with an operating coil and iron coupling poles and return path forming an outer casing to make a sensitive relay
(Reproduced from Gayford, 1969)

Reed relays are normally constructed with a single make contact only, although change-over versions are available. A normally closed situation can be provided by means of a permanent magnet whose flux is cancelled by operating a solenoid. The enclosure of the contacts prevents the ingress of dirt, humidity and fumes which could affect the contact performance.

TRANSFORMERS

When a coil carries a changing or alternating current, in contrast to a steady or direct current, a changing magnetic field results. Consider two separate coils, one wound on top of the other. When a varying current flows in one coil (called the primary coil), a varying magnetic field is produced. The lines of force will intersect the second (secondary) coil. When a coil is cut by a changing number of magnetic lines of force, a voltage is induced in it. The magnitude of the voltage depends on both the number of lines cutting the coil and the number of turns in the coil. Thus if both coils have the same number of turns, the voltage induced in the secondary winding will equal that in the primary, assuming the number of lines cutting the two coils is the same. When the secondary has twice as many turns as the primary, the secondary voltage will be twice the primary voltage. Such a device is known as a transformer. It is usual (though not always at radio frequencies) to wind the coils upon a core made of a suitable magnetic material in order to increase the degree of magnetic coupling between the coils. A transformer can thus be used to raise or lower an alternating (a.c.) voltage, but not a direct (d.c.) voltage. Mains transformers are encountered in the large majority of electronic apparatus. The mains supply voltage is applied to the primary winding and the secondary windings provide the various voltages needed for the circuits.

The transformer does not contain any active elements capable of producing electrical power. Neglecting any losses, the power in the primary should equal the power in the secondary or secondaries. Using the appropriate r.m.s. values (*see* Chapter 5), the electrical power is given by the product (voltage × current), in the circuit concerned. Neglecting power losses,

$$\text{Primary voltage } (V_p) \times \text{primary current } (I_p)$$
$$= \text{Secondary voltage } (V_s) \times \text{secondary current } (I_s)$$

i.e. $V_pI_p = V_sI_s$.

If the secondary voltage is one-fifth of the primary voltage, the secondary current will be five times as large as the primary current.

The use of a Transformer for Matching

Ohm's law (*see* Chapter 4) defines the resistance of a circuit (the opposition offered by the circuit to current flow) as having a value R in ohms given by $R = V/I$. Consider a transformer having a 5:1 step-down ratio. Suppose that when 50 V r.m.s. is applied to the primary, a current of 1 A r.m.s. flows in the primary when V is the voltage in volts applied across the primary and I amperes is the current flowing. The secondary voltage will be 10 V and the secondary current 5 A. The effective resistance of the primary is $50/1 = 50$ ohms. That of the secondary is $10/5 = 2$ ohms. The ratio of primary to secondary resistance is $50/2 = 25:1 = 5^2:1$. The effective resistance in the secondary is related to that in the primary by the square of the turns ratio. Transformers are often used to change the effective resistance of a circuit. Thus a 'matching transformer' is used to match the high resistance circuit of the output stage of an audio amplifier into the low resistance of a loudspeaker voice coil. Matching transformers were much used to obtain the best power transfer between stages in transistor a.c. amplifiers. However, transformers are not the most reliable of components. Apart from the possibility of a break occurring in a winding, they tend to be microphonic and are prone to the effect of unwanted stray magnetic fields. Since the price of transistors has fallen markedly, it is preferable to use more transistors to attain the desired degree of amplification and to effect matching and thus to eliminate transformers (Cherry, 1963).

Losses in Transformers

In practice transformers are not perfect power transfer devices but have losses. These can be divided into four categories: core losses, flux leakage losses, winding losses and self-capacity.

The core losses arise because of the production of induced circulating currents (eddy currents) in the core and the effects of hysteresis in producing heat in the core. In practice, not all the magnetic flux generated in the primary will cut the secondary turns and this represents a wastage. The d.c. resistance of the windings will dissipate heat. At audio and radio frequencies, the self-capacities of the windings may shunt off current and introduce losses.

At power line frequencies, transformer coils are wound on a laminated silicon–iron core. A discussion of the properties of silicon–iron is given by Craik (1971). The thin sheet laminations reduce eddy currents induced in the core which waste power. At audio frequencies, small laminated cores of special alloys are used, such as mumetal. At radio frequencies, the coils are either 'air-cored' or wound on a ferrite core.

EDDY CURRENTS

When a changing current is flowing in a conductor adjacent to a piece of metal, the changing magnetic field induces 'eddy' currents in the metal. The term eddy current arises from the fact that the

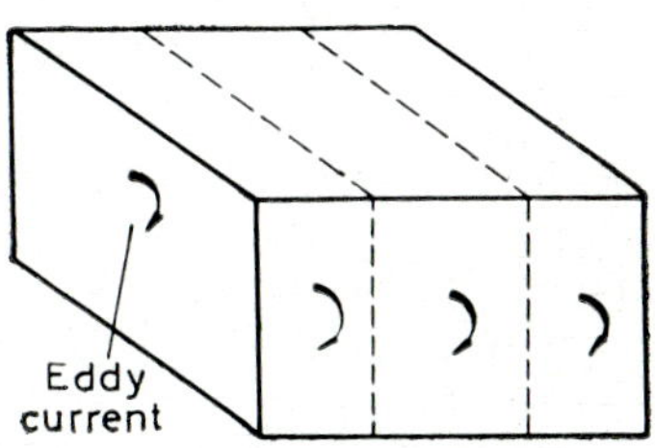

Figure 1.10. Eddy currents circulating in a solid core

induced current whirls around the metal like eddies in water. If an alternating current flows in a coil wound on a solid iron core, eddy currents will flow (*Figure 1.10*) and the core becomes warm if the power involved is sufficient. This heating represents a waste of the electrical power supplied to the transformer. The use of thin laminations, insulated from each other, in the core reduces the losses since the currents can now no longer circulate in the bulk of the material (*Figure 1.11*).

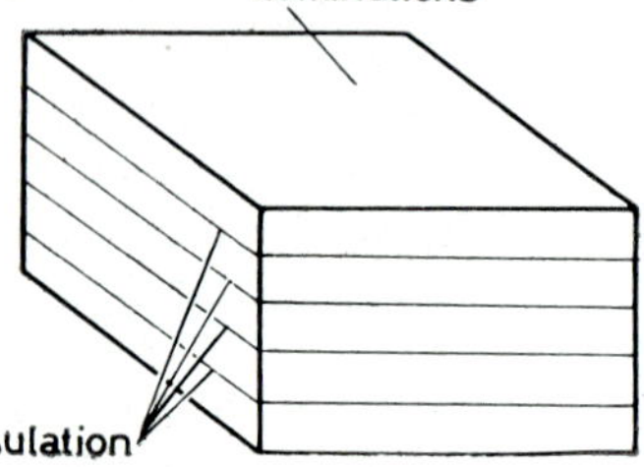

Figure 1.11. A laminated core

In transformer design, attention is paid to means for reducing eddy currents. However, the heating of tissue by induced eddy currents is the basis of treatment by therapeutic diathermy units operating at a frequency of 27 MHz.

REFERENCES

Atkinson, J. (1947). *Telephony*, p. 88. London: New Era Publishing Co.

Bence Jones, H. (1852). *On Animal Electricity, being an Account of the Discoveries of Emil du Bois Reymond*. London: Churchill.

Cherry, E. M. (1963). 'An engineering approach to the design of transistor feedback amplifiers.' *Radio electron. Engng* **25,** 127.

Craik, D. J. (1971). *Structure and Properties of Magnetic Materials*. London: Plan.

Field, J. C. G. (1970). 'Magnetic screening.' *Electron. Engng* **42,** 60.

Gayford, M. L. (1969). *Modern Relay Techniques*. S.T.C. Monograph No. 1. London: Butterworths.

Hill, D. W. and Hook, J. R. (1958). 'A solenoid-operated inspiratory–expiratory valve.' *J. Physiol., Lond.* **145,** 1P.

— and Stone, R. N. (1963). 'A transistor driven gas sampling pump.' *J. scient. Instrum.* **40,** 421.

REFERENCES

Machin, K. E. (1958). 'Relays and related mechanisms.' In *Electronic Apparatus for Biological Research*, p. 510. Ed. by P. E. K. Donaldson. London: Butterworths.

Needham, J. (1962). *Science and Civilization in China*. Vol. 4, p. 230. London: Cambridge University Press.

Watkins, J. (1971). *Modern Electronic Materials*. London: Butterworths.

Chapter 2

Electrostatics

Although much of electronics is concerned with the action of moving electric charges, consideration must also be given to phenomena connected with stationary (static) electric charges. The study of electricity in motion, as when an electric current flows in a circuit, leads to the concept of Current Electricity as opposed to Static Electricity. Many people think of electrostatics in terms of schoolday memories of rubbing a cat skin with an ebonite rod. However, not only has electrostatics a long connection with medicine, but it also has many important present-day applications in therapy and research.

A knowledge of electrostatic phenomena has existed for many years. More than 2,000 years ago, the Greek Thales of Miletos is reputed by Diogenes of Apollonia (624–545 B.C.) to have noted that amber attracted lightweight particles when it was rubbed. When rubbed, the amber is said to be electrified or charged. The effect was known as 'Electricity' from the Greek 'elektron' for amber. About A.D. 500, the Chinese Thao Hung Ching reported that amber rubbed in the palm of the hand, and thus made warm, attracts mustard seeds (Needham, 1962).

POSITIVE AND NEGATIVE ELECTRICITY

Experiment shows that an ebonite rod A rubbed on fur will repel a suspended ebonite rod B which has also been rubbed on fur. However, a glass rod C rubbed on silk will attract both A and B. From this experiment, it is deduced that the electricity resident on A and C is opposite in nature.

In 1745, Benjamin Franklin gave the name of Negative Electricity to the charge on the ebonite rod and Positive Electricity to the charge on the glass rod. The nature of the charge acquired by a rubbed object depends not only on the material of the object but also on that of the rubber. For example, an ebonite rod acquires a positive charge when rubbed with flannel, but a negative charge when rubbed with fur. These experiments with electrically charged rods give rise to the law of electrostatics that Like Charges Repel and Unlike Charges Attract. This is similar to the law of magnetism which states that Like Magnetic Poles Repel and Unlike Poles Attract.

CONDUCTORS AND INSULATORS

Some substances will pass, or conduct, electricity easily and because of this they are known as Conductors. Others, which do not conduct electricity, or at least do so only with difficulty, are known as Insulators. Metals conduct electricity easily, but glass and mica are insulators. There is also another class of substance whose properties of electrical conduction lie between those of conductors and insulators. These are called Semiconductors.

THE ATOMIC STRUCTURE OF MATTER

Arising from the work of the Dane, Niels Bohr, it is possible to consider the structure of the atoms comprising all matter in terms of a central massive nucleus surrounded by one or more orbital electrons. The simplest atom is that of hydrogen. In this there is only one orbital electron and the mass of the nucleus is about 1,840 times that of the orbital electron. Atoms of other substances may have many more orbital electrons, for example, the element germanium (of importance in semiconductor devices) has a total of 32 orbital electrons. The concept of the electrons moving in fixed orbits is of considerable help in explaining the production of x-ray line spectra (Worsnop and Chalklin, 1950) and of optical line spectra as in various forms of laser (Witt, Reed and Tittel, 1964; Goldman *et al.*, 1964; Hall, Hill and Beach, 1971).

However, the concept of rigid electron orbits should not be pushed too far. Modern studies based on the wave mechanics assign a probability to a given electron being in a given orbit at any specified time. Thus since it is based on a statistical approach the view of the structure of an atom becomes much more cloudy, as it were. For many purposes, the simple concept of rigid orbits is very helpful. Electrons have a negative charge and were discovered by Sir J. J. Thompson in 1897 (Tolansky, 1963).

Atoms such as helium contain two kinds of particles in their nucleus. These are Protons and Neutrons. They both have a mass about 1,840 times that of an electron, but the proton carries a positive charge of electricity equal and opposite to that of an electron. A neutron, as its name implies, is electrically neutral. Because of its neutrality it can penetrate into a nucleus without being influenced by the internal electrical binding forces of the nucleus, and it thus represents a potent weapon for splitting nuclei.

A body is said to be in a state of electrical neutrality when it carries equal charges of positive and negative electricity, which then cancel. Normally, substances would exist in a state of neutrality; that is to say the negative charges on the electrons are balanced by an equal number of positive charges on the nucleus. If an atom is caused to lose an orbital electron, it has a net positive charge and is known as a positive ion. An atom acquiring an extra electron becomes a negative ion. Positive and negative ions are of practical importance in gas discharge tubes and Geiger counter tubes for the measurement of radioactivity.

Repeated reference will be made to this concept of atomic structure. The whole subject of electronic engineering is based on the motion of electrons and ions. Conductors derive their property from the fact that they have 'free' electrons in their atoms. These 'free' electrons are mobile and have a greater freedom of motion than the electrons in insulators which are 'bound' to their atoms.

ELECTROSTATIC CHARGING BY FRICTION

When a glass rod is rubbed with silk, the energy generated by the friction removes some of the electrons of the surface glass atoms and transfers them to the silk. As a result, the glass is now left with a net positive charge. On the other hand, the rubbing of ebonite with fur transfers electrons from the fur to the rod. The rod thus acquires a negative charge equal to the positive charge left on the fur.

ELECTROSTATIC INDUCTION

It is possible by using the method of Induction to charge a metal object without making contact with it. In *Figure 2.1* a negative

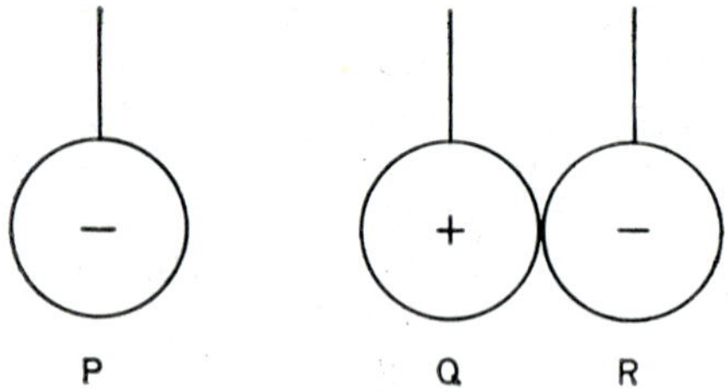

Figure 2.1. Charging by induction

charge P is brought close to a pair of uncharged metal spheres Q and R suspended by insulating threads. With P still present, if Q and R are then separated it is found that Q has acquired a positive charge and R a negative charge. The electrons on the spheres are repelled by the negative charge on P, making R negative and leaving Q with a positive charge.

THE LOCATION OF CHARGE ON A CONDUCTOR

About 1820, Faraday proved in his famous ice pail experiment that the charge on a hollow conductor resides on the outer surface. This also applies to a solid conductor. It is interesting to note that Faraday used an ice pail because this happened to be the most suitable deep hollow container in the Royal Institution of London at that time. The fact that there is no charge inside a conductor enables an apparatus to be screened from possible induced charges by surrounding it with an earthed metal screen as described in Chapter 9. It also allows the use of nylon underwear in the operating room if an outer cotton scrub suit and boots of conducting rubber are worn. Any charge generated by friction of the nylon is conducted to earth by the conduction film of moisture resident in the pores of the cotton and the action of the conducting boots.

THE TRANSFER OF CHARGE BY ACTION AT POINTS

The distribution of the charge on the surface of a conductor depends on the shape, more particularly on the curvature, of the various parts of the surface. The greatest density of charge occurs at the place with the greatest curvature. Thus a charged conductor will have a high charge density at any sharp points on its surface. It is important that conductors and electrodes which have to carry high voltages should be free of any rough edges or points, otherwise sparking might occur from them.

Pointed, insulated conductors are used to take off the charges in electrostatic generators, which are machines for the production of high potential differences by means of electrostatic principles.

In *Figure 2.2*, consider a rubber belt D which is driven by an electric motor upwards past the pointed end of a fixed, insulated conductor PE. This results in a negative charge being induced on the end E and a positive charge on the pointed end P. The high positive charge density on the point ionizes the air around the point, and positive charge streams from P to D and neutralizes the negative charge on the belt opposite P. E is then left with an induced negative

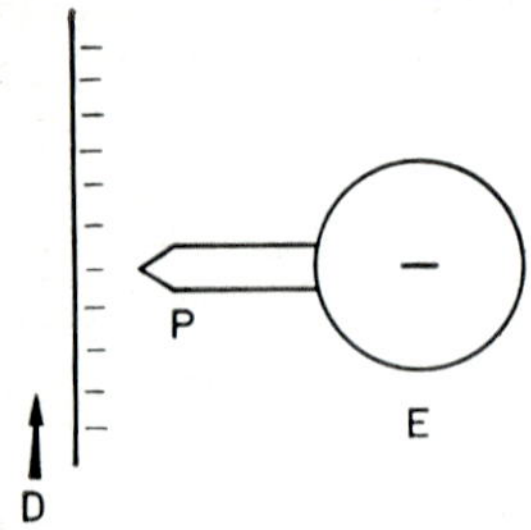

Figure 2.2. The transfer of charge from a point

charge. As the endless belt rotates carrying negative charge past P, the insulated conductor E acquires an increasingly negative charge.

THE VAN DE GRAAF ELECTROSTATIC GENERATOR

This type of machine was invented by Robert Van de Graaf about 1931. The operating principle is illustrated in *Figure 2.3.* The high voltage terminal is a large, smooth metal hemisphere H situated at the top of the insulating column I. An endless rubber belt drives continuously round the pulleys J and K and past the pointed conductors M and N. N is joined to H, and M to the negative terminal of a high voltage supply (30 kV). Negative charge passes from the point M to the belt and is carried until it is opposite N. It then induces a positive charge on N and a negative charge on H. Positive charge streams from the point N to the belt where it neutralizes the negative charge on the belt. Between M and N, the belt carries a negative charge. For the rest of its travel it is uncharged. As the belt rotates, a high negative potential (in a large Van de Graaf this can be as high as two million volts) is built up on the sphere. The high voltage terminal of the generator may be surrounded with a gas mixture, such as a 4 to 1 mixture of nitrogen and carbon dioxide, to prevent a flashover. *Figure 2.4* shows a Van de Graaf generator used in radiotherapy. The generator and its associated x-ray tube are mounted in a housing which can easily be positioned to suit the patient's needs.

APPLICATIONS OF ELECTROSTATICS

Anaesthetic Fires and Explosions

Strict precautions are taken in operating rooms, when anaesthetic agents such as ether or cyclopropane are in use, to prevent the possible build-up of static charge which could give rise to a disastrous

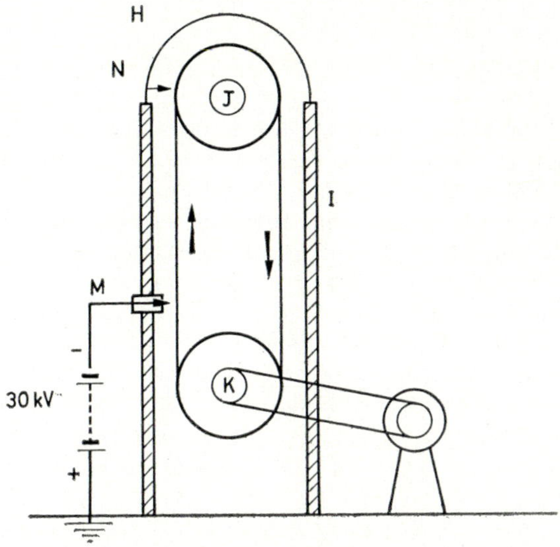

Figure 2.3. The operating principle of a Van de Graaf electrostatic generator

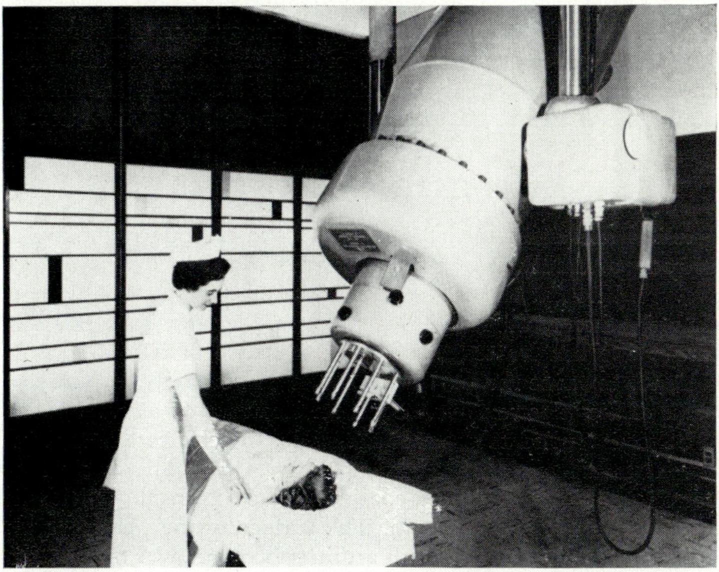

Figure 2.4. A Van de Graaf generator used in a radiotherapy department
(By courtesy of High Voltage Engineering Corporation)

fire or explosion. All rubber items such as anaesthetic circuit hoses, trolley wheels and boots for the theatre personnel are made from conducting rubber. The theatre floor is made from a conducting terrazzo in order to provide a large capacity which can store any charges fed to it without producing a signicant rise in potential. The humidity of the operating theatre atmosphere is also maintained at such a level that an invisible film of moisture forms on all the objects within the room and prevents a build-up of charge. Mackintosh, Mushin and Epstein (1963) deal extensively with the risks connected with anaesthetic explosions, and another useful reference is the leaflet *Report of a Working Party on Anaesthetic Explosions* (London, H.M.S.O., 1956).

Small electrostatic machines have been used therapeutically for the treatment of various muscular and other disorders. In 1855, Guillaume Duchenne of Boulogne published his famous book *De l'électrification localisée et de son application à la pathologie et la thérapeutique.*

X-radiation is produced when a beam of electrons changes its velocity suddenly. In an x-ray tube, a beam of electrons emitted from a heated cathode is accelerated to strike an anode made from some refractory material such as tungsten. A high positive voltage is applied to the anode with respect to the cathode in order to accelerate the electrons. The higher this voltage, the greater the penetrating power of the x-rays produced. For the treatment of deep-seated tumours voltages of several million volts are used, and in some installations these are generated by a Van de Graaf generator.

THE CATHODE RAY TUBE

Figure 2.5 illustrates the basic layout of a cathode ray tube. The electrode assembly is mounted inside a highly evacuated glass envelope. The flat end of the screen is usually made separately and then welded on to the rest of the envelope. Electrons from the heated cathode are accelerated under the influence of a high potential difference to strike the flat screen at the end of the tube. The anode system of the 'electron gun' forms an electrostatic lens. By altering the voltage applied to the second anode, the electron beam can be brought to a focus on the screen (*Figure 2.5b*). This is a pentode electron gun. The phosphor coating of the screen glows with light when it is struck by the beam. The surface of the phosphor distal to the glass is often coated with a thin reflecting layer of aluminium in order to reflect scattered light towards the observer. It also prevents negative ions from striking the centre of the screen and burning it.

The ions are not much deflected because of their larger mass and would strike the screen continuously in the centre. The number of electrons per unit time striking the screen governs the brightness of the spot. Thus the brightness control acts by applying a more negative voltage to the grid of the electron gun and reducing the emission of electrons. In medical laboratories, cathode ray tube oscilloscope

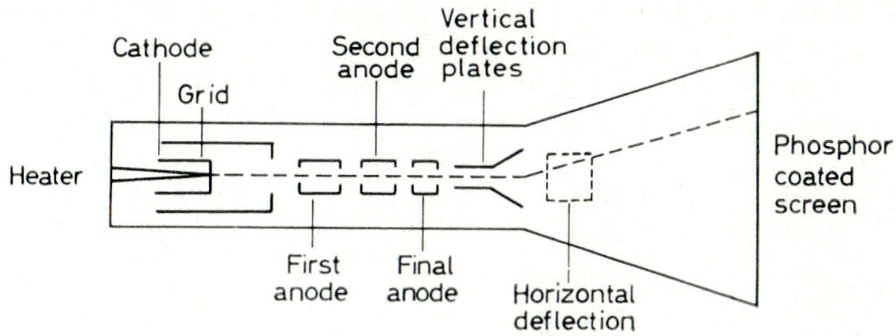

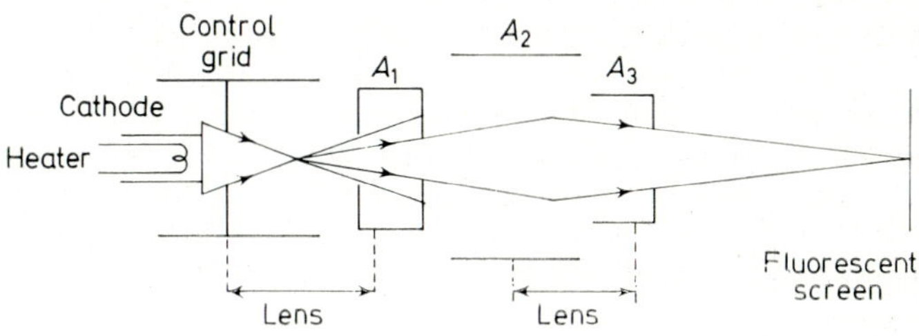

Figure 2.5. The essentials of a cathode ray tube

tubes usually have one of two phosphors. A phosphor which glows green, with an afterglow of approximately 15 milliseconds after the passage of the beam, is used for general purpose observations of circuit waveforms and for the visual and photographic recording of medium speed phenomena such as electromyograms. For the observation of slow speed signals such as the ECG and blood pressure, a phosphor is used which gives an orange-yellow trace with an afterglow lasting about ten seconds. Particularly with long afterglow phosphors, care must be taken to avoid an excessive brightness. This can burn the screen and result in permanent damage. There is usually an interaction between the brightness and focus controls.

A conducting coating on the inside of the cathode ray tube acts to return electrons ejected from the screen by secondary emission to an anode. This prevents the build-up of a negative charge on the screen. Storage oscilloscopes are available in which the image on the screen can be preserved for several hours for subsequent inspection.

The cathode ray tubes used in wideband calibrated oscilloscopes are of the electrostatic type, where the deflection of the electron beam is carried out electrostatically by the influence of signal or time base voltages applied to the deflector plates. The larger screen multi-channel display oscilloscopes used in patient monitoring applications employ an electrostatic accelerating system for the electron beam, but deflect the beam by means of the magnetic field produced by a pair of deflection coils. Focusing is performed by permanent magnets placed around the neck of the tube.

In order to achieve the high brightness level necessary for the observation of transient phenomena, a high value of accelerating voltage is required. However, the resulting high velocity of the electrons in the longitudinal direction makes the beam 'stiffer' and correspondingly harder to deflect laterally. This means that higher deflection voltages will be required and makes it difficult to obtain the high writing speeds of the spot over the screen which are required to delineate, for example, the rise time of a fast pulse. This conflicting set of requirements has led to the development of the PDA (post-deflection acceleration) cathode ray tube. Here the beam is deflected before the final acceleration is performed. The accelerating electrode is a spiral of a graphite material running the length of the inside of the conical end of the tube envelope. In order to obtain a large viewing area in as short a tube as possible, some constructions re-deflect the electron beam between the gun and the screen. To do this a voltage is placed on an 'expansion' mesh to create an electrostatic field to bend the beam further. A 127 mm (5 in) diameter PDA tube can have two stages of distributed post-deflection acceleration through a total of 10 kV and yet have a deflection sensitivity of 1 V per mm (25 V per inch). Golding (1971) provides a close account of PDA systems.

The Cathode Ray Tube Power Supply

In electrostatically deflected cathode ray tubes, the final anode is usually earthed and the grid, cathode and heater are maintained at a high negative voltage relative to earth. For 76 mm (3 in) diameter tubes this might be −1,000 V, and for 152 mm (6 in) diameter tubes −2,000 V.

In many oscilloscopes this e.h.t. (extra high tension) voltage is produced from a secondary winding on the mains transformer via either a full wave rectifier circuit or a voltage doubler. Alternatively, the e.h.t. may be generated from a valve or transistor audio frequency oscillator feeding a step-up transformer. The higher frequency means that the smoothing capacitors can have a lower capacity than is the case at mains frequencies. This reduces the risk of a dangerous shock. Transistorized converters are used in battery-powered portable oscilloscopes and also to supply the 25 kV requirements for the e.h.t. of the large screen magnetically deflected tubes.

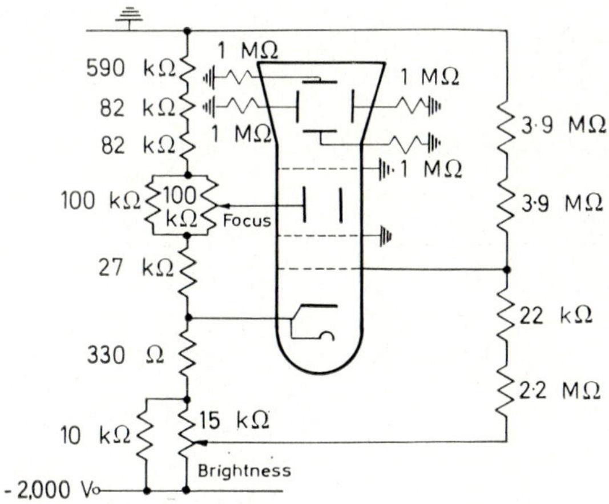

Figure 2.6. A cathode ray tube power supply network

The e.h.t. voltage is applied to a network of resistors forming a potentiometer chain in order to supply the various potentials for the gun electrodes. When measured with respect to the cathode, the grid is a few volts negative and the final anode is highly positive. Since the grid is situated close to the cathode, modest grid potentials can exert a marked influence on the emission of electrons. The circuit for an oscilloscope tube is given in *Figure 2.6*.

Deflection of the Beam

In an 'electrostatic' tube, after leaving the electron gun, the electron beam passes between the first pair of deflection plates. When a voltage difference is maintained between these plates, the beam of negatively charged electrons is repelled from the more negative plate and attracted towards the more positive plate. The angle of deflection of the beam is proportional to the voltage difference between the plates. A second set of deflection plates follows the first, the direction of deflection now being at right angles to that produced by the first pair. The tube is mounted so that on viewing its face, one set of plates produces a horizontal deflection and the other a vertical deflection. Hence they are known as the Horizontal and the Vertical deflection plates. About 50–60 V is required to deflect the beam through 25 mm (1 inch) on the screen. In a 'magnetic' tube, the deflection along the X and Y axes of the spot is accomplished by the fields from pairs of coils mounted around the tube neck. The

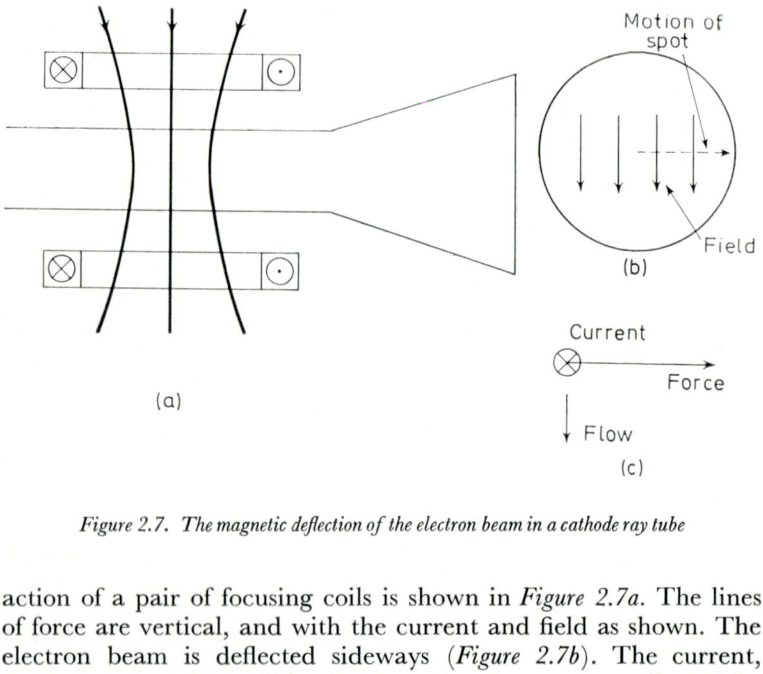

Figure 2.7. The magnetic deflection of the electron beam in a cathode ray tube

action of a pair of focusing coils is shown in *Figure 2.7a*. The lines of force are vertical, and with the current and field as shown. The electron beam is deflected sideways (*Figure 2.7b*). The current, the magnetic field and the force on the electrons are all at right angles to one another (*Figure 2.7c*).

Astigmatism

It is necessary that the average voltage of each pair of deflection plates should be as nearly as possible the same as the voltage on the final anode. If this is not so, a low power cylindrical lens is produced between the plates and the final anode. This gives rise to the aberration known as astigmatism, manifested by the fact that the spot cannot be focused in the horizontal and vertical planes simultaneously. In practice each of a pair of deflection plates is driven from one side of a balanced (push–pull) deflection amplifier. The final anode voltage is usually not fixed at earth potential, but can be varied by means of a potentiometer—the astigmatism control. This makes it possible to adjust the final anode voltage to the average voltage on the deflector plates.

The Timebase Generator

For most purposes, cathode ray tube oscilloscopes are used to plot the variation with time of the amplitude of the input slgnal. The signal is applied via a 'Y deflection amplifier' to the Y plates of the cathode ray tube. Consider a simple alternating input signal as shown in *Figure 2.8a*. Suppose that the signal is applied to the Y plates, with the X plates earthed via high resistances. Positive half cycles of the input signal will deflect the spot upwards and negative half cycles will deflect it downwards. As a result, the spot of light on the tube screen will now trace out a vertical line (*Figure*

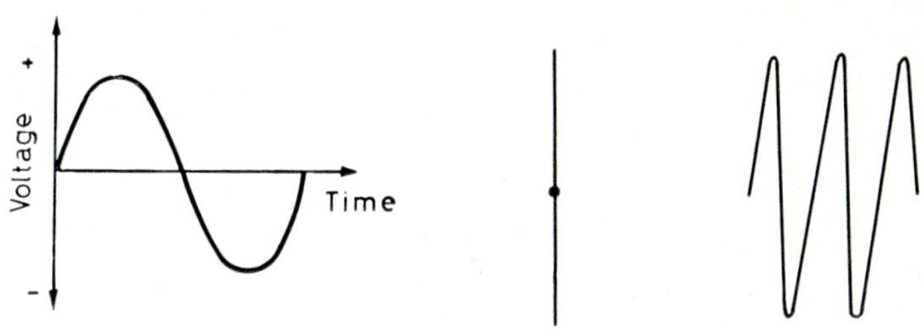

(a) (b) (c)

Figure 2.8. The action of a linear timebase

2.8b). In order to display the variation with time of the signal, the spot must be subjected to a steady deflection in the horizontal direction, conventionally from left to right. In *Figure 2.8c*, each successive cycle is displaced to the right by an equal amount. At the end of each horizontal sweep or scan, the spot is required to return quickly or to 'fly back' to the starting point and recommence scanning. This action can be accomplished by the application of a sawtooth or ramp waveform to the X deflection plates. The waveform is illustrated in *Figure 2.9*.

One simple means of generating a sawtooth is to charge a capacitor via a high value resistor from a high voltage d.c. source. The initial portion of the charging curve, up to approximately one-tenth of the time constant, is almost linear. After a time interval of 0·1 time constants, it is arranged that the capacitor is momentarily shorted out by a switch. The spot then returns to its initial position, the switch is opened, and scanning recommences. On the basis of a deflection sensitivity of 2·4 V per millimetre (60 V per inch),

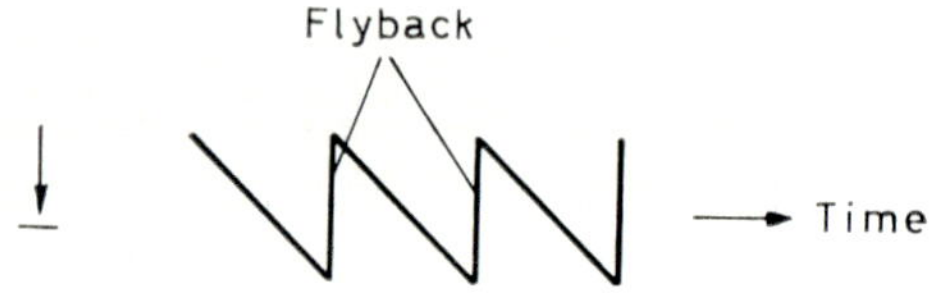

Figure 2.9. A sawtooth timebase waveform

300 V would be needed for a 125 mm (5 in) scan. This is the voltage which must have built up on the timebase capacitor in 0·1 of the charging time constant. This is about one-thirtieth of the charging voltage, which must equal 9,000 V, and this is inconveniently high. For the display of respiratory waveforms, a suitable scan time might be 20 seconds, so that the time constant of the circuit must be 200 seconds. A suitable arrangement is that of *Figure 2.10.* The depar-

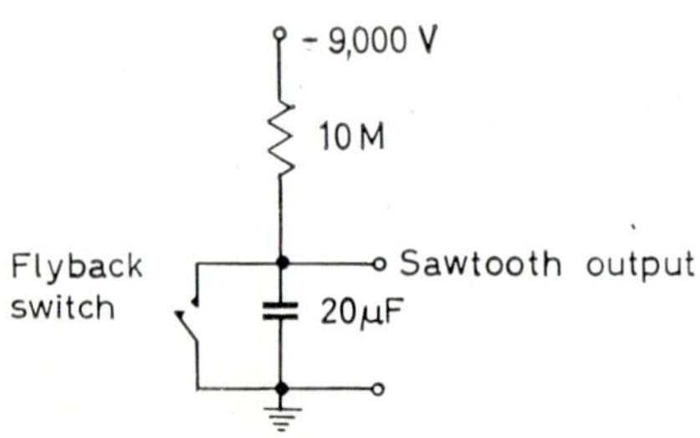

Figure 2.10. The use of the initial linear portion of a capacitor charging curve as a linear timebase

ture from linearity is only 2 per cent if the charging time is limited to one-tenth of the time constant. In practice this system is not used because of the need for a high voltage stable supply and large resistors and capacitors.

A number of bootstrap and operational amplifier integrator circuits are available for the generation of a linearly rising ramp which can be amplified and fed to the deflection plates. A series of coarse timebase speeds is provided by allowing different values of capacitor to be switched into the circuit, and part of the charging resistor is made variable to allow a fine control of the sweep velocity.

Repetitive Timebase Sweeps

Once started, the sweep generator will produce a voltage which sweeps the spot across the horizontal axis of the cathode ray tube. The charging capacitor is normally kept shorted out by means of a conducting diode placed across it. An electronic switching circuit, such as a multivibrator, is made to cut the diode off for a definite time at regular intervals. The period for which the diode is non-conducting and the sweep running determines the distance moved by the spot for a given sweep speed. At the end of the scan, the capacitor is briefly shorted out, causing the spot to fly back to its initial starting position. In this way the timebase now generates sweeps in a repetitive fashion.

The Triggered Timebase

Repetitive timebases are of the free-running type. The start and finish of each scan is determined only by the constants of the switching circuit. Because of this, the sweeps are not linked with, or synchronized to, the signal whose waveform is to be displayed on the cathode ray tube. In order that the waveform should appear stationary for measurement on the screen, the timebase must be synchronized so that it starts each sweep at a definite point of the input signal waveform. This can be accomplished by making the timebase switching circuit monostable in its action instead of astable. Instead of switching continuously, the circuit now only switches when it is actuated by a suitable triggering signal. In the 'External Trigger' mode, the timebase sweep is initiated by an external signal fed into the 'Trigger Input' terminal of the oscilloscope. For example, the timebase scan could be arranged to commence when the shutter of a recording camera is opened. In the 'Internal Trigger' mode, the triggering is derived automatically from the output of the Y amplifier, thus synchronizing the scan to the input signal so that the images from successive scans fall on top of one another. This is the most commonly used mode.

Flyback Suppression

The velocity of the spot is higher during the flyback than during the scan. This fact is utilized in the flyback suppression circuit in order to ensure that the brilliance of the trace is reduced during the flyback so that the reverse motion of the spot is concealed.

Deflection Amplifiers

If the Y plate sensitivity of the cathode ray tube is 2·4 V per millimetre (60 V per inch), then an amplifier gain of 60,000 would be required in order to produce a 25 mm (1 in) high trace from a 1 mV electrocardiogram. For medical applications, it is very convenient if the amplifier is direct coupled. Slowly varying signals such as respiratory waveforms can then be displayed, together with signals having a d.c. component such as a mean pressure. A switch marked 'a.c. or d.c.' is usually provided to give either capacitor or direct coupling to the input of the amplifier concerned. A.C. coupling is used when a varying signal, such as a pulse pressure or ripple, has to be observed superimposed on top of a steady signal or d.c. voltage. The frequency response of the amplifier is quoted in terms of the frequency at which the gain is reduced by a factor of 0·707 (3 db down). The amplifier has a gain bandwidth product. That is to say, the higher the gain the smaller the allowable bandwidth. For example, the input sensitivity could be 200 mV per cm from d.c. to 100 kHz or 20 mV per cm from d.c. to 1 MHz. For the observation of fast pulses a wide bandwidth is necessary to include the higher harmonic frequencies.

When two variables are to be compared using a 'loop figure' with one fed to the Y axis and the other to the X axis, identical amplifiers should be available for each axis. In this way any phase shift observed will be due to the signals alone and not to differences in the phase shift frequency characteristics of the amplifiers. For loop figure work, the time base is stopped and the spot placed at the centre of the screen. Typical examples in respiratory investigations include the plotting of pressure–flow rate and pressure–volume loops, and in cardiology the plotting of vector loops. Two frequencies may be compared by the well-known method of putting one on the X and one on the Y axis and forming Lissajous figures (Golding, 1971).

Z Modulation

Particularly in loop figure work, it may be desirable to modulate the brightness of the spot, for example, with time marker pips. The brightness control is first adjusted either to blank out the trace or to give a reference brightness and the modulation signal applied via a high voltage capacitor to the grid of the electron gun.

Shift Controls and Calibration

Both X and Y shift controls are provided to allow the position of the trace on the cathode ray tube screen to be adjusted along the X and Y axes. These controls unbalance the X and Y amplifiers. It is usual to provide a neon tube across each half of the output stage of the X and Y amplifiers. If the spot has been deflected beyond the edge of the screen, the voltage developed across the amplifier load is sufficient to strike the particular neon and thus draw attention to where the spot has gone. In all measuring as opposed to purely display oscilloscopes, the Y gain control is calibrated directly in terms of voltage sensitivity and the timebase speed control in terms of time. It is usual to provide a voltage calibrator from which a 1 V, 50 Hz square wave can be obtained to check the calibration of the controls.

Double Beam Oscilloscopes

Double beam oscilloscopes are widely used for the comparison of two signals, both of which vary with time. When the cathode ray tube has only one electron gun, it is possible to use a beam splitter plate to divide the original electron beam into two. With this system, since the two beams are derived from one, they must both utilize the same timebase. One Y deflection plate is common to both beams so that the beams are deflected in opposite directions for the same polarity of input signal applied to the Y_1 and Y_2 amplifiers. Because of these limitations, this system has been superseded by cathode ray tubes which have two independent electron guns. The Y deflection directions for each beam are now the same and different timebase speeds can be used for each beam if desired.

The cost of wide band Y amplifiers is considerable, so that a commonly encountered arrangement is that of beam switching. An electronic switch circuit is used to switch the spot between two levels on the tube face. The switching rate is about 100 kHz. One input signal is applied as the spot scans the upper level, and the other whilst it is in the lower position. The persistence of the phosphor fills in the continuity of the tracing. The switching action is shown in *Figure 2.11*. The switching speed severely limits the maximum frequencies which can be observed in the two-trace

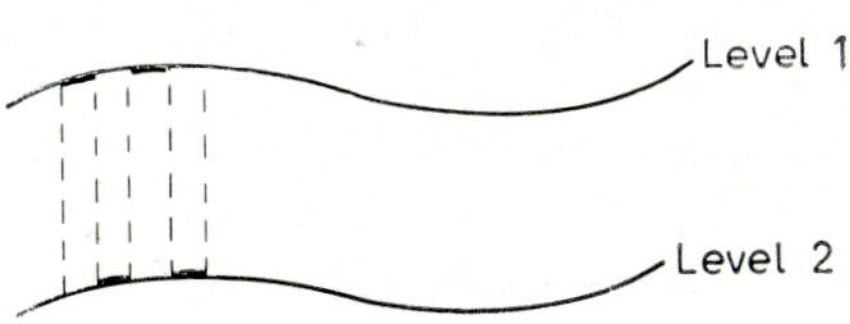

Figure 2.11. The action of a beam switching circuit

mode. At the higher timebase frequencies, the switching action shows up, so that here time-sharing is employed. The timebase is caused to scan across one level on the tube face and is then switched to the second level for the next scan. This limitation does not arise with a double gun tube.

Figure 2.12 illustrates a good general purpose biomedical oscilloscope. It uses a double gun cathode ray tube. Identical amplifiers can be used on the X and Y axes for loop figure work. The maximum sensitivity is 100 microvolts per cm, the accelerating voltage on the tube being 3 kV. The bandwidth at this sensitivity is from d.c. to 100 kHz. The calibrated timebase speeds range from 1 microsecond to 5 seconds per cm.

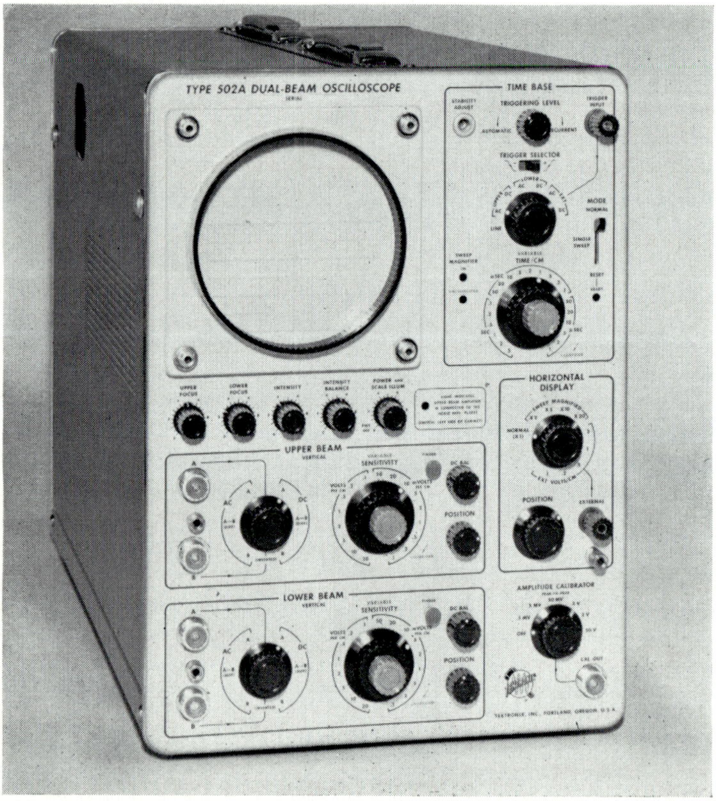

Figure 2.12. A double beam cathode ray tube oscilloscope designed for biomedical applications

(By courtesy of Tektronix U.K. Ltd.)

ELECTRIC POTENTIAL

It is a matter of experience that like charges tend to repel each other. Hence if two like charges are brought nearer to each other, then work must be done to accomplish this. *Figures 2.13* and *2.14* show

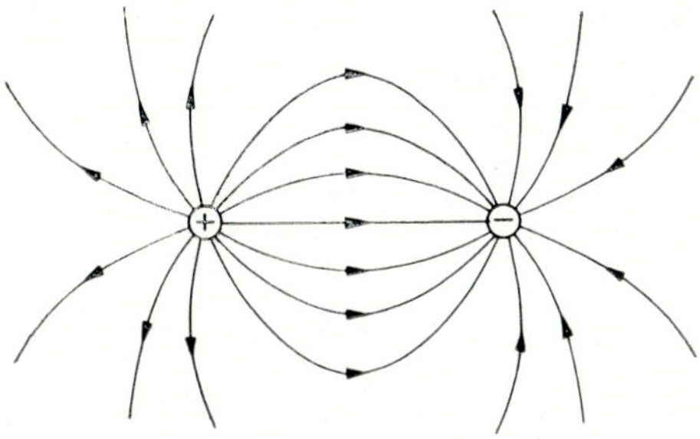

Figure 2.13. The electric field existing between two equal and opposite charges

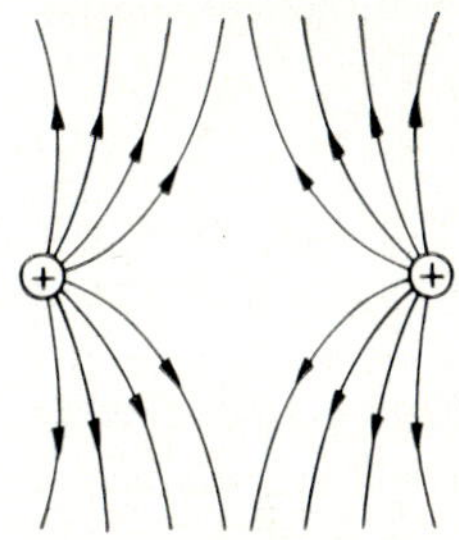

Figure 2.14. The electric field existing between two equal and similar charges

the field existing between a pair of unlike and like charges. The charges in *Figure 2.14* constitute an electric dipole. One or more such generators are used to simulate the production of the electrocardiogram in studies on the origin of the ECG. If one charge A is as far away as possible, that is, it is said to be situated at infinity, then the repulsive force on it from the other like charge B is zero. Then the charge A is said to have zero electric potential. The fact that two electric charges attract or repel each other at a distance, depending on the sign of the charges, shows that there is an area of influence surrounding each charge.

Consider two like charges A and B. Since like charges repel each other, if A is to be moved towards B, work must be done on charge A to move it. Energy is defined as 'the capacity to do work,' so that charge A now possesses energy (potential energy) by virtue of the work that has been done. The potential at a point in an electric field is defined as being numerically equal to the work done in bringing a unit positive charge from infinity to that point.

The practical unit of quantity of electricity is the Coulomb, named after the Frenchman, Charles Augustus Coulomb (1736–1806). It is the quantity of electricity passing a given section of a conductor in one second when the current is one ampere. The ampere is named after the French physicist André Marie Ampère (1775–1836). The practical unit of the potential difference between two points is the Volt, after the Italian Alessandro Volta (1745–1827). The volt is defined as the difference of electric potential between two points of a conducting wire carrying a constant current of one ampere, when the power dissipated between these points is one watt. It can also be defined as the potential difference between two points if one joule of work is done when one coulomb of charge is taken from one point to the other.

ELECTRIC FIELD

Faraday, who first proposed the idea of magnetic lines of force, also thought of the medium surrounding an electric charge as being in a state of electric stress. This region is known as the electric field around the charge. As in a magnetic field, electric lines of force

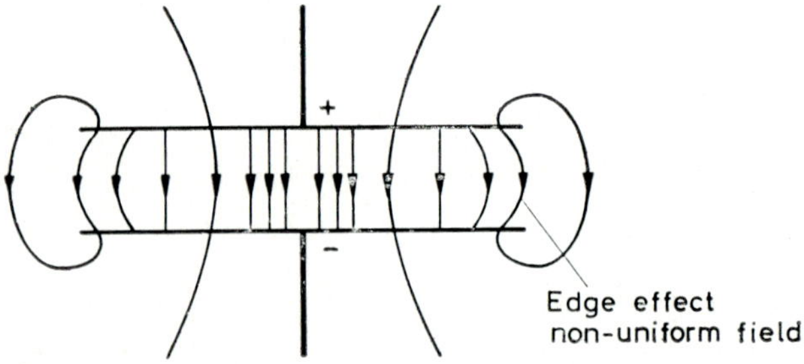

Figure 2.15. The electric field existing between two oppositely charged plane parallel metal plates

represent the strength and direction of the field. The lines of force between two parallel metal plates carrying equal and opposite charges are straight and parallel except at the plate edges, when the field becomes non-uniform (*Figure 2.15*).

THE ELECTROSTATIC VOLTMETER

High values of potential difference can be measured by means of an electrostatic voltmeter. One form of the instrument, fitted with a lamp and scale, is shown in *Figure 2.16.* It is used to measure the potential difference existing between two points, one of which is earthed (at zero potential). The high potential is applied to a well-insulated metal electrode, whilst the earth point is taken to a moving vane mounted on a taut band suspension. The vane and the electrode acquire unlike charges and the vane deflects on its suspension towards the electrode. This motion causes a spot of light

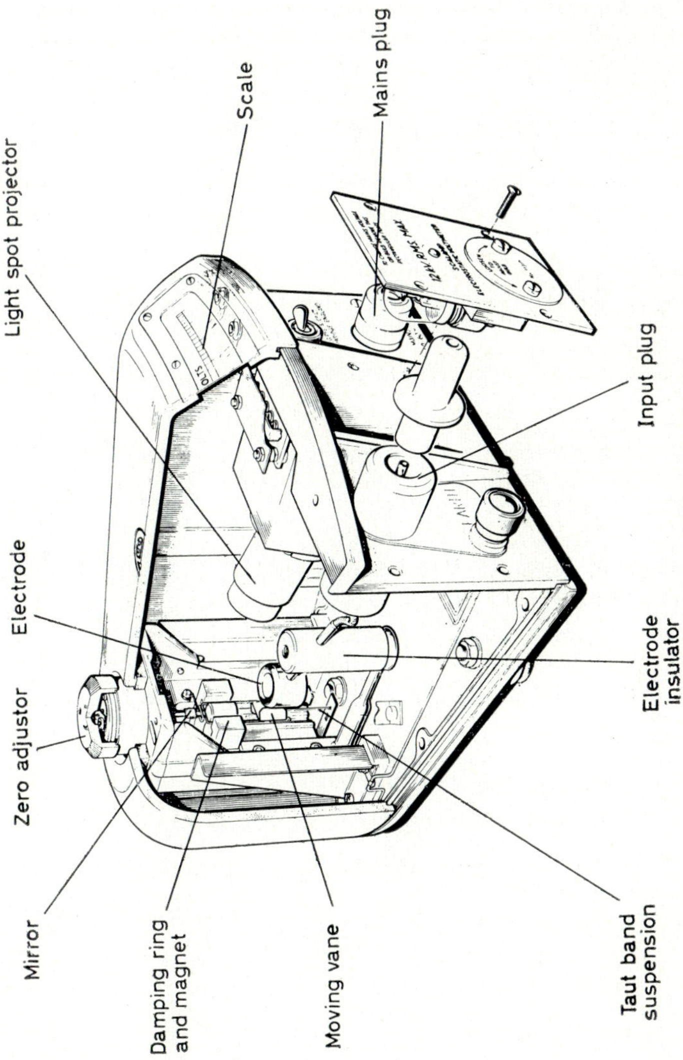

Figure 2.16. An electrostatic kilovoltmeter
(By courtesy of Pye-Unicam Ltd.)

to be deflected by the mirror mounted on the suspension so that it moves across the scale, which is calibrated in kilovolts. It is found that the deflection is proportional to the square of the applied potential difference. Hence, the instrument can be used to measure both d.c. and a.c. potential differences. The instrument has a square law scale, that is, it is cramped at one end and open at the other. Eddy-current damping is provided by means of a copper ring rotating in the field of a permanent magnet. A typical meter would be provided with three d.c. ranges of 0–5, 3–10 and 5–18 kV together with three a.c. ranges of 1–5, 3–10 and 5–12 kV r.m.s. The error at any point of the a.c. or d.c. ranges is plus or minus 2 per cent of the full-scale reading. Panel mounting electrostatic meters are also available in which the moving vane carries a pointer moving over a scale.

REFERENCES

Golding, J. F. (1971). *Measuring Oscilloscopes.* London: Iliffe.

Goldman, L., Blaney, D. J., Freemond, A. and Hornby, P. (1964). 'Biomedical aspects of lasers.' *J. Am. med. Ass.* **188,** 302.

Hall, R. R., Hill, D. W. and Beach, A. D. (1971). 'A carbon dioxide surgical laser.' *Ann. R. Coll. Surg.* **48,** 181.

Mackintosh, R., Mushin, W. W. and Epstein, H. G. (1963). *Physics for the Anaesthetist,* 3rd edn. p. 326. Oxford: Blackwell.

Needham, J. (1962). *Science and Civilization in China,* Vol. 4. London: Cambridge University Press.

Tolansky, S. (1963). *An Introduction to Atomic Physics,* 5th ed. London: Longmans Green.

Witt, P. N., Reed, C. F. and Tittel, F. K. (1964). 'Laser lesions and spider web construction.' *Nature, Lond.* **201,** 150.

Worsnop, B. L. and Chalklin, F. C. (1950). *X-rays.* London: Methuen.

Chapter 3

Cells and Other Portable Power Sources

The desire to study the effects of drugs and exercise in experimental animals and man has led to the development of miniature transducers and their associated circuitry including radio telemetry systems. A range of therapeutic devices has also emerged such as hearing aids, e.m.g. controlled lockable knee joints, and stimulators for the treatment of incontinence of urine and faeces. Possibly some of the most spectacular developments have taken place with cardiac pacemakers.

The demand for inconspicuous devices which can be worn continuously for extended periods of time focuses attention on the need for efficient cells capable of providing electrical power for the circuitry and for actuators such as solenoids. Where only circuitry is involved, it may be sufficient to use non-rechargeable primary cells. The constancy of their output voltage with time renders mercury cells attractive from the circuit viewpoint. However, their cost is not negligible, particularly when a circuit may use perhaps three such cells at a time. Old age pensioners are likely to form a population group requiring therapeutic aids, and here cheapness and ease of purchase are important considerations. When power has to be available for actuators, emphasis will be placed on the use of rechargeable cells. Many users will be women, and care must be taken to see that they understand the perils of overcharging and can use the charger. Particularly in country districts, not all homes have electricity!

The advent of microconsumption integrated circuits is making it feasible to implant increasingly more sophisticated circuitry within tissue. Biological rejection problems seem largely to have been overcome by the use of an outer encapsulation of a medical grade silicone rubber. However, care is still needed in the fabrication to avoid disruption of the circuit function resulting from the leakage of battery materials, the ingress through epoxy resin of body fluids, or mechanical fracture arising from strains developed during the curing of the epoxy resin encapsulation. Considerable study has been made of factors conducive to the premature failing of batteries which are implanted with their circuits, and of the use of induction systems to enable the primary source of power to be kept outside the body. The manufacture of improved artificial limbs has provided a stimulus to the choice of both gas and electric powered systems, and perhaps the greatest challenge comes from the demand for cardiac support devices. The need for the provision of portable sources of electric power is urgent, and the field is rapidly expanding, embracing as it does bio-electric power sources and fuel cells.

PRIMARY CELLS

In contrast to the new developments discussed above, it is interesting to recall that in 1791, Luigi Galvani of Bologna published his work *Commentary on the effects of electricity in muscular motion*. His observations concerned the muscles of a dissected frog's leg which lay on a table on which there was an electrostatic generator. Violent contractions of the limb occurred when an assistant touched the inner crural nerve with the point of a scalpel. It was apparent that the contractions occurred simultaneously with the discharge of a spark from the electrical machine, and only if the scalpel was earthed by the assistant touching with a finger the iron nails which held the blade to the bone handle. Galvani varied the experimental conditions by using the electrical charges from thunderclouds rather than those from an electrical machine. As a result he found that his frog preparations, hanging by copper hooks from an iron railing, contracted not only during the thunderstorms but also in calm weather. Impatient at the long wait occurring between contractions, Galvani began to scrape and press the copper hook fixed to the frog's backbone against the iron railing. This action produced contractions independent of variations in the weather. Similar effects were found with an iron plate and a brass hook. Some of Galvani's experiments with dissimilar metals are illustrated in *Figure 3.1*.

There was no effect observed when insulating substances such as glass and stone were used. A detailed account is given in Foley's (1953) translation of Galvani's work from which *Figure 3.1* is taken. Galvani suggested that an electric fluid must be in the animal itself and introduced the concept of Animal Electricity.

In 1800, Alessandro Volta published his paper *On the electricity excited by the mere contact of conducting substances of different kinds*. He did not completely discard the idea of 'animal electricity',

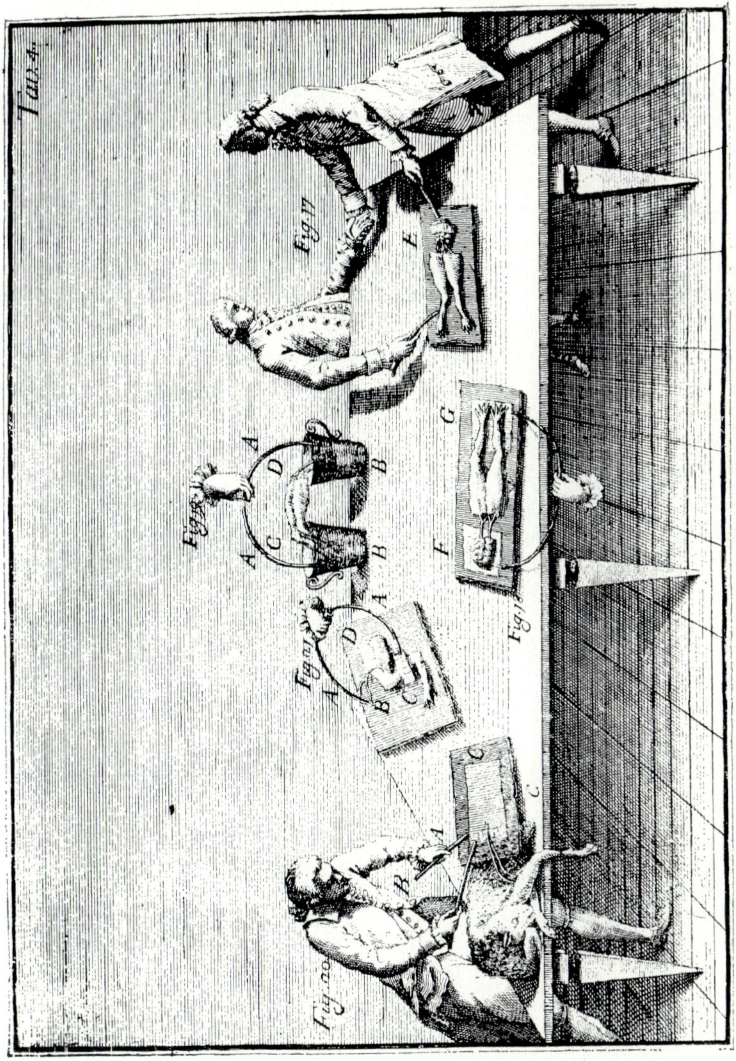

Figure 3.1. Galvani's experiments on animal electricity

but made it clear that the contact of the metals with the moist frog 'could excite and dislodge the electric fluid from its state of rest, so that the organs of the animal act only passively'.

A year after Galvani's death, Volta described an arrangement for producing a stronger galvanic effect. He used a number of pairs of metal discs of copper and zinc placed in line, each pair separated from the next by a cardboard disc moistened with salt water. This arrangement is called a 'Pile'. When the outermost plates, one of copper and one of zinc, were connected to the frog preparation, a strong contraction resulted. Volta's pile was the first battery of cells to be invented. Volta described in great detail the effect of allowing a steady current to pass through his body. The passage of current through the body has aroused considerable attention in studies on the production of electro-sleep and electro-anaesthesia. Smith (1963) reports that a combination of a d.c. current with a square wave pulsation superimposed is satisfactory. Smith also pays tribute to the pioneer work in this field of Leduc in France. Leduc was publishing in the *Archives d'Electricité Médicale* of Bordeaux in 1902.

The Simple Cell

When two dissimilar metals which are spaced well apart in the electrochemical series are immersed in an electrolyte (generally an acid, an alkali or a metal salt), the more electropositive of the plates reacts chemically with the electrolyte. Positive ions are displaced from the plate, leaving it negatively charged. The positive ions move to the other plate, which is lower in the electrochemical series, and give it a positive charge. The potential difference now existing between the plates depends not on their size but on their composition, and is approximately 1·5 V.

The Electrochemical Series

Most electropositive	Potassium
	Sodium
	Magnesium
	Aluminium
	Manganese
	Zinc
	Cadmium
	Iron
	Nickel
	Hydrogen
	Copper
	Mercury
	Silver
	Platinum
Least electropositive	Carbon

On connecting an external circuit across the plates, a current of electrons flows externally from the negatively charged to the positively charged plate. This process is accompanied by a flow, inside the cell, of positive ions to the positive plate, where they tend to neutralize the electrons flowing in the external circuit. As a result, a neutral layer soon forms around the positive plate.

Polarization

The formation of this neutral layer produces two serious unwanted effects. The film lowers the charge acquired by the positive plate by reducing the attraction for positive ions in the electrolyte. The film also reduces the area available for the positive ions. This has the effect of increasing the internal resistance of the cell and reducing the current which can be drawn from it. The action of the film is thus to reduce the amount of power available from the cell. A cell which has such a layer is said to be polarized.

The Capacity of a Cell

The time for which a cell can provide a given current is related to the type and quality of the materials used in the cell construction and to the operating temperature of the cell. The capacity of a cell is quoted in terms of milliampere-hours (mAh). The greater the

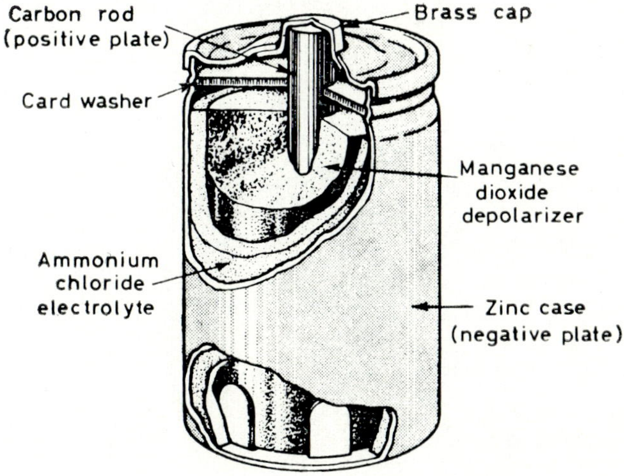

Figure 3.2. Cylindrical low voltage Leclanché cell

(By courtesy of Mallory Batteries Ltd. and *Electronics Manufacturer*)

current drawn, the shorter the life. The end of the useful cell life is marked by the terminal voltage falling to a specified low value, the rate of decline of the voltage usually being more rapid near the end of life. A cell is useful only when its chemical components are active. However, impurities in the zinc react with metal and this action continues even when a current is not being drawn from the cell. This effect is known as 'local action' and it reduces the shelf life of a cell. In a Leclanché cell, it is impurities in the zinc plate which react with the zinc and electrolyte in a local action.

The Leclanché Cell

This form of cell is commonly used to power portable transistorized equipment and in h.t. batteries. In comparison with other types it is relatively inexpensive, but the terminal voltage falls markedly with life. The positive electrode is made from carbon and the negative electrode from zinc. The depolarizing agent is manganese dioxide. *Figure 3.2* illustrates the usual cylindrical type of low voltage cell, whilst *Figure 3.3* shows the series of flat 'layer type' cells used in high tension batteries. Small 300 V batteries of this type form convenient voltage sources for the polarization of devices such as

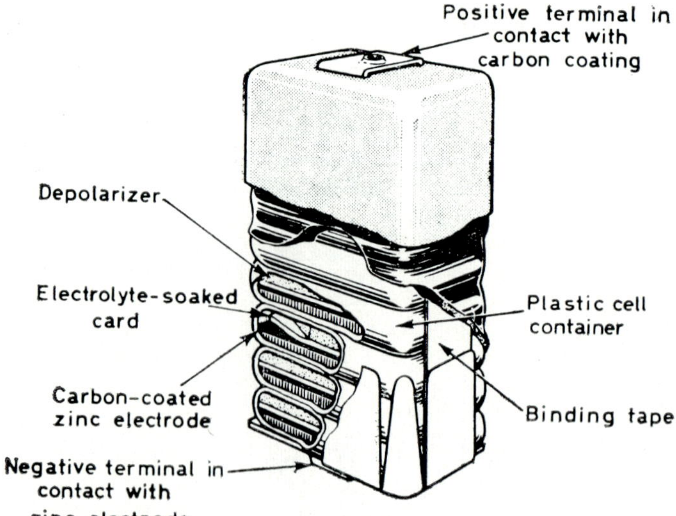

Figure 3.3. Layer type Leclanché cells used in h.t. batteries
(By courtesy of Mallory Batteries Ltd. and *Electronics Manufacturer*)

ionization chambers. The depolarizing action of the manganese dioxide results from a reaction with the neutralized hydrogen layer formed around the carbon rod to produce water. In practice, the hydrogen film forms faster than it can be removed by the depolarizer. As a result, the e.m.f. falls fairly rapidly with continuous use. The local action in a Leclanché cell is increased, and the shelf life correspondingly shortened, at a higher ambient temperature. Leclanché cells are best suited to intermittent load applications, especially if a heavy current is to be drawn.

Leclanché cells are not suitable for miniaturization, for example, for use with implanted cardiac pacemakers. This follows because of their temperature dependence and the inability to handle a continuous load. Versions of Leclanché cells are available which are fully sealed to avoid the leakage of their corrosive contents.

The Alkaline–Manganese Cell

In comparison with the conventional Leclanché, the construction of an alkaline–manganese cell is 'inside out'. The potassium hydroxide electrolyte is placed at the centre of the cell in the form of pressed powder cylinders. Both the manganese dioxide depolarizer and the positive carbon conductor material are combined into one 'mix' which is pressed into a cylindrical form to fit around the electrolyte. The complete cell is housed in a double steel case which plays no part in the electricity-producing reactions. The positive terminal, in contact with the depolarizer via the steel cases, is a stud at the top of the cell. The negative terminal, at the bottom of the cell, is in direct contact with the inner zinc anode cylinders (*Figure 3.4*).

For applications which do not require a high voltage stability and where miniaturization is not so important, the alkaline–manganese battery is the first choice. The same long shelf life and corrosion-free construction are possible as with mercury batteries. Compared with the Leclanché zinc–carbon type, the alkaline–manganese type offers the following advantages: a life longer by a factor of at least three times for light current loads to over ten times for heavy current loads, together with a long storage life and a lower internal resistance. The shelf life is $2\frac{1}{2}$ years under normal storage conditions. *Figure 3.5* shows the percentage of the original capacity retained with time of storage at $-20°C$ and $+45°C$. Satisfactory operation is possible from $-20°C$ to $+70°C$. Normal values of the internal resistance are less than one ohm. Local action has been minimized by the use of high purity zinc for the anode and by the addition of zinc oxide to the

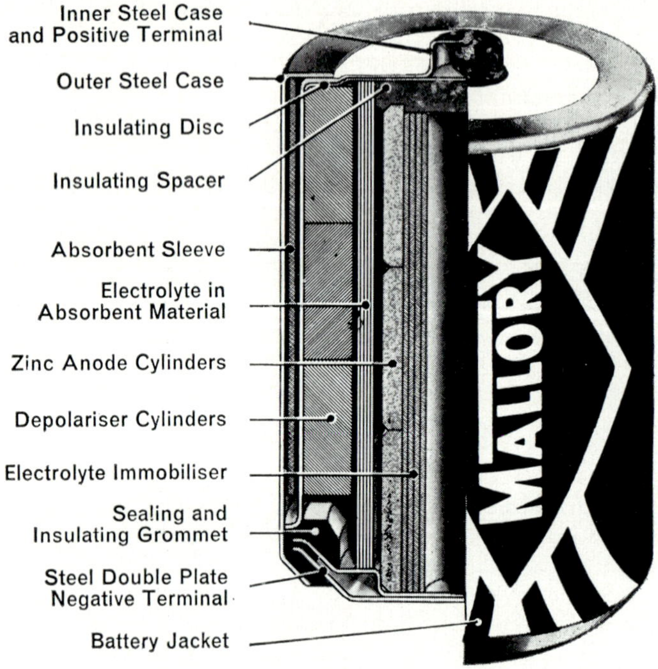

Figure 3.4. Construction of an alkaline–manganese cell
(By courtesy of Mallory Batteries Ltd. and *Electronics Manufacturer*)

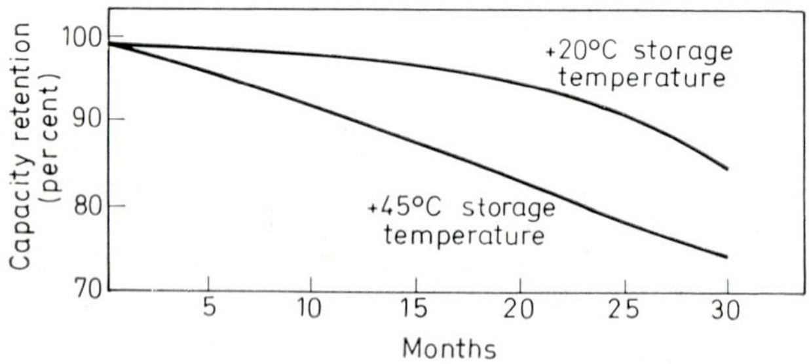

Figure 3.5. A typical capacity retention curve for a Mallory alkaline–manganese system
(By courtesy of Mallory Batteries Ltd.)

electrolyte. This reacts with the potassium hydroxide to form potassium zincate, the high concentration of which inhibits the solution of the anode. The ability of the alkaline–manganese cell to provide a better heavy current performance arises from the compression into a 'mix' of the carbon and depolarizer. This renders the action of the depolarizer more effective and lowers the internal resistance of the cell. Like the Leclanché, the nominal cell voltage is 1·5 V.

The Mercuric Oxide Cell

The mercury cell is suitable for miniaturization and offers the advantages of a long life and stability of its e.m.f. As compared with a Leclanché, an 'inside-out' construction is again used (*Figure 3.6*). The inner negative electrode consists of zinc in the form of either a foil or a powder. The positive electrode consists of mercury, liberated from mercuric oxide which acts as a depolarizer. A small percentage of micronized graphite is added to the mercuric oxide in order to improve its physical characteristics and to reduce the internal resistance of the cell. The high stability of the e.m.f. of mercury cells is attributed to the saturation of the electrolyte with potassium zincate, formed by reaction between the zinc oxide and potassium hydroxide. The zincate inhibits attack of the zinc by the potassium hydroxide. Thus the possibility of forming hydrogen during storage or normal discharge is limited.

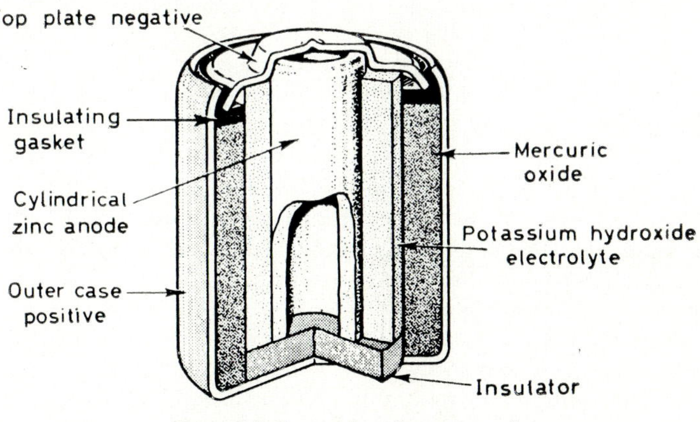

Figure 3.6. Construction of a mercury cell
(By courtesy of Mallory Batteries Ltd. and *Electronics Manufacturer*)

When a mercury cell is connected across an external circuit, zinc ions enter the electrolyte to displace positive ions of hydrogen, which in turn move to the mercuric oxide. Here positive ions of mercury are displaced, the hydrogen combining with the oxygen to form water. The displaced mercury ions take up the incoming electrons from the external circuit and are neutralized. Polarization does not occur since mercury is itself the electrode material. Mercury primary cells are available in both cylindrical (*Figure 3.6*) and button construction (*Figure 3.7*). The outer case of the cell is made from a passive material such as stainless steel. A self-venting

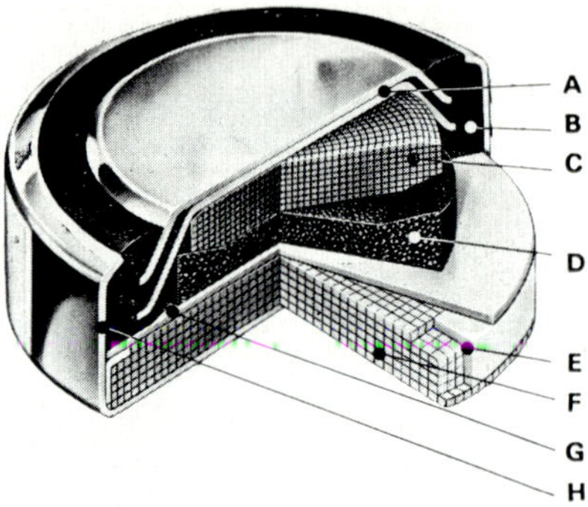

A	Double top	E	Depolarizer sleeve
B	Plastic sealing grommet	F	Depolarizer pellet
C	Zinc anode pellet	G	Synthetic barrier
D	Electrolyte in absorbent	H	Cell can

Figure 3.7. Button stucture mercury cell
(By courtesy of Mallory Batteries Ltd.)

arrangement allows any gas generated in discharging to escape. The nominal cell voltage of industrial type mercury cells is 1·35 V, and these are designed for instrumentation and scientific duties where the battery performance is critical. A commercial range is available with a nominal cell voltage of 1·4 V where voltage precision is not so critical. Cell capacities range from 16 to 14,000 mAh. Considering equal amounts, the chemicals of a mercury cell have six to seven times the capacity of those in a Leclanché cell. For a mercury cell, it is possible to quote an accurate capacity in mAh which will hold over the entire range of current drains. *Figure 3.8* compares the discharge performance of a Leclanché cell with that of an equivalent mercury cell.

Because of the flatness of the curve relating e.m.f. to discharge time, little warning is available of the sudden failure of the cell at the end of its life. In the event of a sudden malfunction of a piece of equipment which contains a mercury cell, it is worth checking the cell at an early stage. Naylor (1970) discusses zinc–carbon, alkaline–manganese and mercuric oxide cells.

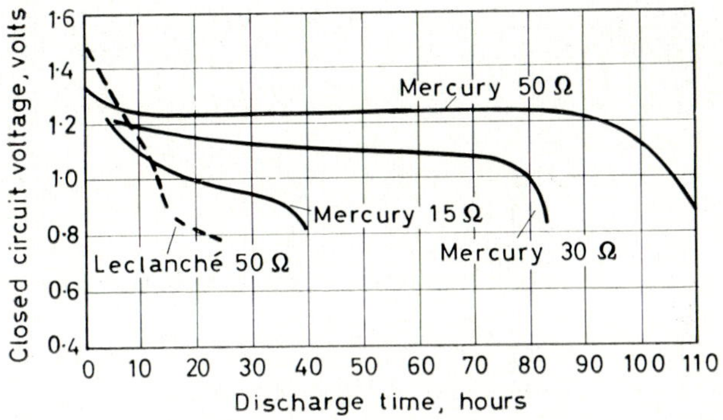

Figure 3.8. A comparison of the discharge performance of a Leclanché cell with that of an equivalent mercury cell

(By courtesy of Mallory Batteries Ltd. and *Electronics Manufacturer*)

The Lithium Cell

The average life of implantable cardiac pacemakers powered by mercury batteries has been estimated by Furman *et al.* (1969) to be less than two years, whilst Chardack (1968) estimates the life expectancy of a pacemaker patient to be about five years, so on this basis the average patient is likely to require three changes of pacemaker. Hence the current interest in the development of pacemaker power supplies with a ten-year life expectancy. As will be described later, one approach is based on the use of a radioactive plutonium source, but the shielding problems associated with the radiation and gas pressure build-up make this an expensive method.

An interesting alternative approach is the lithium battery described by Greatbatch *et al.* (1971). This is a solid state battery with a single cell voltage of 2·8 V. The anode is made from metallic lithium and the cathode from a proprietary iodide. The electrolyte is a crystal, lithium iodide, and not a corrosive liquid. The cell produces electricity by migrating lithium ions through the electrolyte. Elemental iodide is stripped from the cathode via the absorption of an electron. The positive lithium ion migrates through the salt and combines with an iodine ion at the cathode electrolyte interface. The great advantage is that no gas is liberated, so that the battery can be hermetically sealed in a welded stainless steel enclosure. Greatbatch *et al.* (1971) estimate the 10 per cent failure point of a 4 ampere-hour capacity cell as being in excess of five years.

The Standard or Weston Cadmium Cell

The advantage of this type of cell is that its e.m.f. can be accurately calibrated and it can thus be used to supply a 'standard' voltage for calibration purposes. The construction of the Weston standard cell is shown in *Figure 3.9*.

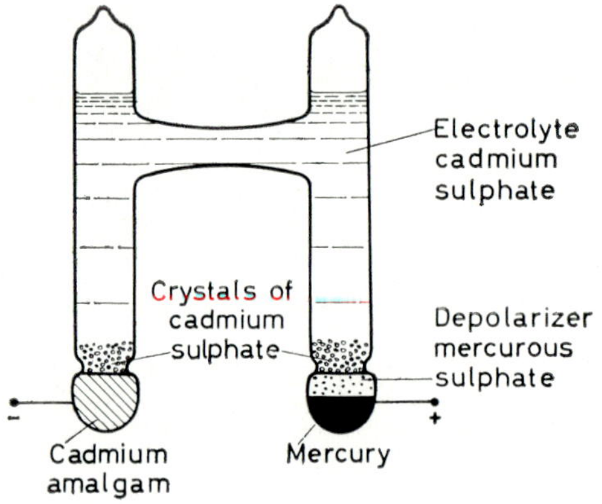

Figure 3.9. Construction of a Weston standard cell

The electrolyte is a saturated solution of cadmium sulphate and the positive pole is a cadmium amalgam. The depolarizer is mercurous sulphate. The e.m.f. E of the cell in volts is given to a close approximation by $E = 1{\cdot}0186 - 0{\cdot}000037\ (t - 20)$ where t is the temperature of the cell in degrees centigrade. Thus the e.m.f. is little dependent upon temperature. For accurate work with a precision d.c. potentiometer, a temperature compensation coil is placed in series with the Weston cell. The internal resistance of the cell is relatively high, of the order of a few hundred ohms. If the cell is called upon to supply a current of more than a few micro-amps, its e.m.f. alters markedly and the condition of the cell deteriorates. Hence, in practice, the cell should be placed in series with a high resistance to limit the current which can be drawn. Standard cells are encountered in precision d.c. potentiometers used for the measurement of thermocouple e.m.f.s and for the calibration of meters. They are also used in electrocardiographs in conjunction with a voltage dividing network to provide a standard millivolt for calibration purposes. A similar application occurs in digital voltmeters where the instrument is first set up to indicate the cell voltage.

A description of the manufacture of standard cells is given by Muirhead (1964).

SECONDARY CELLS

The Lead–Acid Accumulator

Primary cells can be recharged to some extent (Hallows, 1953, 1955), but the process requires care and is not often employed. Secondary cells, on the other hand, can be readily recharged and are used where substantial currents must be provided. The most common, and least expensive, type is the lead–acid accumulator as used in cars. The usual battery consists of a series of 2 V cells. The voltage of a freshly charged cell may rise to 2·2 V, remaining steady around 2 V during normal discharge and falling to 1·8 V when recharging is required. In precision d.c. potentiometers, a series rheostat is provided to take up the voltage variation with discharge of the accumulator used to power the slide wire. To preserve their efficiency, the batteries should be subjected to a regular cycle of charge and discharge. A set of four 6 V 'motor scooter' type accumulators makes a convenient portable power source for laboratory applications. Although mains power units are nearly always used, on many occasions a hum-free, steady low voltage source is a convenient item to have available in experimental work.

Manufacturers quote a recommended charge and discharge current based on a ten or twenty hour rate. The capacity of an accumulator is quoted in terms of the number of ampere-hours (Ah) of electricity it can provide. It should be remembered that the sulphuric acid spray from a charging lead–acid cell can be quite corrosive to nearby apparatus.

Nickel–Cadmium Accumulators

For some applications such as portable electrocardiographs, portable d.c. defibrillators for use in ambulances and radio-telemetry transmitters, it may be desirable to power the apparatus from rechargeable accumulators. Another application arises with portable stimulators used in the electronic control of urinary incontinence. Although these are normally powered by mercury batteries, the cost of battery replacement is relatively high and the use of a pair of accumulators with one in use and one on charge has been appreciated by the patients concerned. For this class of work, the completely sealed nickel–cadmium accumulator is used. Commercially, one version is known as the DEAC accumulator after the Deutsch-Edison Akkumulatoren Company. Being hermetically sealed, they need no maintenance other than regular charging and they cannot damage nearby circuits. They are mechanically rugged and have a long life if they are not seriously overcharged. A low-voltage charging circuit is often built into the apparatus and the cells are designed to withstand a considerable degree of overcharging. At the ten-hour discharge rate, DEACs can be obtained with capacities as low as 20 mAh and as high as 1,500 Ah.

Three other types of rechargeable cells that have been used in implanted devices are the silver–cadmium cell, the silver–zinc cell and the rechargeable mercury cell. Greatbatch (1970) states that the useful life of rechargeable cells with charging has generally been less than that of primary mercury cells without recharging. The action of cells evolves gas, and this must be consumed as it is produced in a fully sealed cell. In the nickel–cadmium accumulator the rate of production of oxygen at the negative electrode equals the rate of recombination with the cadmium.

ELECTRIC FISH

A phenomenon which has been known for thousands of years is that of 'electric fish'. Aristotle (384–322 B.C.) mentions the shock produced by the Torpedo fish (*Historia Animalium*, **20B**, 18–29). The Greek Paul of Aegina (A.D. 650) states that in cases of headache the Torpedo, when applied to the head while still alive, produces relief to pain, probably by its peculiar property of producing torpor. Scribonius recommended the use of the Torpedo to cure both headaches and gout. A good review of the subject is that of Keynes (1956). He mentions a report by Michael Adanson in 1751 from West Africa of the powerful electric shock experienced on touching the electric catfish, *Malapterurus electricus*. Another powerful electric fish is the electric eel, *Electrophorus*, formerly *Gymnotus*. John Hunter (1773) examined the anatomical structure of the *Gymnotus* and reported that it contained a total of 96 piles, giving 4,000 cells in series, forming a prodigiously powerful voltaic 'pile'. In the early days of the study of electricity and living matter, electric fish aroused a great deal of interest. *Figure 3.10*, taken from Du Bois Reymond (1887), shows the use of frog nerve–muscle preparations as primitive relays in the measurement of the initial shock delivered by an electric fish.

IMPLANTABLE POWER SOURCES

The basic mercury cell consists of a mercury–zinc system with

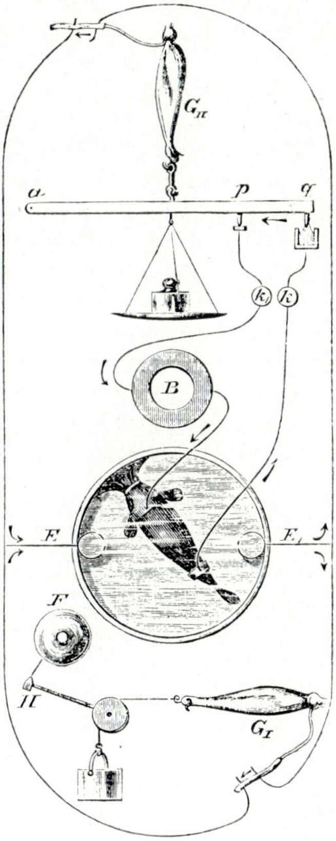

E and *E*,, zinc electrodes in the trough containing the fish. *F*, *H*, *G*,, the bell, hammer, and muscle arranged to form an alarum. *a*, *p*, *q*, lever of the frog-interrupter. *G*,,, its muscle. *p*, the platinum point which rests upon the supporting plate. *q*, amalgamated copper wire which dips into mercury. *K*, *K*,, keys. *B*, galvanometer. The action of the interrupter is such, that only one shock can pass through the galvanometer, for by the contraction of the muscle *G*,, the galvanometer circuit is broken at *q* and not again closed. The alarum of course goes on ringing.

Figure 3.10. Frog alarum

(By courtesy of The Clarendon Press)

a potassium hydroxide electrolyte. For use in implanted circuits, a special type of cell is preferred in which sodium hydroxide is substituted for potassium hydroxide in order to give a less active electrolyte. This reduces the available short-circuit current, but this does not matter at the low current drains encountered in practice. Manganese dioxide has also been added to the mercuric dioxide cathode. Greatbatch (1970) states that during the first 16 per cent of the cell life, the manganese dioxide is reduced to manganese oxide and the residue locks up on a matrix which then supports the liquid mercury evolved during the remainder of the cell life. These factors are responsible for shelf lives of up to 10 years at body temperature. Greatbatch (1970) goes on to say that the e.m.f. of the medical mercury cell remains at approximately 1·45 V until the 16 per cent of manganese dioxide is exhausted, when it falls to 1·35 V. The addition of a slug of silver to the cell structure absorbs excess mercury evolved into a harmless amalgam. Greatbatch (1965) has described an x-ray method for checking the amount of life left in a mercury cell.

A considerable effort has been put into the development of various types of implantable power sources with the aim of achieving a longer life than is possible with mercury batteries. The approaches have included the use of piezoelectric crystals which are activated by body movements such as pulsation of the aorta (Enger and Kennedy, 1964; Lewin *et al.*, 1968). The arrangement of Myers *et al.* (1964) is shown in *Figure 3.11*.

The generation of electricity by a galvanic cell comprising two electrodes of dissimilar metals, with the body fluids as the electrolyte, has also been employed (Strohl *et al.*, 1966; Massie *et al.*, 1968).

Massie and his colleagues were able to obtain 50–75 μW of power from a 16 cm² platinum black–aluminium cell implanted subcutaneously for 200 days. The electrodes were bare and the power available diminished gradually with time. It was concluded that this was due to an extensive tissue–electrode reaction and the accumulation of insoluble aluminium oxidation products on the surface of the cathode. Roy *et al.* (1970) have investigated the use of a platinum–zinc pair, and Schaldach (1970) a silver–silver chloride–zinc pair. Neither of these systems used protected electrodes. Wolfson *et al.* (1968) made use of a fuel cell fed with a continuous supply of fuel and oxidant from the body fluids.

Massie *et al.* (1968) also experimented with a hybrid cell in which the anode was consumed whilst oxygen from the body fluids was reduced at the cathode. Tseung, King and Wan (1971) have produced an encapsulated, implantable aluminium–platinum black electrochemical cell. It is covered with a silicone rubber membrane, and the anode and cathode compartments are separated by an anionic ion exchange membrane. This is a hybrid cell, the silicone membrane allowing through the oxygen from body

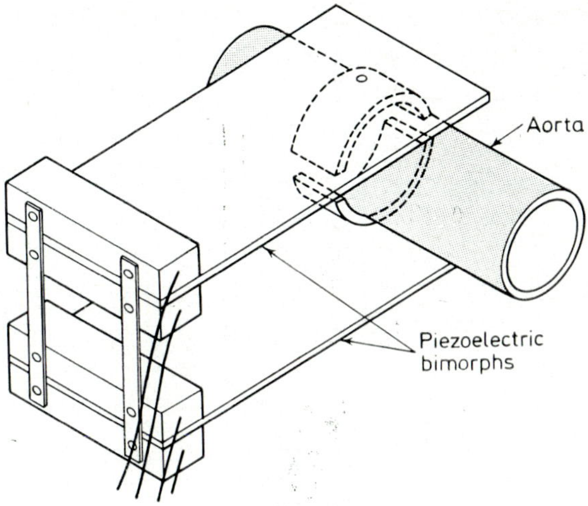

Figure 3.11. Ceramic bimorph power source

(Reproduced after Myers *et al.*, 1964, by courtesy of the Editor of *American Journal of Medical Electronics*)

fluids required for reduction at the cathode. Tseung and his co-workers gave the electrode reactions as

Anodic reaction

$$2\,Al + 6\,OH' = 2\,Al\,(OH)_3 + 6\,e = Al_2O_3 + 3\,H_2O + 6\,e$$

Cathodic reaction

$$6\,e + 3\,H_2O + 1\tfrac{1}{2}O_2 = 6\,OH'$$

Overall reaction

$$2\,Al + 1\tfrac{1}{2}\,O_2 + Al_2O_3$$

The anionic ion exchange membrane is relatively impermeable to oxygen and is not permeable to large molecules or corrosion products of aluminium whilst allowing the OH′ ions to diffuse. The cell does not use the body fluids as its conducting medium, but has a 0·9 per cent sodium chloride solution as its electrolyte. Tseung, King and Wan (1971) found that a cell of 5·5 cm^2 area gave a continuous power output in excess of 70–100 μW at 0·9 V into a 10 k Ω load with implantation in different rats over a period of more than 12 months.

An interesting development is the use of a radioactive source of about 0·2 grammes of plutonium-238 (virtually a pure alpha emitter) as a source of heat. This is used to drive a semiconductor thermopile giving an open circuit output voltage of 0·4 V, and a power of 400 μW into a 100 ohm load. This is then stepped up in a

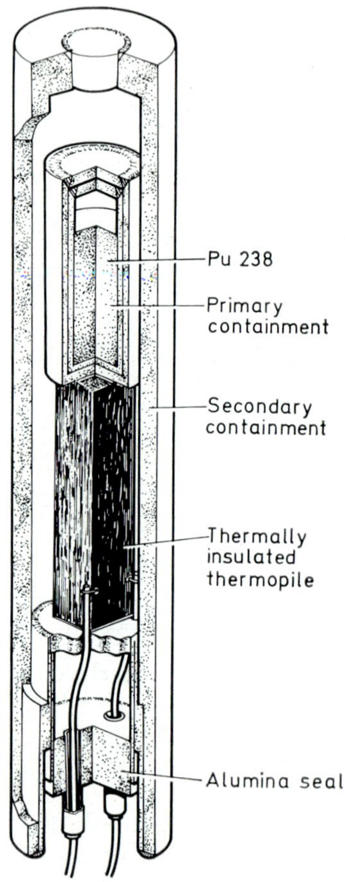

Figure 3.12. Isotope battery
(By courtesy of the United Kingdom Atomic Energy Authority)

transistorized d.c.-to-d.c. converter to supply 5–6 V to the pacemaker circuitry. Since the plutonium is highly toxic to the patient, the sealing of the nuclear battery must be of a very high standard.

Helium is evolved in the radioactive decay process. Pressures greater than 500 kg wt/cm^2 (7,110 lbf/in^{2}g, 49 MN/m^2) can build up and the sealing must be able to withstand this. The gas build-up sets the life of the nuclear battery at about 10 years. The construction is shown in *Figure 3.12*.

Another approach is the use of a radioactive beta particle source of tritium which irradiates a semiconductor junction to provide a power supply.

REFERENCES

Du Bois Reymond, E. (1887). 'Observations and experiments on malapterurus brought to Berlin alive.' In *Translations of Foreign Biological Memoirs*. 1. *Memoirs on the Physiology of Nerve, of Muscle, and of the Electrical Organ*. Ed. by J. Burdon-Sanderson. Oxford: Clarendon Press.

Chardack, W. (1968). 'The current status of implantable pacemakers.' *J. Electrocardiography* **1,** 135.

Enger, C. and Kennedy, J. (1964). 'An improved bio-electric generator.' *Trans. Am. Soc. artif. internal Organs* **10,** 373.

Furman, S., Escher, J. W., Parker, B. and Solomon, N. (1969). 'Clinical analysis of pacemaker function.' *Am J. Cardiol.* **23,** 112.

Galvani, L. (1791). *Commentary on the Effects of Electricity on Muscular Motion*. Translation by M. G. Foley, and Notes by I. B. Cohen. Burndy Library, Norwalk, U.S.A.

Greatbatch, W. (1965). 'X-ray techniques for evaluation of exhaustion and detection of mechanical defects in implantable mercury batteries.' *Med. Electron. biol. Engng* **3,** 305.

— (1970). 'Physiological stimulators for clinical use.' In *Biomedical Engineering Systems*, p. 412. Ed. by M. Clynes and J. H. Milsum. New York: McGraw-Hill.

— Lee, J., Mathias, W., Eldridge, M., Moser, J. and Schneider, A. (1971). 'The solid-state lithium battery: a new improved chemical power source for implantable cardiac pacemakers.' *IEEE Trans. bio-med. Engng* **37,** 99.

Hallows, R. W. (1953). 'Re-activating the dry cell.' *Wireless Wld* **59,** 344.

— (1955). 'Dry-cell reactivator.' *Wireless Wld* **61,** 503.

Hunter, J. (1773). *The Works of John Hunter, F.R.S.*, p. 398. Ed. by J. F. Palmer. London: Longmans Green.

Keynes, R. D. (1956). 'The generation of electricity by fishes.' *Endeavour* **15,** 215.

Leduc, S. (1902). 'Production of sleep and general and local anaesthesia by intermittent current of low voltage.' *Archs Élect. méd.* **10,** 617.

Lewin, G., Myers, G., Parsonnet, V. and Raman, K. (1968). 'An improved biological power source for cardiac pacemakers.' *Trans. Am. Soc. artif. internal Organs* **14,** 215.

Massie, H., Racie, P., Parker, R., Hanh, A. W. and Sun, H. H. (1968). 'Study of power generating implantable electrodes.' *Med. biol. Engng* **6,** 503.

Muirhead & Co. (1964). 'Standard cells by Muirhead.' *Technique, Beckenham* **18,** 19.

Myers, G. H., Parsonnet, V., Zucker, I. R. and Cotman, H. (1964). 'Biologically energized cardiac pacemakers.' *Am. J. Med. Electron.* **3,** 233.

Naylor, D. (1970). 'New primary cells help to reduce equipment size.' *Electron. Engng* **42,** 74.

Roy, O. Z., Wahnert, R. W., Heggvett, H. A. and Waddell, W. G. (1970). 'Bioelectrical energy sources.' *Ann. N.Y. Acad. Sci.* **167,** 645.

Schaldach, M. (2970). 'A pacemaker driven by a biogalvanic element.' In *Cardiac Engineering*, p. 321. Ed. by Y. Nosé. New York: Interscience.

Smith, R. H. (1963). *Electrical Anaesthesia.* Springfield, Ill.: Thomas.

Strohl, T. L., Scott, R. O., Freelel, W. J. and Wolfson, S. K. Jnr. (1966). 'Studies of bioelectric power sources for cardiac pacemakers.' *Trans. Am. Soc. artif. internal Organs* **12,** 318.

Tseung, A. C. C., King, W. J. and Wan, B. Y. C. (1971). 'An encapsulated, implantable metal–oxygen cell as a long-term power source for medical and biological applications.' *Med. biol. Engng* **8,** 1.

Volta, A. (1800). 'On the electricity excited by the mere contact of conducting substances of different kinds.' *Phil. Trans. R. Soc.* **90,** 403.

Wolfson, S. K. Jnr., Gofberg, S. L., Prusiner, P. and Nanis, L. (1968). 'The bioauto fuel cell. A device for pacemaker power from direct energy conversion consuming autogenous fuel.' *Trans. Am. Soc. artif. internal Organs* **14,** 198.

Chapter 4

D.C. Circuits, Resistors and Capacitors

In the previous chapter, several forms of primary and secondary cells together with fuel cells were described. These devices are characterized by the fact that when they are in an active state a potential difference exists between their terminals. If a length of wire is connected across the terminals, then the wire becomes warm. This is because the action of the potential difference is to cause a current to flow through the wire, that is, through the external circuit connected across the battery. Although many pieces of medical electronic apparatus are powered from batteries, others employ a power unit to convert the alternating mains voltage into suitable d.c. voltages for use by the circuits.

ELECTRIC CURRENT

The flow of electric current arises from a drift of electrons from the atoms of the material of the wire in one direction on connection of the battery. If a more powerful battery having a higher voltage is substituted, the electrons drift at a faster rate, and a larger current flows. The practical unit of current is the ampere (A). It is equal to a flow of 6×10^{18} electrons per second past a given point on the wire.

QUANTITY OF ELECTRICITY

The practical unit of quantity (amount) of electricity is the Coulomb. It is equal to the amount of electricity carried past a given point on a wire in one second when the current flowing is one ampere. It is apparent that if a current of I amperes flows past a given point of the wire for t seconds, then the quantity of electricity carried in that time is given by $Q = I \times t$ Coulombs.

UNITS OF CURRENT

Currents of the order of amperes are commonly found in the power output stages of medical electronic apparatus. In many earlier stages, the currents are much smaller. The more common units are milliamperes (mA), where 1 mA=1/1,000 of an ampere (10^{-3}A) and micro-amperes (μA) where 1 μA=1/1,000,000 of an ampere (10^{-6} A). Transistors operating with collector currents of a few micro-amperes are often used in the first stages of low-noise amplifiers. In the use of polarographic electrodes for the measurement of oxygen tension in blood and tissue and in ionization chambers for the measurement of radioactivity, even smaller currents of the order of 10^{-9} (nano-amperes) and 10^{-12} A (pico-amperes) are commonly encountered.

Conventionally, current is depicted as flowing from the positive to the negative terminal of a battery. However, the flow of electrons forming the current is actually in the opposite direction, from the negative to the positive terminal.

POTENTIAL DIFFERENCE

In order for an electric current to flow, a potential difference must be established across the ends of the conductor. It is helpful here to think in terms of a water analogy, where a pressure difference must be produced across the ends of a pipe in order to force water to flow through it. As discussed in Chapter 2, the concept of an electric potential difference is based upon an energy concept. The practical unit of potential difference is the volt, and two points in an electrical circuit are said to have a potential difference of one volt if one joule of energy is released when one coulomb of electricity passes between the points. Smaller units are the millivolt (1 mV=1/1,000 V) commonly encountered in cardiology and the microvolt (1 μV=1/1,000,000 V) in electroencephalography. Larger units are the kilovolt (1 kV=1,000 V) encountered in Geiger counter, scintillation counter and cathode ray tube power supplies, and the megavolt (1 MV=1,000,000 V) encountered in radiotherapy.

RESISTANCE

In 1826, George Simon Ohm (1787–1854) completed a long series of measurements on the flow of electricity along metals. From this work he deduced the following statement, known as Ohm's law: 'The ratio of the P.D. (V) between the ends of a conductor to the current (I) flowing in it is always constant, provided that the physical conditions of the conductor, such as temperature, remain constant'. The constant V/I was called by Ohm the resistance (R) of the conductor. It can be seen that the resistance is high when a large applied voltage will produce only a small flow of current. Ohm's law gives the following relationships: $R=V/I$, $V=IR$ and $I=V/R$. R is in ohms when V is in volts and I is in amperes. The larger units of resistance, the kilohm ($1\ k\Omega=1{,}000\ \Omega$) and the megohm ($1\ M\Omega=1{,}000{,}000\ \Omega$), are frequently encountered in electronic circuits. Low resistances, such as contact resistances, are often quoted in terms of milliohms ($1\ m\Omega=1/1{,}000\ \Omega$). The micro-ohm ($1\ m\Omega=10^{-6}\ \Omega$) often occurs in the measurement of resistivity.

Specific Resistance (or Resistivity)

In Chapter 7 it will be seen to be convenient to compare the resistance of various types of material in terms of their specific resistance or resistivity. The specific resistance is given by $R=ls/A$ where R is the resistance in ohms of a piece of the material of specific resistance s, cross-sectional area A and length l. It follows that if l and A are both equal to unity, then s is numerically equal to the resistance of a unit cube of the material. The units of resistivity are ohm-cm and micro-ohm-cm.

Pure copper, which has a very low resistivity (approximately $1{\cdot}7\ \mu\Omega$-cm), is generally used for current-carrying conductors. However, copper alloys such as Constantan (60 parts copper, 40 parts nickel), used as one of the components of thermocouples for measuring body temperature, Nichrome (an alloy of copper, nickel and chromium), used for electric heater windings, and Manganin (an alloy of copper, manganese and nickel), used for resistance windings, have a much higher resistance. The resistance of Nichrome, for example, is about 98 $\mu\Omega$-cm. The resistance of these alloys remains fairly constant when their temperature changes. Hence wire-wound resistors are constructed from Nichrome. Precision resistances used in decade resistance boxes are wound from a material such as Manganin (Price, 1964).

Variation of Resistance with Temperature

The temperature variation of the resistance of a metal is given over a wide temperature range by the equation $R_t=R_o\ (1+\alpha_t+\beta_t^2)$ where R_t and R_o are the resistances at $t°$ C and 0° C. For platinum, a typical value of α would be $+0{\cdot}0038$, and for β $-0{\cdot}000\ 000\ 58$. The variation in the resistance of a coil of nickel or platinum wire made up in the form of a rectal probe is used to measure body temperature (Hill, 1959a) in some forms of apparatus. Although the characteristics of a batch of such probes are very reproducible, they require a sensitive bridge circuit to measure the small changes in resistance, and the probes are relatively large. For these reasons most body temperature probes are based upon the use of thermistors.

THERMISTORS (N.T.C. RESISTORS)

A thermistor (negative temperature coefficient resistor) is a thermally sensitive resistor whose resistance decreases as its temperature increases. In other words, it is a resistor having a negative temperature coefficient of resistance. The coefficient has a high value, typically −4 per cent per degree centigrade at 20° C. The thermistor material is a semiconductor, often a mixture of nickel, cobalt and manganese oxides. There are three main types of thermistors in regular use—bead types, disk types and rod types. They are available in a number of different forms and cover a range of resistance from a few ohms to megohms. A good description of thermistors is that of Hyde (1970).

Bead Thermistors

Where a fast speed of response is required, bead thermistors are commonly used. A tiny bead of the material is fused on to fine platinum wires, in many cases the bead itself being fused into the tip of a glass envelope. This provides mechanical protection for the fragile bead as well as preventing the ingress of moisture, chemicals and gases. If the glass layer is thin, the speed of response can still be sufficiently rapid for the thermistor to be used as a temperature probe capable of responding to respiratory gas flows. When the bead is mounted in an evacuated or gas-filled glass bulb, it becomes sensitive to self-heating and will demonstrate a marked fall in resistance for a small power dissipation. For example, the type R thermistor by I.T.T. Ltd. will increase its bead temperature by 1° C for a power dissipation of only 0·016 mW. The fact that the resistance decreases as the applied power increases enables a thermistor to function in a feedback path in such a way as to hold the output amplitude from an oscillator sensibly constant. Some types of glass bead thermistors are indirectly heated—that is, they are provided with a separate heater enabling the thermistor resistance to be controlled from an isolated supply.

Disk Thermistors

Disk thermistors are constructed from a disk of semiconductor material which has silvered sides and soldered connections. They can handle a higher power dissipation than bead types since they are not hermetically sealed and have a relatively larger mass. They are also cheaper, but are slower acting than bead types. Disk thermistors are employed in both temperature measurement and control applications.

Rod Thermistors

Rod thermistors generally have a large mass of semiconductor material compared with bead or disk types. They are rod-shaped in order to provide a large surface area for heat dissipation purposes, and are mainly used in current surge suppression and time delay applications.

Thermistor Characteristics

Figure 4.1 shows a typical resistance–temperature characteristic for a thermistor. The equation to the curve is $R=A\exp(B/T)$

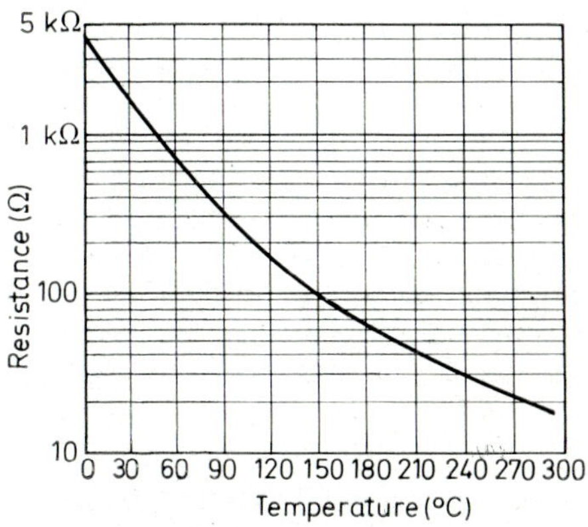

Figure 4.1. Resistance–temperature characteristic of a typical negative temperature coefficient thermistor

(By courtesy of I.T.T. Components Goup Europe)

where R is the resistance of the thermistor, T is the temperature of the thermistor in kelvins (°K), B is the 'characteristic' temperature of the thermistor in °K (this is an arbitrary constant not related to any specific value of R or T) and A is a constant. Thus

$R_1 = R_2 \exp(B/T_1 - B/T_2)$ where R_1 and R_2 respectively are the thermistor resistances at absolute temperatures T_1 and T_2 °K. The temperature coefficient of a thermistor is given approximately by $-(B/T^2)$. Typical values of B lie in the range 2,500–5,000 °K.

Figure 4.2 illustrates a typical voltage–current characteristic for a thermistor. As the current through the thermistor is increased from zero, the voltage drop developed across the thermistor will at first be linearly related to the voltage drop. However, as the current is further increased, self-heating in the thermistor will cause its

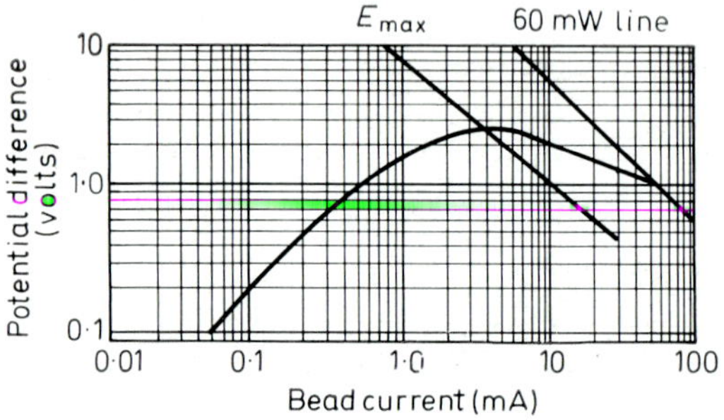

Figure 4.2. Typical voltage-current characteristic for a thermistor having an E_{max} of approximately 2·5 V

(By courtesy of I.T.T. Components Group Europe)

resistance to fall, resulting in a non-linear curve. The voltage drop reaches a maximum E_{max}, after which the thermistor exhibits a negative slope resistance. The thermistor resistance at the voltage maximum is approximately one-third of its room temperature resistance. The combination of voltage and current corresponding to a power dissipation of 60 mW is also shown.

Thermistor Linearization

Bead thermistors are commonly used in temperature measuring instruments and their exponential resistance–temperature characteristics prevent a direct linear calibration in terms of temperature for each instrument. Not only is it desirable to have a linear calibration, but it is also necessary to be able easily to interchange probes or to switch in a number of probes in sequence whilst still maintaining the calibration. It has been found that a linear temperature–resistance characteristic can be achieved over a limited temperature range if the thermistor is shunted with a suitable value of fixed resistor. A thermistor plus shunt resistor network exhibits a point of inflection in its graph of total resistance against temperature where the rate of change of the resistance of the combination with temperature is a minimum. It is about this point of inflection that a more linear change of resistance is obtained. *Figure 4.3* illustrates the effect of shunting a thermistor with a resistor of negligible temperature coefficient and having a resistance value of 1,346 Ω. The resistance of the thermistor alone is 2,000 Ω at 20° C and it has

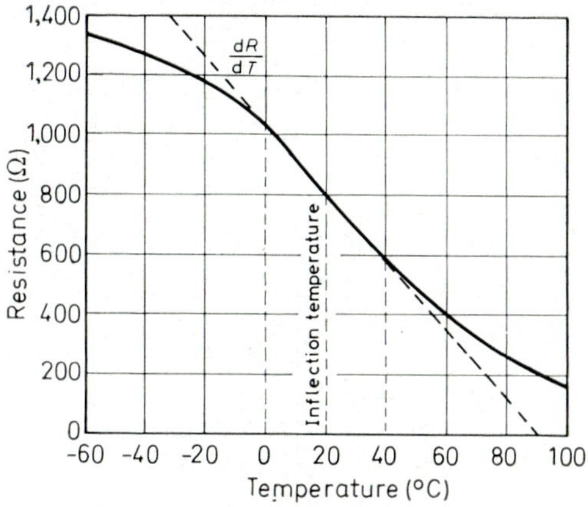

Figure 4.3. Resistance–temperature characteristic of the combination of a 1,346 Ω resistor and a thermistor whose resistance is 2,000 Ω at 20°C

(By courtesy of I.T.T. Components Group Europe)

a *B* value of 3,000° K. The characteristic of the combination is substantially linear over the temperature range 0–40° C. A simple rule is that when the thermistor has the same resistance as its shunt, the temperature coefficient of the combination is half that of the thermistor alone. With regard to the production of matched probes, Godin (1962) has shown that similar thermistors can be adjusted to have nearly identical resistance–temperature characteristics by the addition of both a series and a parallel resistor.

Nordon and Bainbridge (1962) have designed a bridge circuit (*Figure 4.4*) which can be adjusted to linearize the change in thermistor resistance with temperature. The shunt resistances R_1 and R_2 are chosen to linearize the change in thermistor resistance with temperature, and then the differing values of the linear temperature sensitivity for each thermistor are made equal by adjusting R_3 and R_4. These values are made high in comparison with those of the thermistor shunt resistor combinations. This ensures that each thermistor is fed with a sensibly constant current. It is the magnitude of these currents which is adjusted so that for a given temperature change the same potential difference will appear across a given thermistor–shunt resistor combination. In this way, drifts in the bridge output voltage with changes in the ambient temperature are eliminated. Only one thermistor is mounted in the temperature

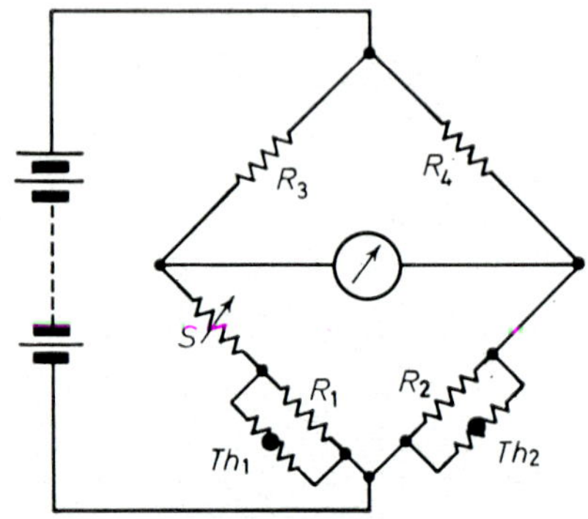

Figure 4.4. The use of a bridge circuit to linearize the resistance–temperature characteristic of a thermistor

(Reproduced after Nordon and Bainbridge, 1962, by courtesy of the Editor of *Journal of Scientific Instruments*)

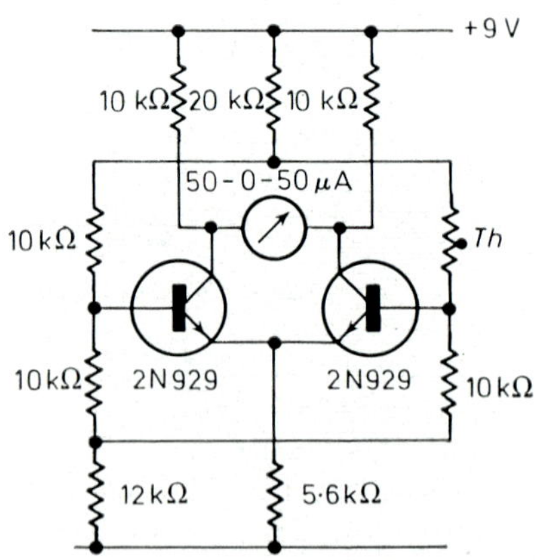

Figure 4.5. The use of a thermistor in a bridge circuit with a transistor amplifier to measure temperature

(By courtesy of I.T.T. Components Group Europe)

probe, the other being in the control box. Care must be taken to ensure that the current passing through each thermistor is insufficient to produce any significant degree of self-heating. The sensitivity of a thermistor bridge can be increased by feeding the bridge output into a d.c. amplifier as in *Figure 4.5.* With this circuit, a full-scale sensitivity of $\pm 0{\cdot}5°$ C at 20° C can be obtained using a 50–0–50 μA meter.

ELECTRICAL POWER AND HEATING EFFECTS

If a current of I amperes is caused to flow through a resistance of R ohms, then the electrical power dissipated in the wire is $W = I^2R$ where W is in watts. From Ohm's law, the power can also be expressed as $W = V^2/R = IV$. The manufacturers of resistors for use in electronic circuits quote maximum permissible wattage dissipation figures for each type of resistor. Commonly encountered values for wire-wound types are 3, 5 and 10 W. Carbon composition resistors are available with 1, $\frac{1}{2}$, $\frac{1}{4}$ and $\frac{1}{8}$ W ratings at 70° C. In order to obtain a stable operation of a circuit, it is important to see that a generous margin is allowed in regard to the wattage ratings of individual components. A maximum voltage which can be applied to particular types of resistor is also quoted. If this is exceeded, tracking or flash-over may occur. When the applied voltage is high, a series of lower value resistors is used instead of just one resistor in order to provide a longer insulation path.

TYPES OF RESISTOR

Carbon Composition Resistors

These are the most commonly encountered resistors in electronic circuitry for general purpose use. The resistive element is cylindrical in form and composed of a hot-moulded mixture of carbon powder and a resin binder. The whole is placed in a ceramic tube and leads

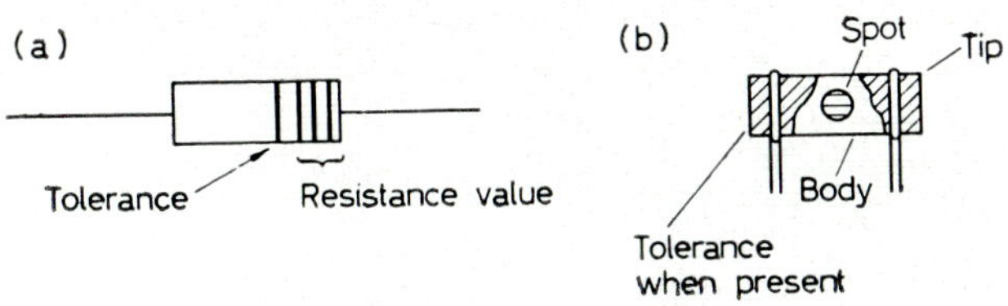

Figure 4.6. Colour coding of resistors

are led out at each end. The nominal value in ohms of each resistor, together with the tolerance on this value, is indicated by a series of coloured bands painted around the body of the resistor as shown in *Figure 4.6a.* A typical manufacturer's range would be from 10 Ω to 22 M Ω with a ± 10 per cent tolerance. The relationship of the colours to numerals is shown below.

Black	0	Blue	6
Brown	1	Violet	7
Red	2	Grey	8
Orange	3	White	9
Yellow	4	Gold	± 5 per cent tolerance
Green	5	Silver	± 10 per cent tolerance

The colours in order of increasing numerical value can be remembered by the mnemonic '*B*illy *B*rown *R*evives *O*n *Y*our *G*in *B*ut *V*alues *G*ood *W*hisky'. The first band, that closest to one end of the resistor, gives the first digit of the resistance value, the second band gives the second digit and the third band gives the number of zeros. If a fourth band is present it indicates either a ± 5 per cent or a ± 10 per cent tolerance. If it is absent, the tolerance is ± 20 per cent (*Figure 4.7a*).

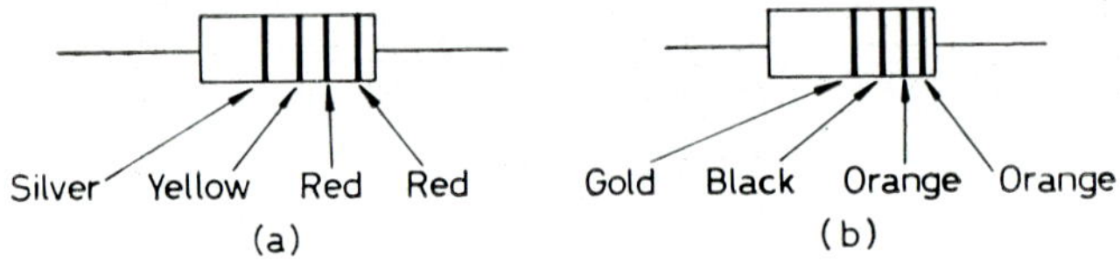

Figure 4.7. Colour coding of resistors

On uninsulated resistors the value is indicated not by bands but by paint applied to the body of the resistor as shown in *Figure 4.7b*. In this case the value is read as follows: the body colour indicates the first digit, the tip at one end the second digit, and the number of zeros is shown by a spot in the centre of the body. If the tolerance is ± 5 per cent or ± 10 per cent, this is shown by gold or silver paint applied to the remaining end of the body, or it is left blank to indicate a ± 20 per cent tolerance. Thus *Figure 4.7a* indicates a 220,000 Ω ± 10 per cent resistor, and *Figure 4.7b* a 330 Ω ± 5 per cent resistor.

A component supplier's catalogue will quote a range of available values of resistance. These values are chosen so that if each forms the centre value of a group of width equal to the specific tolerance range, successive groups will overlap to cover the whole available range. *Figure 4.8* shows the overlapping of 10 and 20 per cent tolerances on the preferred resistor values between 100 and 1,000 Ω.

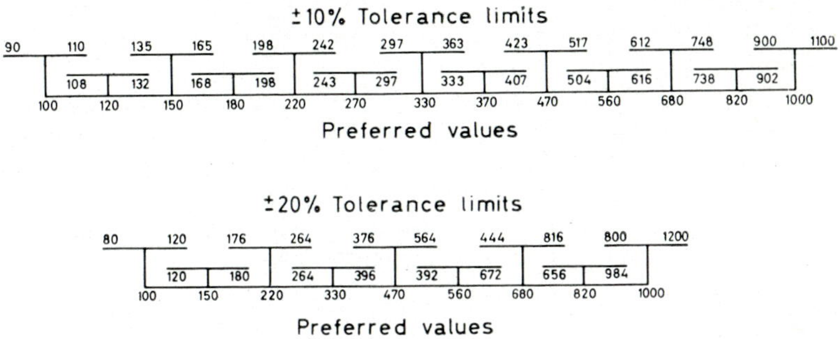

Figure 4.8. Preferred resistor values, together with ±10 per cent and ±20 per cent tolerances in the range 100–1,000 Ω

High Stability Resistors

High stability resistors are made by forming a layer of 'cracked' carbon on a ceramic rod. The carbon is 'cracked' by exposing it to a hydrocarbon vapour at about 1,000° C. 'Hi-Stab' resistors are commonly available in the range 10 Ω to 33 M Ω, with a tolerance of ±5 per cent, ±2 per cent or ±1 per cent. The resistive element is completely sealed and insulated to withstand arduous operating conditions. The maximum permissible working voltage is quoted as 350 V for values of 330 kΩ and above only. The carbon film is cut in the form of a helix to give the required resistance value. Stanley (1971) discusses both the reliability and the stability of carbon film resistors.

An improved form of high-stability resistor is the metal oxide film type (Hayden, 1962). The resistive film normally consists of tin oxide doped with oxides such as those of antimony, indium, bismuth or phosphorus laid down on a high-purity glass substrate. This has to be alkali-free and of optical quality. The metal oxide film resistor is superior to the cracked carbon type in respect of stability under arduous environmental conditions, long-term storage and operating conditions of many years' duration. This type is also to be preferred for low-noise operation. An average figure for noise is 0·05 μV per volt applied across the resistor. A good account of resistive materials and resistor construction is that of Watkins (1971).

Variable Resistors and Potentiometers

For use in electronic circuits where space is not limited, these components usually consist of a metal wiper arm connected to, but insulated from, a 6 mm diameter metal shaft. The angle of rotation is approximately 300 degrees, the arm sweeping over a resistive track. The device is provided with three terminals, the centre one connecting to the wiper arm, and the ends of the resistive track to the other two. In medical instrumentation, reliability is important and wire-wound potentiometers and variable resistors are to be preferred where possible. They are formed by winding a coil of Nichrome wire around a flat strip of insulating material and then bending the strip into a circular form, the wiper arm now rubbing along the edge. The oxide coating of the wire separates adjacent turns. A typical range available for wire-wound types is from 50 Ω to 100 kΩ with a ±20 per cent tolerance and a 3 W rating. The fact that there must be a gap between adjacent turns can cause discontinuities, for example, jerkiness of the trace when a motor-driven potentiometer is used as a slow speed time base for a cathode ray tube display (Scott and Cumming, 1960). *Figure 4.9* illustrates the circuit symbols for variable and preset rheostats and potentiometers.

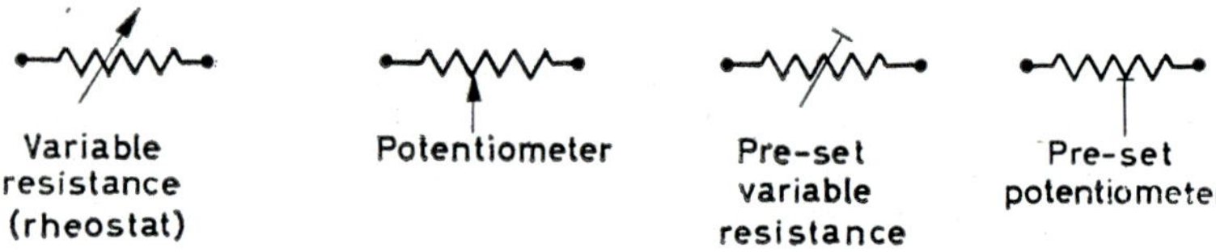

Figure 4.9. Circuit symbols for variable resistors (rheostats) and potentiometers

A linear arrangement can be used instead of a circular track, a lead screw now moving the variable contact along the track. For preset applications the end of the lead screw shaft is fitted with a screwdriver slot. The slim, rectangular form of this type lends itself to mounting on printed circuit boards.

Instead of wire, carbon is often employed as the resistive element, particularly for the higher values of resistance. A typical range would be from 10 kΩ to 2 MΩ with a ±20 per cent tolerance and a $\frac{1}{2}$ W rating. The main drawback to carbon potentiometers lies in the fact that after a considerable amount of use they are liable to become electrically 'noisy'. This occurs when there is an intermittent contact between the track and the wiper. If this arises from 'bald' patches in the track, then the component must be changed. If it is due to loose particles of carbon forcing the slide away from the track, a temporary cure can sometimes be effected by squirting the track with a proprietary cleaning fluid. Miniature preset carbon track potentiometers are available in convenient forms for mounting on printed circuit boards. Both linear and rotary types are available with a Cermet (a ceramic-based resistive element) track rather than carbon.

Linear and Logarithmic Law Potentiometers

In linear potentiometers, the resistance between the wiper arm and an end of the track will vary linearly with the rotation of the shaft. Carbon potentiometers can also be ordered with a graded track such that a linear rotation of the shaft produces a logarithmic variation of resistance. These were originally intended for volume controls in audio circuits, where they produced a linear variation of the sound heard by the logarithmic response of the ear with rotation of the control. They are of course useful in applications where a large change in resistance is required per rotation.

Loading of Potentiometers

The law of a linear potentiometer is only accurately obeyed if the device is subjected to negligible loading. That is to say that no appreciable resistance is placed in parallel with the output from the potentiometer. In *Figure 4.10*, this means that R_L must be consider-

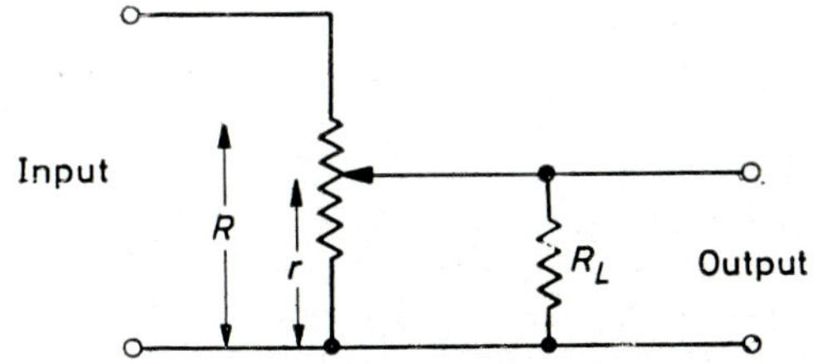

Figure 4.10. The loading of a potentiometer by an external resistance

ably greater than r. In order to achieve this it may be necessary to work the potentiometer into an emitter follower or source follower. Although they are expensive, 'cam-corrected' potentiometers are available in which, by means of cams, individual segments of the wire-wound track are adjusted to give the best linearity. They find application in analogue computers.

Potentiometers are usually operated in the form of a voltage dividing network. *Figure 4.11* shows the variation of the output voltage for various degrees of rotation of the shaft when a constant voltage source is used. In the case of a heavy loading, when $R_L = \frac{1}{10}R$,

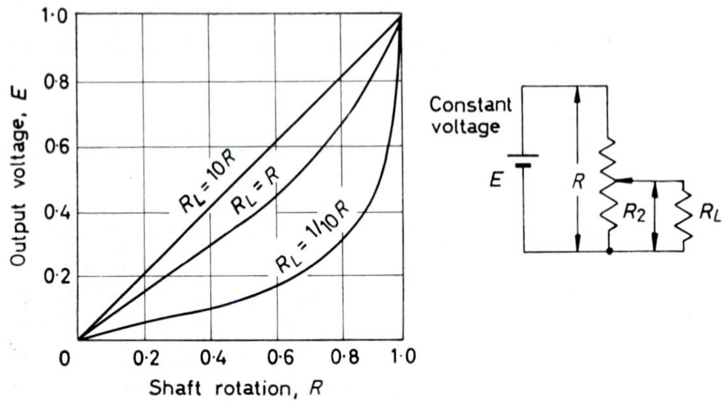

Figure 4.11. The variation of the loading effect with the value of the external resistance
(Reproduced from Donaldson, 1958)

it is seen that now nearly all the variation of the output voltage occurs during the last 20 per cent of rotation.

Multi-turn Potentiometers

A greater degree of voltage division accuracy can be obtained by the use of a longer resistive track. Wire-wound resistances are available having three, ten, fifteen, twenty-five or forty turn helical tracks. The resistance wire is covered in varnish and wound around the turns of a helical copper coil (*Figure 4.12*). The insulation on the inner surfaces of the turns is bared to enable a sliding contact to rotate around the turns. The contacts and slip ring are made from precious metal to increase the operating life and to minimize electrical noise and contact resistance. The standard tolerance is ± 5 per cent for resistance and $\pm 0{\cdot}5$ per cent for linearity. Ten-turn helical potentiometers are commonly used with a turns counting dial. Using this it is possible to divide the ten turns of the potentiometer into 1,000 parts for the setting of the sliding contact. Such an arrangement can be used to replace decade resistance boxes, to form an accurate voltage divider, as a fine adjustment in bridge circuits and for the setting up of analogue computer circuits. It is also widely used for setting the 'pulse height' and 'window' conditions for pulse amplitude analysers used in radioactive counting systems. Standard ten-turn potentiometers are available in 15 resistance values ranging from 25 Ω to 300 kΩ.

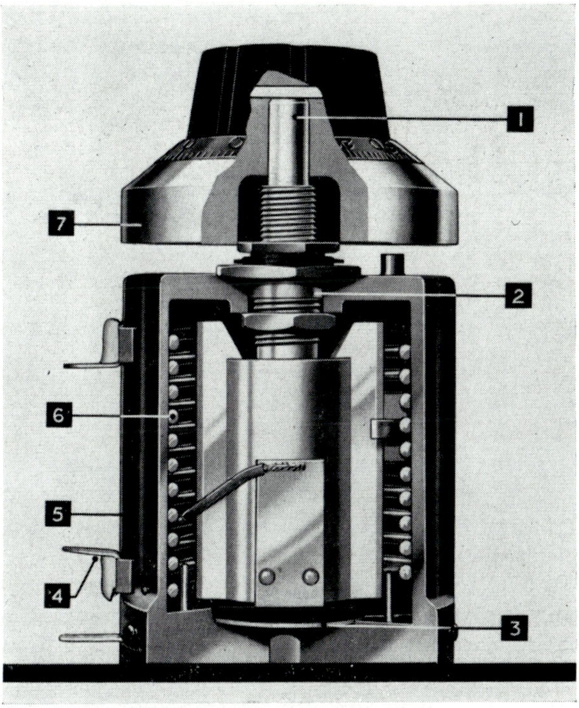

1 Stainless steel shaft.
2 Cadmium-plated brass bearing.
3 Contacts and slip ring.
4 Gold-plated brass terminals.
5 One-piece moulded phenolic housing.
6 Coil, made from carefully selected resistance wire.
7 Turns-counting dial.

Figure 4.12. Construction of a multi-turn helical potentiometer
(By courtesy of Beckman Instruments Ltd.)

INTERNAL AND EXTERNAL RESISTANCE

In *Figure 4.13*, a cell is shown connected to an external resistance R. The current flowing I is measured with an ammeter and the potential difference V appearing across R is measured with a voltmeter.

The electromotive force E of the cell is the potential difference appearing across the terminals of the cell when no current is drawn from it, that is, it is the 'open-circuit voltage' of the cell. The e.m.f. depends only on the nature of the chemicals used in that particular cell, and not on the amount of them used. When the circuit is completed and current flows, it is found that the potential difference V across R is smaller than the e.m.f. E. It is assumed that the voltage drop appearing across the ammeter is negligible. The fact that the voltage produced across the cell terminals falls on connecting the

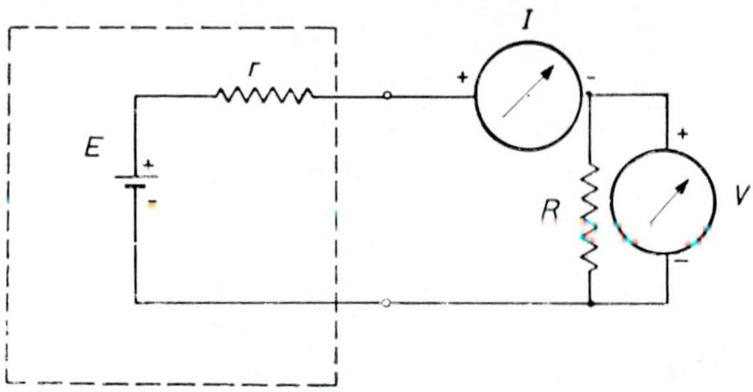

Figure 4.13. The concept of internal and external resistance

load R is due to the voltage drop across the internal resistance r of the chemicals of the cell. Thus $V=E-Ir$. It is apparent that if a cell is required to be able to deliver high currents, whilst still maintaining the value of the voltage between its terminals, the internal resistance must be made to be very small. This arises in the case of accumulators where the internal resistance is low, of the order of one hundredth of an ohm.

On the other hand, some cells such as pH or pCO_2 electrodes possess a very high internal resistance, of the order of 100 MΩ. It is the e.m.f., or open-circuit voltage, of these electrodes which is related to the pH or pCO_2 being measured. For this reason, it is essential that the output voltage be measured with a device that draws only a negligible current from the cell. Such an arrangement is known as an Electrometer. Electrometers are frequently encountered in medical electronics, and will be dealt with in more detail in Chapter 13.

RESISTANCES CONNECTED IN SERIES

Figure 4.14 illustrates a simple voltage-dividing circuit. Here the same current I flows through both resistors R_1 and R_2 and the voltage drop across R_1 is proportional to the value of R_1. Similarly the voltage drop across R_2 is proportional to R_2. Hence the applied voltage E is now divided down in the ratio of the resistances. The

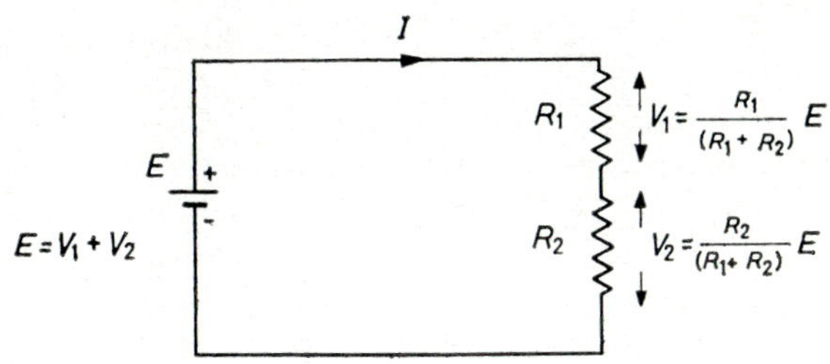

Figure 4.14. A simple voltage-dividing circuit

resistors R_1 and R_2 are said to be connected in series. In general, if resistors R_1, R_2, R_3 and R_4 are connected in series, the total resistance of the combination is equal to $R_1+R_2+R_3+R_4$.

RESISTANCES CONNECTED IN PARALLEL

In *Figure 4.15*, the two resistors R_1 and R_2 are connected in Parallel or in Shunt. Here, the voltage applied across each of the resistors is equal to E. Then by Ohm's law $I_1R_1=I_2R_2$. Therefore $I_1/I_2=$

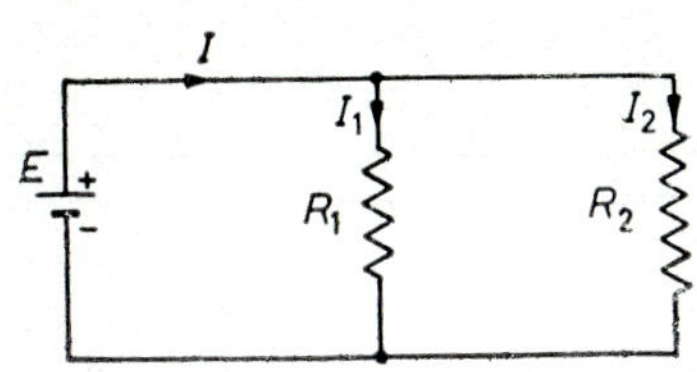

Figure 4.15. Resistors connected in parallel

R_2/R_1. The total circuit current thus divides inversely as the resistance in each branch of the circuit. Let R be the equivalent resistance of R_1 and R_2 in parallel. Then $E=IR$.
$R=E/I=E/(I_1+I_2)=E/(E/R_1+E/R_2)$. Therefore, $1/R=1/R_1+1/R_2$. That is, $R=R_1R_2/(R_1+R_2)$.

This formula is conveniently remembered by the phrase 'Product over Sum'. It is obvious that placing a second resistor in parallel with an existing resistor can only reduce, and not increase, the resistance offered by the first resistor. Thus the equivalent resistance offered by two resistors in parallel is always less than the resistance of the smaller of the two individual resistors.

MOVING COIL METERS

When an electric current is passed through a coil of wire suspended in a magnetic field, a force acts on the coil in such a way as to form a couple which tends to rotate the coil. If the field is uniform, the extent of the rotation is proportional to the strength of the current. Hence this principle is widely used for the measurement of currents from a few tens of micro-amperes upwards in the case of moving coil meters fitted with pointers. *Figure 4.16* shows the basic construction

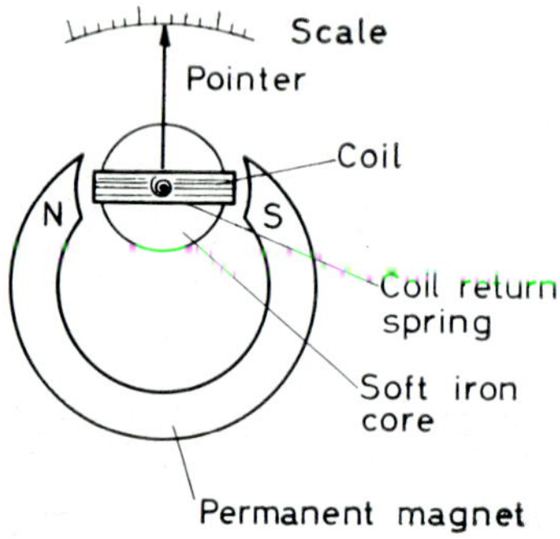

Figure 4.16. The basic construction of a pivoted moving coil meter

of a moving coil meter. A coil of fine wire is mounted on a lightweight former and this is pivoted between the poles of a powerful permanent magnet. The coil assembly carries a metal pointer which sweeps over a calibrated scale as the coil is deflected. The coil is caused to return to its rest position when the current is removed by a pair of spiral springs. The resting or 'zero' position can be adjusted using a screwdriver by means of a mechanical adjustment, and the setting should be checked before the meter is used. For the angle through which the coil turns to be proportional to the coil current, the magnet lines of force must be radial in direction. This is ensured by the use of a soft iron core (*Figure 4.17*).

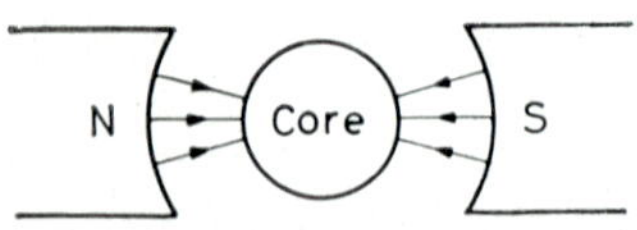

Figure 4.17. The use of a soft iron core to produce a radial magnetic field

The moving coil meter is essentially a current-measuring device, and in electronic practice basic full-scale sensitivities of 50 or 100 μA are commonly encountered.

The resistance of a 1 mA movement is about 75 Ω whilst that of a 100 μA movement would be about 1,000 Ω. Currently (1972), there is a tendency on the part of meter manufacturers to replace pivoted meter movements with taut band suspensions. *Figure 4.18* illustrates the principle of the taut band suspension. The moving coil is suspended between two taut metal strips kept in tension by the spring. The suspension strips are made from a special alloy

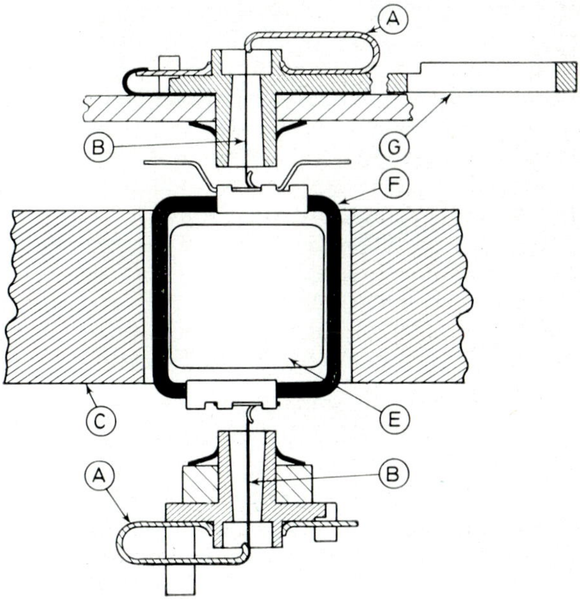

A	Suspension spring	E	Core piece
B	Gold alloy ligament	F	Coil
C	Magnet	G	Zero adjustment lever

Figure 4.18. The taut band suspension
(By courtesy of Sifam Instruments Ltd.)

which is both strong and resistant to corrosion. It is also resistant to shock. Since no conventional pivots or jewel bearings are employed, it is thus completely free from errors caused by pivot and jewel friction, wear or deterioration. Hysteresis effects have been reduced to a negligible level, so that the pointer returns to within 0·25 per cent of the true zero, even after long periods of continuous deflection. Thus repeated accurate measurements of extremely small currents can be made.

Instruments for measuring small currents, down to a fraction of a microamp, can be constructed on the moving coil principle. They are known as Galvanometers, after Galvani. A beam of light is usually used in place of a metal pointer. The beam is reflected from a small mirror carried on the moving coil assembly and this forms an image of a cross-wire on the ground glass scale. A longer path for the beam can be obtained by folding the path with mirrors in order to increase the sensitivity.

Figure 4.13 illustrates the positions of an ammeter and a volmeter in a simple circuit. Whenever a meter is introduced into the circuit, it is important that the meter should not significantly affect the quantity being measured. Thus a current-measuring meter should possess a low resistance and a voltmeter should have a high resistance. Consider a moving coil meter having a full-scale deflection of 1 mA. If the movement were to be modified so that it could read full scale for 1 V, then by Ohm's law, 1 V at a current of 1 mA means that the effective resistance of the meter must be 1,000 Ω/V. This value is suitable for use with general electrical measurements, but it is too low for work with electronic circuits. A full-scale current of 50 μA, giving an effective resistance of 20,000 Ω/V, is commonly used in electronic measurement practice.

MULTI-RANGE METERS

Voltage Ranges

If a moving coil meter movement has a coil resistance of 1,000 Ω and a full-scale current of 100 μA, a potential difference of 100 mV will exist across the coil when the deflection is full-scale. The voltage range of the basic movement can be extended by placing a 'multiplier' resistance in series with the coil. Suppose that the meter is required to read full-scale for 10 V, then 9·9 V must be dropped across the multiplier and 0·1 V across the coil at full-scale (*Figure 4.19*). Since

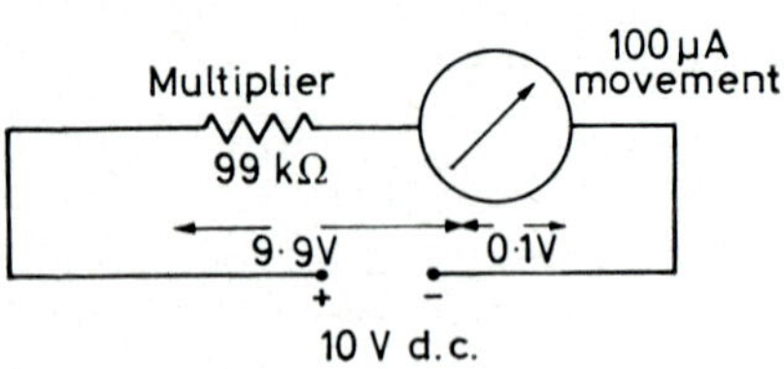

Figure 4.19. The use of a multiplier resistor with a voltmeter

the full-scale current is 100 μA, the multiplier resistance must be 99 kΩ. Similarly, if the range is to be extended to 100 V f.s.d., the multiplier resistance must be increased to 990 kΩ.

Current Ranges

In order to extend the current-measuring range of the basic movement, 'shunt' resistances are used. Suppose that a 1 mA full-scale movement is required to measure 10 mA full-scale, then 1 mA will flow through the coil and 9 mA through the shunt (*Figure 4.20*). Since the resistance of the basic movement is 75 Ω, the resistance of the shunt is 75/9=8·33 Ω. For a full-scale current of 1 A, the shunt resistance has to be 75/999 Ω=0·075 Ω.

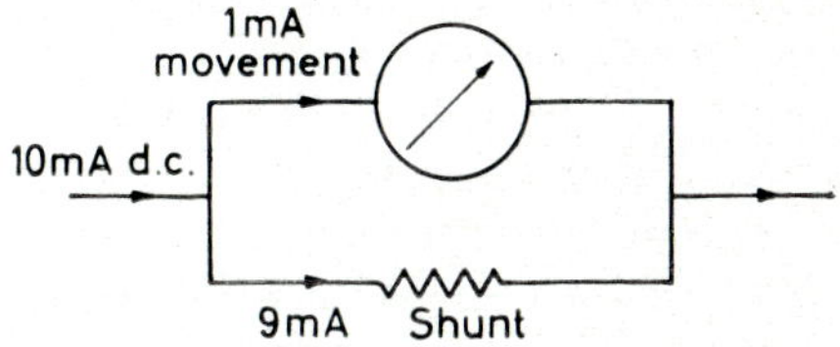

Figure 4.20. The use of a shunt resistor with a current meter

Multi-range test meters use a combination of switched multiplier and shunt resistors to give the required ranges of voltage and current.

Resistance Ranges—The Ohmmeter

Multi-range testmeters usually embody at least one resistance-measuring range. In use, the external leads of the meter are first shorted together at their far ends, and the rheostat adjusted to give full-scale deflection (100 μA) on the meter. This procedure has taken into account the resistance of the leads. The resistance to be measured is then connected to the leads as shown in *Figure 4.21.*

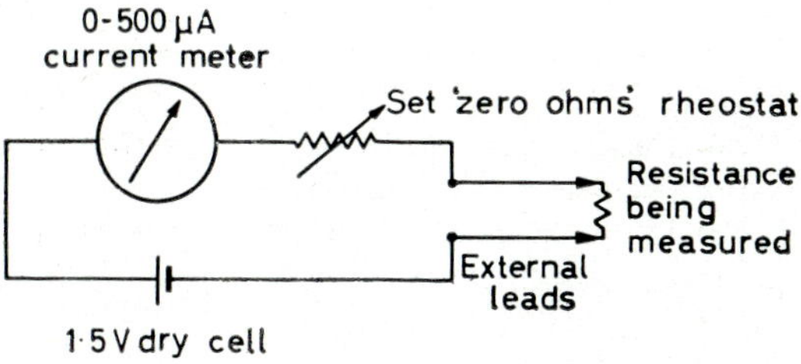

Figure 4.21. The ohmmeter

As a result, the current flowing in the circuit falls, and the current scale of the meter is recalibrated in terms of the external resistance added. The ohmmeter thus reads in the reverse direction to normal, the scale being open at the low resistance end and cramped at the high resistance end. The method is not as accurate as a bridge network, but it is exceedingly convenient for quick checks. It is handy for checking the resistance of the skin electrodes used for stimulating, or the recording of electrocardiograms or electroencephalograms. The d.c. current should not be allowed to flow for long in order to avoid polarization effects.

EFFECT OF VOLTMETER RESISTANCE ON CONDITIONS IN A CIRCUIT

In *Figure 4.22*, the 20 V battery drives a current of 1 mA through the two 10 kΩ resistors in series. Neglecting any effect due to the presence of the voltmeter, 10 V is dropped across each resistance. Suppose that the voltmeter has a resistance of 1,000 Ω/V. On a 10 V f.s.d. range, the meter has an effective resistance of 10,000 Ω. When the meter is connected in the circuit, it will reduce the 10,000

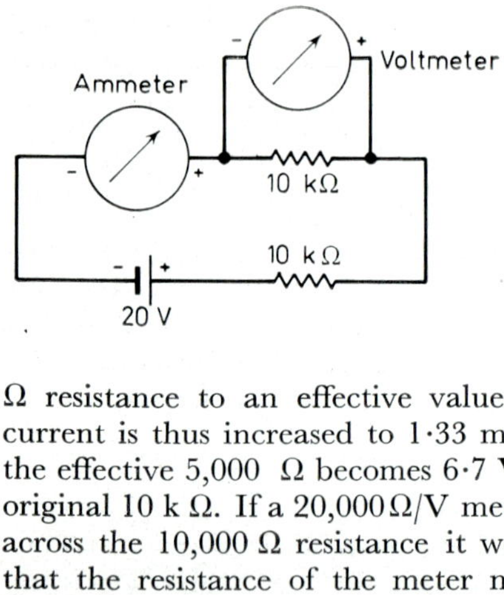

Figure 4.22. The effect of the voltmeter resistance in a circuit

Ω resistance to an effective value of 5,000 Ω. The total circuit current is thus increased to 1·33 mA, and the voltage drop across the effective 5,000 Ω becomes 6·7 V instead of the 10 V across the original 10 k Ω. If a 20,000 Ω/V meter was employed, when placed across the 10,000 Ω resistance it would record 9·75 V. It follows that the resistance of the meter must be much higher than the resistance in the circuit across which it is placed. It may be better to use a higher voltage range on the meter in order to increase the effective value of the meter resistance.

THE D.C. PRECISION POTENTIOMETER

In this device, a 2 V accumulator is connected across 17 standard resistance coils (R_1, R_2, R_3 . . . R_{17}) and a slidewire (*Figure 4.23*). When the current flows through the chain, 0·1 V is dropped across each resistor, making a total of 1·8 V. The e.m.f. E to be measured is connected as shown. By adjusting the coarse tapping S and the fine tapping Q, if E is less than 1·8 V it is possible to make the potential at points S and P identical. When this occurs, the galvanometer deflection will fall to zero, and the voltage indicated on the calibration of the coils and slidewire will be numerically equal to that of the unknown E. The calibration of the d.c. potentiometer in terms of

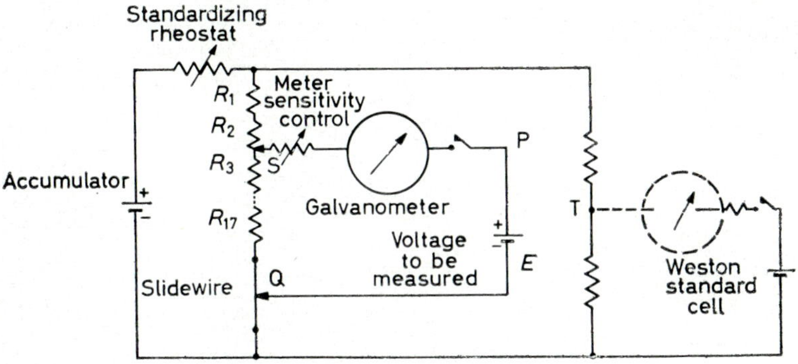

Figure 4.23. A precision d.c. potentiometer

voltage can be accurately adjusted by means of a built-in standard cell. A special tapping point T is provided and the standardizing rheostat is adjusted to give a zero galvanometer deflection when the standard cell is connected to T. The calibration of the dials and slidewire is then correct.

By passing the current through a standard resistance and measuring the resulting potential difference with the potentiometer, the technique can be used to verify the calibration of ammeters. Voltmeters can be checked by using a pair of standard resistances to divide the voltage down by an accurately known ratio to a value where it can be measured by the potentiometer. The d.c. potentiometer also provides a useful source of voltage down to 100 μV for the calibration of d.c. amplifiers.

The normal d.c. precision potentiometer suffers from the disadvantage that it can only measure up to 1·8 V. By using a temperature-stable Zener diode as a voltage reference source and amplifying this 50 times with a d.c. amplifier it is possible to measure voltages up to 500 V.

THE D.C. WHEATSTONE BRIDGE CIRCUIT

The Wheatstone bridge circuit is conventionally drawn in the form of a diamond configuration (*Figure 4.24a*). The operation of the circuit can be easily seen from *Figure 4.24b*, where it is drawn as two voltage-dividing networks, *P*, *R* and *Q*, *S*, in parallel across the energizing battery *E*. If a sensitive current-measuring instrument is connected between points A and B it will not show a deflection if the points A and B are at the same potential. This condition occurs when the voltage-division ratios of the two arms are equal, that is, when $P/R=Q/S$. If *R* is the resistance to be measured, and *S* is a known variable resistance, such as a decade resistance box, then $R=(P/Q)S$. *P* and *Q* are a pair of standard resistances whose ratio

(*a*)

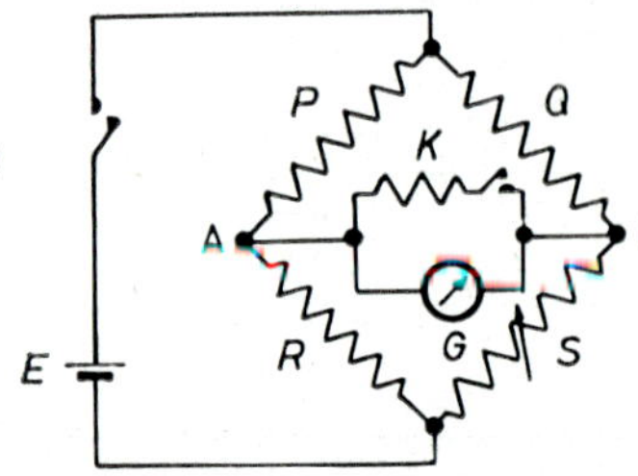

(*b*)

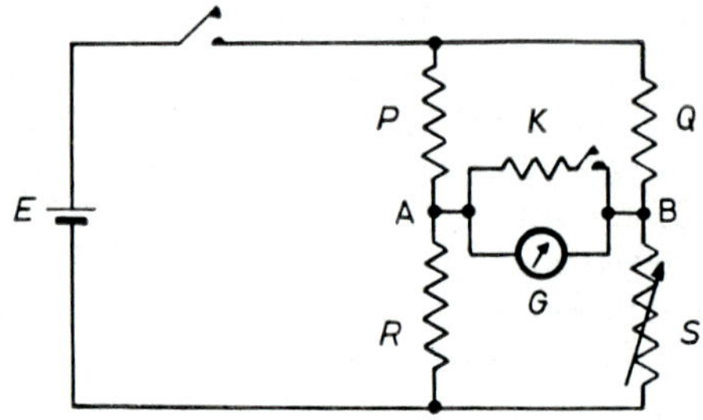

Figure 4.24. The d.c. Wheatstone bridge circuit

is accurately known. They constitute the ratio arms of the bridge. If the ratio P/Q is made equal to unity, the value of *R* can be read off directly from the calibration of *S* when *S* has been adjusted to cause the galvanometer deflection to become zero. The bridge is then said to be 'balanced'. The galvanometer or meter is normally of the centre-zero type and is fitted with a shunt so that its sensitivity can be reduced when the bridge is markedly off balance. Key *K* is spring-loaded to be normally closed, and is opened whilst the final balance point is obtained. For maximum sensitivity, the resistances of the four bridge arms and the galvanometer *G* should be approximately equal. Mitvalsky (1964) discusses the conditions necessary to obtain the maximum sensitivity from an unbalanced Wheatstone bridge. Wheatstone bridge networks are commonly encountered in laboratory component bridges for the measurement of resistances, and in connection with the use of strain gauges. Another important class of bridge circuit occurs when the energizing source supplies a.c. rather than d.c., and this is dealt with in Chapter 5.

CAPACITORS

A capacitor (formerly known as a condenser) is basically an arrangement for storing a quantity of electrical charge. The simplest type of capacitor consists of two parallel metal plates separated by air. An electrical charge can be placed on the plates by connecting a battery across them. The storage property of such a 'parallel-plate' capacitor is directly proportional to the common area between the plates and is inversely proportional to the separation of the plates. The tuning control of a radio receiver and some types of oscillator alters the overlapping areas of a multi-plate capacitor. The capacitance also depends on the nature of the substance between the plates, known as the dielectric material and characterized by a 'dielectric constant'. The capacitance of a given parallel-plate capacitor will be increased by a factor k if a substance such as polystyrene or paraffin wax of dielectric constant k is substituted for air between the plates.

The capacitance of a parallel-plate capacitor is directly proportional to the dielectric constant of the material between the plates. Thus with mica, the capacitance is about five times greater than for a similar arrangement with air spacing. If a quantity Q coulombs of electrical charge is placed on a capacitor, a potential difference of V volts will appear across the plates if the capacitance is C farads, where $Q=VC$. The farad is too large a unit for general electronic practice and the usual sub-units are the microfarad μF (10^{-6} farads) and the picofarad pF (10^{-12} farads), sometimes written as μμF. The capacitance of a parallel plate capacitor is given by

$$C = \frac{kA}{4\pi d \times 0{\cdot}9 \times 10^{6}} \quad \mu\text{F}$$

where d is in cm and A in cm^2.

Impregnated Paper Capacitors and Plastic Film Capacitors

The common tubular metallized paper capacitors found in many circuits consist of a length of paper impregnated with paraffin wax, mineral oil or petroleum jelly, sandwiched between two lengths of paper metallized with a layer of aluminium. Lengths of aluminium foil may also be used. The sandwich of three sheets is then rolled up into a tubular form. Leads are fixed to the inner and outer metallized strips, and the whole is placed in a metal can or a resin moulded case. The metal can is often provided with a transparent insulating sheath. Typically, the power factor for this type is less than 2 per cent at 1 kHz and 20° C, and operation is possible from $-55°$ C to $+100°$ C. The inductance is extremely low, not exceeding that of a solid piece of metal the size of the unit. The insulation resistance is likely to be greater than 200 MΩ/μF at 20° C.

An improved performance is available with metallized plastic film capacitors such as metallized polycarbonate capacitors which have power factors of less than 0·3 per cent. The wound units of metallized polycarbonate are moulded in a thermosetting resin. Working voltages for paper and polycarbonate types range from 100 to 1,000 V.

Polystyrene dielectric capacitors possess a very high insulation resistance, typically greater than 10^{12} Ω, and are used in electrometer circuits. The power factor is extremely low, being less than 0·05 per cent at 1 MHz.

Mica Capacitors

Silvered mica capacitors consist of a stack of mica plates covered with a layer of silver. They are very efficient and reliable devices, but are usually only used up to capacities of about 10,000 pF because of their size and expense. They are being replaced in oscillator circuits by polystyrene types. These are available with a 2·5 per cent tolerance, mica being available with a ±2 per cent tolerance. Stability and accuracy are important in the construction of twin-T filter circuits and R–C oscillators. Because of their stability, mica capacitors are often used as standards in a.c. bridge circuits.

Electrolytic Capacitors

Electrolytic capacitors are employed where a high value of capacitance is required in a reasonable volume. There are two main types: the low voltage—high capacity type (capacities up to 1,000 μF, d.c. working voltages up to 100 V), and high voltage types (capacities from 1 to 50 μF, d.c. working voltage 300 to 600 V). High capacities are available, e.g. 15,000 μF at a working voltage of 6·3 V. The common type of electrolytic capacitor is the aluminium foil type. However, increasing emphasis is being placed on the tantalum types.

Aluminium Foil Electrolytic Capacitors

Figure 4.25 shows the construction of a 'dry' aluminium electrolytic capacitor. The high purity aluminium foils are separated by paper tissues impregnated with the electrolyte. One foil acts as the positive electrode (anode). The dielectric consists of a thin oxide layer, formed by electrolysis, on the anode. The other foil is the negative electrode (cathode). This foil serves to make contact with the electrolyte which is the true negative electrode of the capacitor. The foil

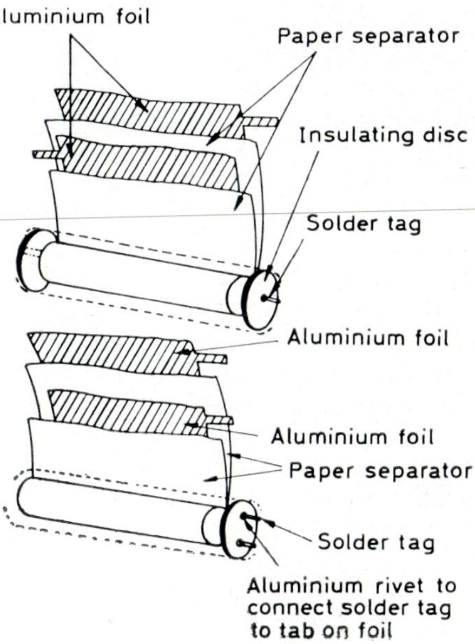

Figure 4.25. The construction of a dry aluminium electrolytic capacitor

(By courtesy of I.T.T. Components Group Europe)

assembly is normally hermetically sealed inside a metal case. The foils are etched to provide extra area for the oxide film. The electrolyte might consist of a paste of glycol and lead tetraborate. A good account of aluminium electrolytic capacitors is that of Pitt (1969).

Electrolytic capacitors achieve their high values of capacity by virtue of the fact that their dielectric layer is very thin. However, because of this, their leakage current is rather high. Thus, when a d.c. voltage is applied across the capacitor, a steady leakage current flows. In one manufacturer's range the leakage current is given by

0·08 $CV+100$ μA on units up to and including 100 V working, and 0·05 $CV+250$ μA on units above 100 V, both at 25° C ±5° C, where C is the capacitance in μF and V is the working voltage.

It is also necessary to specify the maximum ripple voltage allowable on the applied d.c. voltage. The peak value of the ripple voltage plus the d.c. voltage should not exceed the working voltage of the capacitor.

One major factor affecting reliability in miniature electronic circuits is the risk of sudden failure in high capacitance, low voltage electrolytic capacitors. This failure is usually caused by the development of an excessive leakage current. This risk has been greatly reduced by the development of solid aluminium electrolytic capacitors. These use wound aluminium foil electrodes, interleaved with glass fibre instead of paper. By means of a pyrolysis process, a solid manganese dioxide electrolyte is formed as the dielectric on the electrodes. Each capacitor is housed in, for mechanical protection, a metal case which is sealed with a ceramic disk. Hermetic sealing is not necessary as the capacitor is impregnated to withstand severe humidity conditions. This approach avoids the high cost of a solid tantalum capacitor and the leakage problems of wet aluminium types. A failure rate of only 0·02 per cent per 1,000 hours at the rated voltage and 25°C is possible. The solid aluminium type can also withstand higher reverse voltages (up to 15 per cent of the rated forward voltage for 125 hours) than solid tantalum or wet foil types. There is no limit to the discharge current, so that a series resistance is not required in the circuit.

Tantalum Foil Electrolytic Capacitors

The substantial leakage current of aluminium foil electrolytic capacitors can be prohibitive in transistor circuits, and attention has been concentrated on the tantalum types. These also produce a lower value of electrical noise than do aluminium electrolytics. The construction consists of a tantalum anode, a tantalum pentoxide dielectric, and a silver cathode. The electrolyte is an inner cathode of fine silver with an outer case of nickel. The tantalum anode is a porous sintered compact of high purity tantalum powder. The careful control of the powder size and the density of the compact result in a large surface area per unit volume. The dielectric film is formed on this surface. The outer case is of nickel with a seal consisting of a PTFE gasket clamped between coined plates of tantalum and silver by a work-hardened nickel ring (*Figure 4.26*). The wet tantalum capacitor has the widest temperature range

(−55° C to +200° C) and the lowest leakage current of an electrolytic unit. Solid tantalum capacitors are also available. Tantalum foil capacitors are similar in construction to the aluminium type,

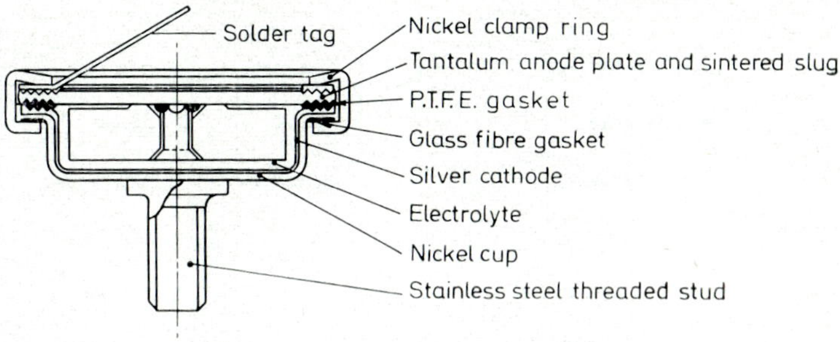

Figure 4.26. The construction of a wet tantalum electrolytic capacitor

(By courtesy of Plessey Ltd.)

with the electrodes made of tantalum (*Figure 4.27*). The stability of the oxide layer, together with the fact that little gas is produced during the operating life of the capacitor, enables the case to be fully hermetically sealed. The purity of the assembly is ensured by inorganic seals and a silver case (Walton, 1965).

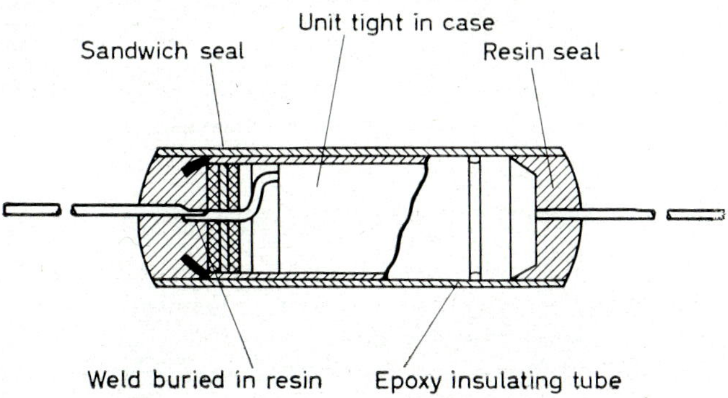

Figure 4.27. The construction of a tantalum foil electrolytic capacitor
(By courtesy of I.T.T. Components Group Europe)

Although they are more expensive in the first instance than aluminium electrolytes, tantalum electrolytic capacitors offer the advantages of lower leakage currents, less noise, a longer shelf life, and a smaller size for a given capacity. *Figure 4.28* compares the characteristics of various types of capacitor.

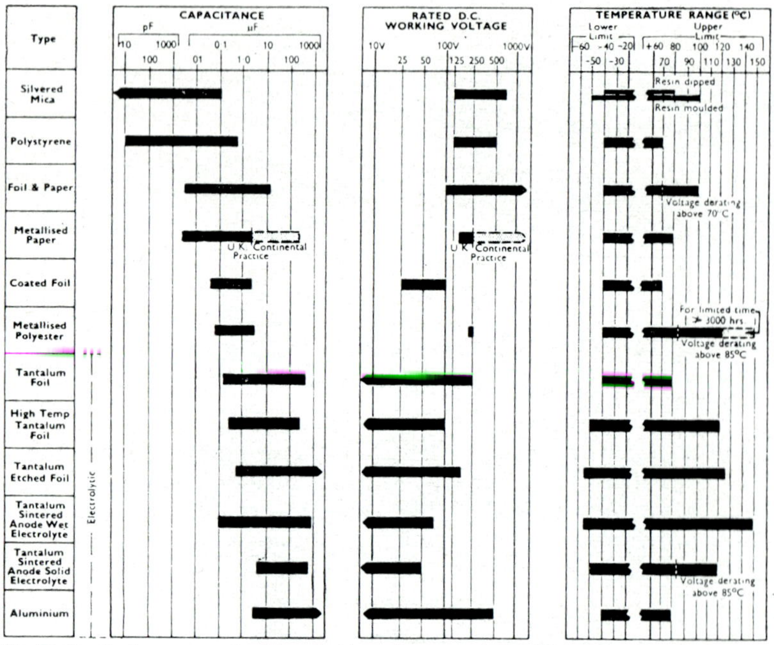

Note The voltage rating shown is not necessarily available over the whole range of capacitance, e.g. A 6000μF 400V aluminium capacitor would not be available

Figure 4.28. A comparison of the characteristics of various types of capacitor

(By courtesy of I.T.T. Components Group Europe)

THE POLARITY OF ELECTROLYTIC CAPACITORS

The polarity of the positive and negative terminals of an electrolytic capacitor must be respected when it is connected in a circuit. Otherwise, the oxide film will be removed in use and the capacitor will break down. Non-polarized electrolytics are available, having two anodes housed in a common can. This construction effectively provides two separate capacitors connected back to back in series.

THE CHARGE AND DISCHARGE OF CAPACITORS

In the circuit of *Figure 4.29a*, the capacitor C is connected to a battery E via a resistance R and a switch S. When the switch is closed, the capacitor starts to charge. *Figure 4.29b* shows a plot of the voltage V across the capacitor against time. Initially V is zero and it then rises, rapidly at first and then more slowly. If sufficient time is

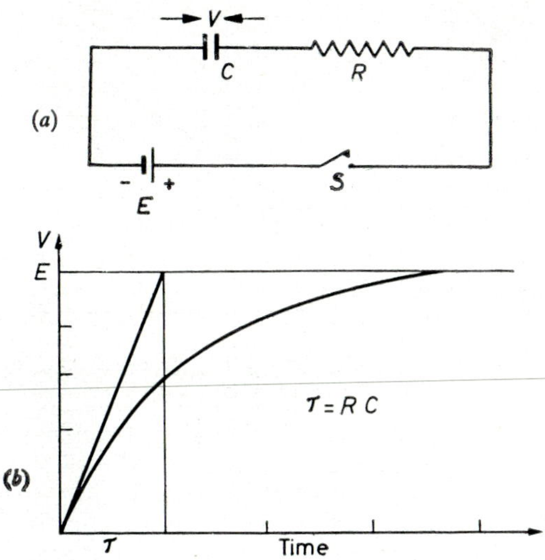

Figure 4.29. The charging, with time, of a capacitor

allowed, V will eventually rise to a value equal to E and the current flow will stop. The charging relationship is given by $V = E(1 - e^{-t/RC})$ where e equals 2·718 (the base of natural logarithms), and t is the time of charge in seconds. The product $RC = \tau$ is known as the time constant of the circuit. If R is in megohms and C is in microfarads, τ is in seconds. If the initial slope of the charging curve is projected, it will cut the line corresponding to the battery voltage at a time equal to one time constant. After a period equal to one time constant, the capacitor will have charged up to 63 per cent of its final value. After two time constants, it will have reached 86·5 per cent of its final value, and after four time constants, 98 per cent of the final value.

Taking logarithms of both sides of the charging equation gives $\log_e V = \log_e E + t/RC$. Hence a plot of $\log_e V$ against t will yield a straight line. This is called a 'semi-log plot' since V is plotted logarithmically on one axis and t is plotted linearly on the other axis (*Figure 4.30*).

In *Figure 4.31a*, the switch S_1 allows the capacitor C to be charged up to the battery voltage E. S_1 is then opened and S_2 is closed, allowing C to discharge through the resistance R. *Figure 4.31b* shows a plot of the voltage V across the capacitor as a function of time. The discharge equation for this curve is $V = Ee^{-t/RC}$. The projection of the initial slope cuts the time axis at a time $\tau = RC$, i.e. at one time

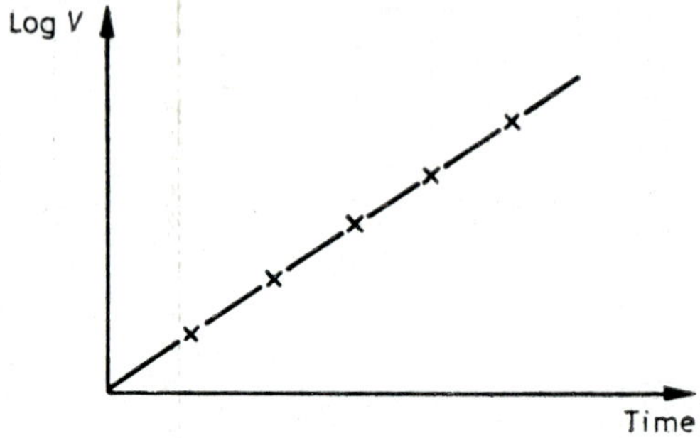

Figure 4.30. The semi-log plot of the voltage appearing across the charging capacitor with time

constant. A semi-log plot of $\log_e V$ against t yields a straight line. (In both the charge and discharge cases, a plot of $\log_{10} V$ against t will also yield a straight line, but the slopes will be different from those found when $\log_e V$ is plotted.)

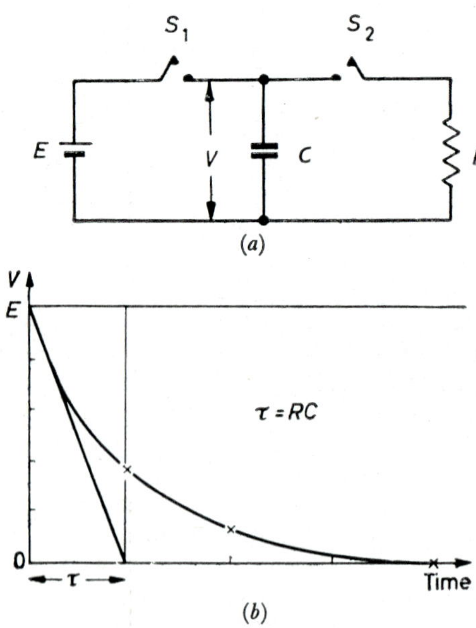

Figure 4.31. The discharging, with time, of a capacitor

Exponential curves occur in a number of medical situations, for example, in the decay of radioactive isotopes used in diagnostic tests, in the uptake and elimination of volatile anaesthetic agents from body compartments, and when the volume of gas in the lungs is plotted against time when ventilation is performed with a constant pressure ventilator. The concept of a time constant is of practical importance in considering the uptake and elimination of volatile anaesthetic agents (Nunn and Pincock, 1957) and the ventilation of different regions of the lungs.

INTEGRATING CIRCUITS

An integrating circuit consists of a resistor and a capacitor in series, and an output signal is taken from across the capacitor, as shown in *Figure 4.32*. Let V_I be a step input signal and V_1 and V_2 be the

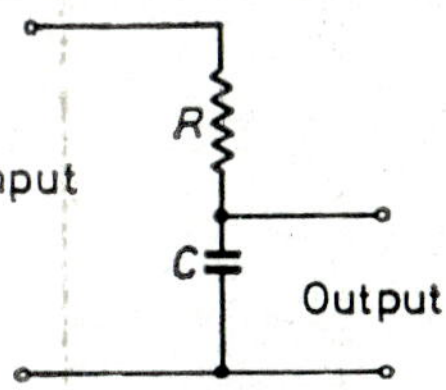

Figure 4.32. A simple integrating circuit

resultant voltages appearing across R and C respectively. Then $V_I = V_1 + V_2$. $V_1 = iR$ and $V_2 = Q/C = \int i\,dt/C$ where Q is the instantaneous value of the charge on C and i is the current which flows. Since $V_1 = iR = RC(dV_2/dt)$, then $RC(dV_2/dt) + V_2 = V_I$. The solution of this equation is $V_2 = V_I\,[1 - \exp(-t/CR)]$. *Figure 4.33* shows the

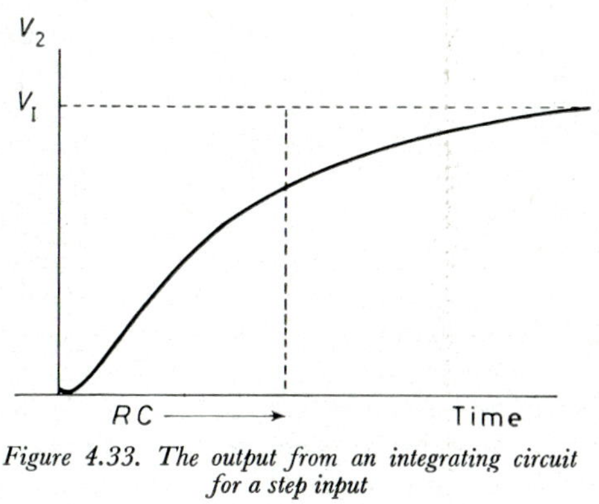

Figure 4.33. The output from an integrating circuit for a step input

output waveform appearing across C for a step change input. This circuit is known as an integrating circuit because it provides for small values of t an output $(1/CR)\int V_1 \mathrm{d}t$. This relationship holds for any input, not necessarily a step, provided that V_2 is insignificant compared with V_1. The rise time of the circuit can be expressed in terms of one time constant. The rise time of the pointer of an instrument is commonly expressed in terms of the 10–90 per cent rise time, that is, the time taken for the deflection to rise from 10 per cent to 90 per cent of its final value. This is equal to 2·2 time constants.

It is of interest to consider the effect of passing a train of rectangular pulses through the circuit of *Figure 4.32*. When the circuit time

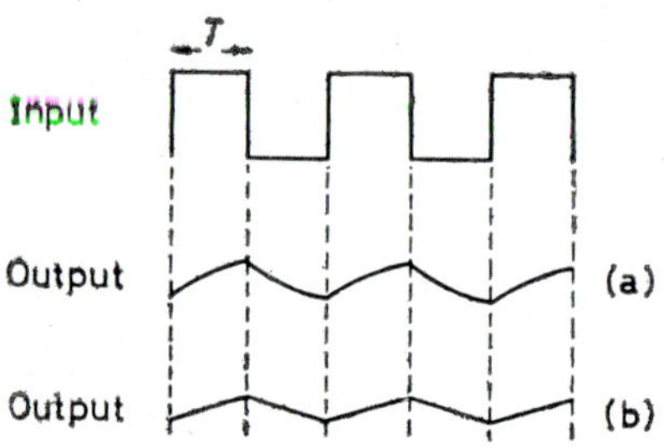

Figure 4.34. The effect of applying rectangular pulses to an integrating circuit

constant RC is small compared with the pulse width, then the exponential charge and discharge curves of the capacitor markedly distort the input rectangular pulses as shown in *Figure 4.34a*. When the time constant is long compared with the pulse width t, the initial portions of the charge and discharge curves are virtually linear. The output waveform is then triangular in shape (*Figure 4.34b*). Under these circumstances, the maximum value of the output voltage is proportional to the area under the input pulse waveform. A case of practical importance in respiratory investigations occurs in the integrating pneumotachograph (Hill, 1959b). The function of a pneumotachograph is to produce a voltage signal which is proportional to the instantaneous value of a subject's respiratory volume flow rate in litres per minute. This voltage is then fed into an integrating circuit and integrated over each half of each respiratory cycle in order to yield an output which is proportional to the volume of gas in litres passed in that period, that is, to the inspiratory and expiratory tidal volumes.

The simpler types of heart-rate meter (cardiotachometer) also employ an integrating circuit. Each R-wave of the subject's electrocardiogram is caused to trigger a pulse-forming circuit which then produces a standard rectangular voltage pulse for each heart beat. These pulses are fed into a diode pump circuit (Kitchen, 1959), which is a form of 'leaky' integrator circuit. The output voltage from this circuit is proportional to the number of standard pulses fed into it per minute, and it is displayed on a meter graduated in beats per minute. Relative to the input waveform, integrating circuits essentially possess a long time constant and thus act to smooth or iron out short-term fluctuations in the input signal. An example occurs in the smoothing of the output signal from an arterial blood pressure transducer to yield a signal proportional to the mean pressure.

The charging of a large capacitor via a resistor can form the basis of a simple time delay circuit. An end-tidal sampler for use with a colorimetric CO_2 analyser in respiratory studies has been described by Nunn (1957).

More sophisticated integrating circuits with provision for setting the initial conditions can be conveniently constructed with the help of operational amplifiers, and this approach is dealt with in Chapter 7.

DIFFERENTIATING CIRCUITS

In the charge and discharge curves of *Figures 4.29* and *4.31* ample time was allowed for the charge or discharge to take place. Now consider the application of a series of rectangular voltage pulses to a circuit consisting of a capacitor C in series with a resistor R as shown in *Figure 4.35*.

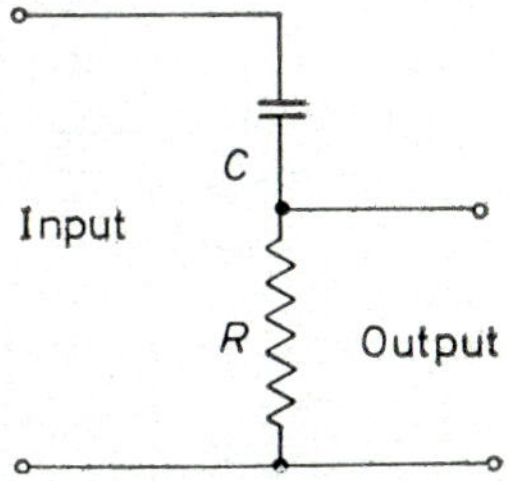

Figure 4.35. A simple differentiating circuit

Rectangular pulses, in which the voltage suddenly increases from one value to another and then returns after a definite interval, are commonly generated by many stimulator circuits used in neurophysiological investigations. Suppose that the pulse width and spacing are each equal to T seconds, and that the output waveform is taken from across R. If the time constant RC is long compared with

T, then the shape of the input pulses is transmitted in a more or less faithful fashion. As the time constant CR is progressively reduced, distortion is introduced until finally each rectangular pulse is reduced at the output to a pair of sharp pulses, as shown in the bottom line of *Figure 4.36*. The first of the spikes, corresponding with the leading edge of the input pulse, is positive going. The second pulse, corresponding with the trailing edge of the input pulse, is negative going. A voltage output only appears across R when the capacitor charge or discharge current is flowing. Once the charge or discharge process is completed, the voltage across R falls to zero. The progressive introduction of exponential curvatures into the output signal arises from the fact that, with a short time-constant circuit, the capacitor has time to become almost charged during

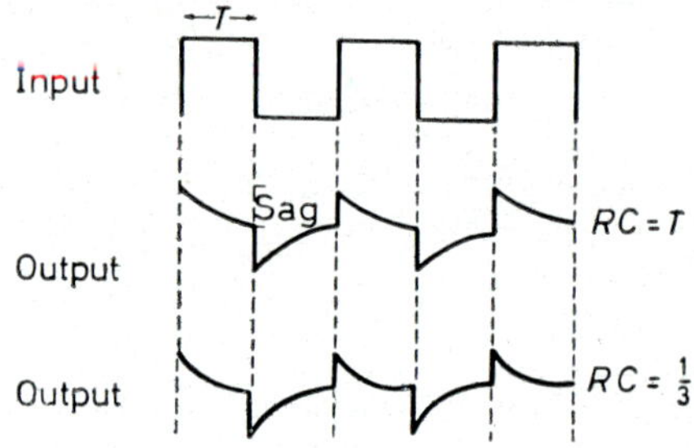

Figure 4.36. The effect of applying rectangular pulses to a differentiating circuit

the leading positive-going edge of the input pulse and almost discharged on the trailing negative-going edge. Towards the end of charge or discharge, the current flowing through the capacitor falls to a low value and the voltage appearing across R falls off markedly. When the time constant is small compared with the pulse width, the amplitude of the output pulse is approximately proportional to the rate of change of the input voltage. Referring to *Figure 4.35*, let V_I be a step input signal and V_1 and V_2 be the resultant output voltages appearing across R and C respectively. $V_2 = \int i\mathrm{d}t/C = \int V_1\mathrm{d}t/RC$ and since $V_I = V_1 + V_2$, $V_1 + \int V_1\mathrm{d}t/RC = V_I$. Differentiating, $\mathrm{d}V_1/\mathrm{d}t + V_1/RC = \mathrm{d}V_I/\mathrm{d}t = 0$. The solution of this differential equation is $V_1 = V_I \exp(-t/CR)$. Thus the voltage developed across R decays exponentially with time since the charging current of C decays in a similar fashion. $V_1 = -RC(\mathrm{d}V_I/\mathrm{d}t)$ provided that V_1 is small compared with V_I so that $\mathrm{d}V_1/\mathrm{d}t$ can be neglected. Differentiating circuits are frequently used to generate short, sharp pulses for the triggering of other circuits and to pick out the point of maximum amplitude change in an electrical waveform. Because they respond to time rates of change, differentiating circuits accentuate noise components of the input signal since these are rapidly varying. Hence it is usual to precede a differentiating circuit with a low pass filter to remove unwanted high frequency components. The maximum rate of change of left ventricular pressure $(\mathrm{d}p/\mathrm{d}t)_{max}$ is one index of myocardial contractility and this can be generated by passing the output from the pressure transducer through a differentiating circuit. A greater degree of flexibility can be obtained with operational amplifier differentiating circuits, and these are mentioned in Chapter 7.

THE C–R COUPLING OF AMPLIFIER STAGES

When the time constant *R–C* is considerably greater than the width of the applied rectangular pulse, the normally flat top of the pulse suffers only a small droop or sag. As an approximation, the percentage sag appearing in the output pulse is equal to the percentage of the time constant that equals the pulse width. Thus for a two-second time constant, typical of those used in electrocardiographs, a pulse of width 0·02 seconds (20 ms) would have its amplitude at the trailing edge reduced by 1 per cent from that which existed at the leading edge. If a 5 per cent sag is allowable, then the time constant can be decreased to 100 ms. An adequately long time constant is essential if clinical significance is to be placed, for example, on changes seen in the *S–T* segment of an electrocardiogram. EEG amplifiers are often provided with the facility for changing the principal coupling time constant in the circuit.

Particular care is needed in the design of the interstage couplings of pulse amplifiers designed to handle pulses with fast rise times. Stray capacitors which slow the rise time must be minimized and the gain of the stages limited to reduce the enhancement of the input capacities by the Miller effect. It is possible to obtain some additional improvement in the rise time of the circuit by placing an inductance in series with the load resistance of each stage; this is known as a peaking circuit. Having achieved the best compromise of rise time and gain, it is then necessary to pass the top of the pulse as faithfully as possible; this requires the longest possible fall time, but then difficulties may be experienced with pulse pile-up in the amplifier—that is to say, pulses cannot be transmitted at a sufficiently fast rate. If it is required simply to count the number of pulses, it may be possible to increase the throughput of pulses by introducing a degree of pulse shaping within the amplifier. A useful introductory account of some of these considerations is that of Delaney (1969).

There must exist a connection between the requirements for the amplification of voltage steps and sinewaves. In fact, there is a great deal of similarity in designing a wideband sinusoidal amplifier and a pulse amplifier. Delaney (1969) makes the point that if an imperfect step output having a rise time of one microsecond and a fall time of one millisecond can be accepted, this can be handled by an amplifier which handles accurately a range of frequencies from 1 kHz to 1 MHz.

REFERENCES

Delaney, C. F. G. (1969). *Electronics for the Physicist.* Harmondsworth: Penguin.

Donaldson, P. E. K. (1958). *Electronic Apparatus for Biological Research.* London: Butterworths.

Godin, M. C. (1962). 'A method for equalising thermistors.' *J. scient. Instrum.* **39,** 241.

Hayden, J. D. (1962). 'Metal oxide film resistors.' *Electron. Engng* **34,** 804.

Hill, D. W. (1959a). 'The measuring and recording of temperatures during hypothermia.' *Brit. J. Anaesth.* **31,** 22.

— (1959b). 'Rapid measurement of respiratory pressures and volumes.' *Brit. J. Anaesth.* **31,** 352.

Hyde, F. J. (1970). *Thermistors.* London: Iliffe.

Kitchen, L. D. (1959). 'A cardiac ratemeter using transistors.' *Electron. Engng* **31,** 44.

Mitvalsky, V. (1964). 'The maximum sensitivity of the unbalanced Wheatstone bridge.' *J. scient. Instrum.* **41,** 454.

Norden, P. and Bainbridge, N. W. (1962). 'The use of unmatched thermistors for the measurement of temperature difference under varying ambient conditions.' *J. scient. Instrum.* **39,** 399.

Nunn, J. F. and Pincock, A. C. (1957). 'A time phased end-tidal sampler suitable for use during anaesthesia.' *Brit. J. Anaesth.* **29,** 98.

Pitt, A. T. (1969). 'Performance characteristics of aluminium electrolytic capacitors.' *Electron. Engng* **41,** 33.

Price, J. R. (1964). 'Improvements in the design of precision wirewound resistors.' *Electron. Engng* **36,** 474.

Richards, J. C. S. (1967). 'Sensitive thermistor thermometer.' *Electron. Engng* **39,** 674.

Scarr, R. W. A. and Setterington, R. A. (1960). 'Thermistors, their theory, manufacture and application.' *Proc. Instn elect. Engrs* **107,** 395.

REFERENCES

Scott, R. P. W. and Cumming, C. A. (1960). 'Cathode ray tube presentation of chromatograms.' In *Gas Chromatography*, p. 117. Ed. by R. P. W. Scott. London: Butterworths.

Stanley, K. W. (1971). 'Reliability and stability of carbon film resistors.' *Mullard tech. Communs* **11,** 223.

Walton, B. (1965). 'Capacitors with thin oxide film dielectrics.' *Electron. Engng* **37**, 384.

Watkins, J. (1971). *Modern Electronic Materials*. London: Butterworths.

Chapter 5

A.C. Circuits

THE CONCEPT OF AN ALTERNATING VOLTAGE

The plot of a direct, or steady, voltage against time is shown in *Figure 5.1*. For example, the voltage produced by a stabilized power unit, or the voltage of a mercury cell before it starts to run down, will be constant with respect to time. From Ohm's law, a direct voltage applied to a circuit where the resistance is constant will give rise to a direct or steady current. It is usual to refer to 'd.c. circuits' where the voltages and currents concerned are essentially unidirectional.

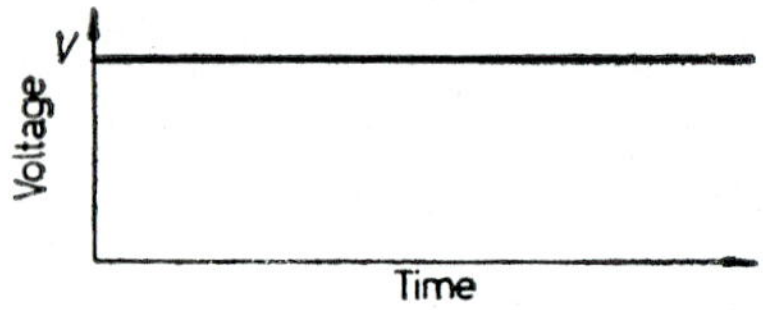

Figure 5.1. The constancy with time of a d.c. voltage

In addition to direct voltages and currents, alternating voltages and currents occur frequently in electronic engineering. An alternating voltage is one which acts alternately in opposite directions, and whose instantaneous values undergo a definite cycle of changes at regular intervals of time. The most commonly encountered alternating voltages (and currents) follow a sinusoidal waveform. A plot of a typical sinusoidal voltage against time is shown in *Figure 5.2*. It is seen that at regular intervals of time, the voltage falls to zero. In between, it attains alternately a positive and then a negative maximum value. One complete cycle of this periodic waveform occurs between alternate zeros or between successive positive and negative maxima. The time taken to complete one cycle is called the Periodic Time. The number of cycles completed per second is called the Frequency, and this is numerically equal to the reciprocal of the

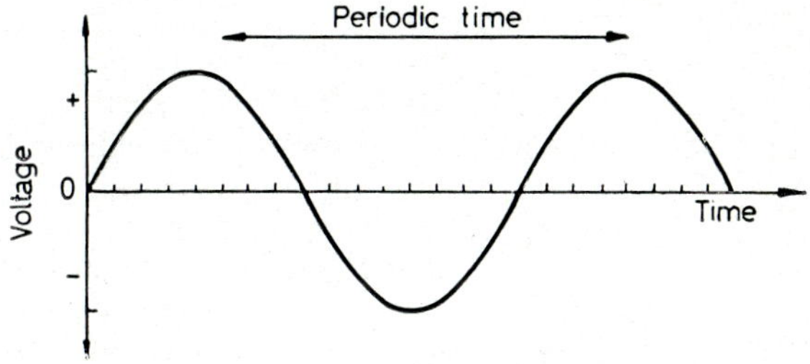

Figure 5.2. The variation of the amplitude of an alternating voltage with the position of the generating coil

periodic time in seconds. One cycle per second is known as one Hertz. The normal mains supply in the United Kingdom is of an alternating nature, having a frequency of 50 Hz and thus a periodic time of 20 ms. In the U.S.A. and Canada, the mains frequency is 60 Hz with a periodic time of 16·67 ms.

POWER, ROOT MEAN SQUARE AND PEAK VALUES

Many applications of electricity are concerned with its use to perform work, that is, to supply power. Electrical energy is just another form of energy, and it can be converted into other forms, such as heat energy in an electric fire or light radiation in a lamp. Energy is defined as 'the capacity to do work', and Power as 'the rate of doing work'. The basic unit of electrical power is the watt. If a direct current of I amperes flows through a resistance of R ohms, an electrical power of I^2R watts is dissipated. This is equivalent to I^2R joules of energy per second. The energy is dissipated in the form of heat and it is important to choose a resistor of an adequate wattage rating. From Ohm's law, the power P in watts dissipated in a resistor of R ohms is $P=I^2/R=V^2/R=I\times V$ where V is the voltage dropped across the resistor. The energy delivered per pulse by a d.c. defibrillator is usually expressed in joules (watt-seconds), for example 50 joules.

The payment of an electricity bill in respect of the amount of kilowatt hours of electricity used, pays for the supply of a given amount of work. Taking a simple case, if a consumer's mains supply were changed from direct current (d.c.) to alternating current (a.c.), he would want to be assured that the a.c. supply would produce the same heating effect in his electric fire. It turns out that a sine wave voltage having a peak amplitude of $\sqrt{2}$ (1·414) times that of the original direct voltage will give the same heating power. The power dissipated as heat in a resistor depends upon the square of the voltage and thus will always be positive, whether the instantaneous value of the voltage is positive or negative. The square of the instantaneous value of the voltage will be proportional to the power dissipation at that instant. The mean value of the square of the voltage throughout a cycle will lead to a power value which is constant throughout the cycle. It will be equivalent to a direct voltage. To find the voltage associated with this power, the square root is then taken of the mean voltage squared value. This is called the Root Mean Square or r.m.s. value. Consider a 230 V d.c. supply. The 230 V a.c. supply which produces the same heating power will have a 230 V r.m.s. value. Since the peak value of tl is sine wave is $\sqrt{2}$ times the r.m.s. value, a 230 V r.m.s. mains supply will have a peak value of 325 V. The magnitude of the peak value should be borne in mind when considering the provision of electrical insulation in circuits and the safe working voltage of any capacitors which may be used. Many low voltage pilot lamps are rated at 6·3 V a.c., which is 6·3 V r.m.s. If the voltage waveform is observed on a cathode ray tube oscilloscope, the positive and negative peak values can easily be observed.

THE CONCEPT OF A PHASE DIFFERENCE

A.C. mains supplies are produced by alternators in the power stations. Basically, a coil of wire is rotated about a diameter in a strong magnetic field (*Figure 5.3a*). One complete revolution of the coil produces one complete cycle of a sine wave. In *Figure 5.3b*, the peak voltages are produced in the positions CC, where the coil is cutting the maximum number of lines of force because it is then moving at right angles to them. At positions AA, the voltage generated falls to zero since here the coil is moving parallel to the lines of force and not cutting them. Faraday's law, after Michael Faraday (1791–1867), states that the induced e.m.f. in the coil is proportional to the rate of change of the lines of force linking the coil. Lenz's law, due to H. Lenz in 1833, states that the direction of the induced e.m.f. is always such that it opposes the direction of the change producing it.

It is convenient to discuss the development of a sine wave cycle in terms of the angle of rotation of the generating coil, each cycle now being divided up into 360 degrees corresponding to one revolution of the coil.

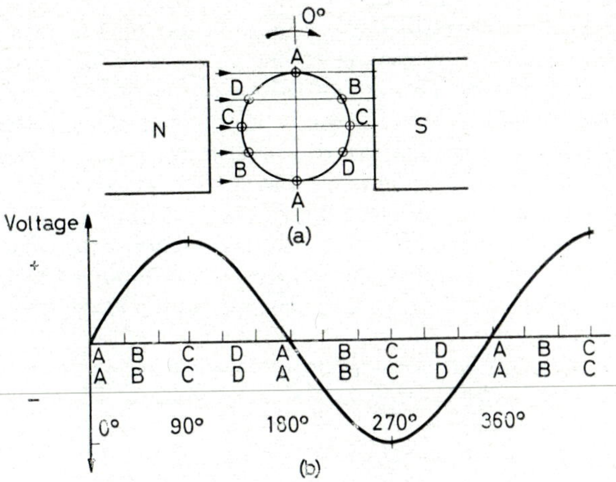

Figure 5.3. The rotation of a coil in a magnetic field to generate an alternating voltage

On this basis, the coil will have turned through 90 degrees at one quarter of a revolution, 180 degrees at one half and 270 degrees at three-quarters of a revolution.

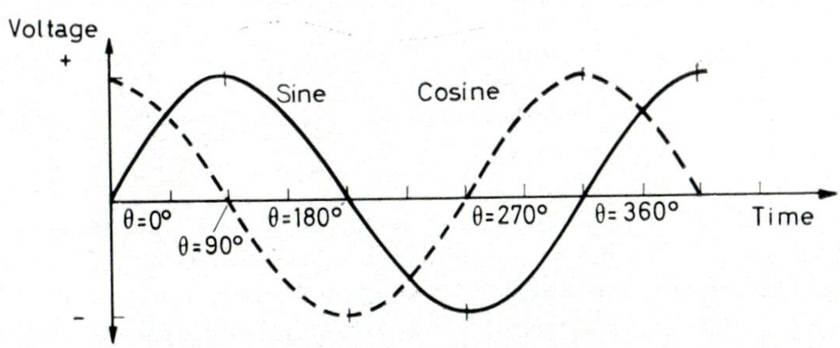

Figure 5.4. The variation of the amplitude of a sine and cosine waveform with time

In *Figure 5.4* is shown a simple alternating voltage having a sine waveform plotted against time. It is characterized by an equation of the form $V = V_{max} \sin \theta$ where θ (the angle of rotation) is a function of time.

Let θ be the angle the plane of the coil makes with a line at right angles to the magnetic lines of force. Trigonometric tables show that $\sin 0°=0$, $\sin 90°=1$, $\sin 180°=0$, $\sin 270°=-1$ and $\sin 360°=0$. From these figures it can be seen that the shape of the sine waveform is traced out, V alternating between zero and plus or minus V_{max}. The second waveform shown in *Figure 5.4* (broken line) corresponds with $V=V_{max} \cos \theta$. The cosine values are $\cos 0°=1$, $\cos 90°=0$, $\cos 180°=-1$, $\cos 270°=0$ and $\cos 360°=1$. It can be seen that a cosine wave starts with a positive maximum at $\theta=0°$ whilst the amplitude of the sine wave is zero at $\theta=0°$. The two waves are a quarter of a wave out of step. They are said to differ in phase by 90 degrees. The concept of a phase difference between two electrical signals is very important in considering the function of feedback in oscillators and amplifiers and the action of electromagnetic flowmeters.

Two waveforms are said to be in quadrature when they differ in phase by 90 degrees, that is, one is a quarter of a cycle behind or in front of the other.

ANGULAR FREQUENCY

As well as being expressed in degrees, an angle can be expressed in circular measure, that is, in radians. In *Figure 5.5*, the angle θ in radians is given by $\theta=a/r=\text{arc}/\text{radius}$. Considering a circle of radius r, its circumference will have a length $2\pi r$. Thus the angle

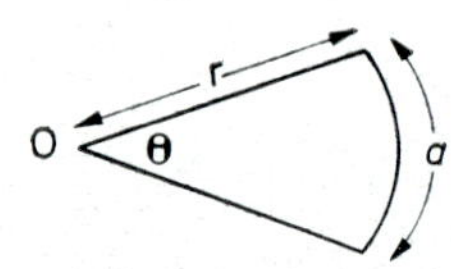

Figure 5.5. The expression of an angle in circular measure (radians)

corresponding to 360 degrees will be $2\pi r/r=2\pi$ radians. In the case of a coil rotating in a uniform magnetic field and generating a sine waveform, the angle turned through in 1 sec will be $2\pi \times f$ radians, where f is the frequency of rotation. Since the waveform is periodic, the angle turned through will be a function of time. Hence it is possible to write $E=E_{max} \sin \theta=E_{max} \sin 2\pi ft=E_{max} \sin \omega t$ where $\omega=2\pi f$ is the angular frequency.

If a phase difference of 180 degrees exists between two waves, then at any given instant in time the voltage amplitudes of each will be of opposite sign. On adding them together, cancellation will tend to occur. Under these conditions, the cancellation would be complete if the amplitude were equal. When the two waveforms are exactly in step (in phase), they will add up to produce a wave having an amplitude equal to the sum of the individual amplitudes.

When a sine waveform is passed into a differentiating circuit, it is differentiated to give a cosine wave. Thus R–C networks introduce a phase shift. Under some circumstances this could give rise to a positive overall phase shift round a circuit and hence oscillation. For the phase shift produced to be small (less than 5 degrees), the time constant should be greater than twice the period of the lowest frequency to be passed.

POWER FACTOR

In a d.c. circuit, the product of the current and voltage represents power available for doing work. Electrical power is measured in watts if the current is measured in amperes and the voltage in volts. In an a.c. circuit, the product of the r.m.s. values of the current and voltage gives the Apparent Power, measured in volt-amperes (VA). This is the maximum value of the power which the circuit can provide, and it occurs when the current and voltage are in phase. If they are not, the True Power in watts is given by the expression $V_{r.m.s.} \times I_{r.m.s.} \times \cos\varphi$ where φ is the phase angle between the voltage and current waveforms. Cos φ is called the Power Factor of the circuit. In a purely resistive circuit, the voltage and current will be in phase, so that $\varphi=0$ and $\cos\varphi=1$. In the case of a purely reactive component, such as an ideal capacitor, the voltage and current will be 90 degrees out of phase, $\varphi=90°$ and $\cos\varphi=0$. Hence no power would be dissipated in a pure capacitance or inductance. In practice, however, power is dissipated in the resistance associated with capacitors and inductors. Devices such as fluorescent lamps which use chokes (inductances) incorporate a power factor correction capacitor to bring the power factor of the device back to nearly unity.

It should be mentioned that inductors and capacitors are known as reactive components because they react to an impressed current change by giving rise to a voltage of such a polarity that it opposes the original current change.

HARMONICS

Apart from a d.c. signal, a sinusoidal waveform is the simplest type of signal encountered. Sine wave signal generators are in common use for the provision of test signals for the evaluation of the frequency response of amplifiers, filters and recorders. In a number of designs it is possible to set up frequencies directly in the range 1 Hz to 1 MHz by setting up the required value on a bank of switches; this is the so-called decade oscillator. Many electrical signals can be shown to be made up of a series of sine waves having related frequencies: this applies to the electrocardiogram and the pneumotachogram. In addition to the sine waves, the signal may also contain a d.c. component. An obvious example occurs with the arterial blood pressure waveform where a mean pressure is associated with the pulse pressure. The related sine wave frequencies are known as harmonics, and music provides many examples. If a tuning fork is gently sounded it produces a pure audio tone. If this is picked up by a microphone and displayed on a cathode ray tube, a pure sine wave is observed. The same note produced by the bowing of a violin string will sound differently. This is due to the simultaneous production of harmonic frequencies of the note. These are responsible for the quality or timbre of the note. The tuning fork produces the fundamental frequency alone, the actual frequency depending on the construction of the fork. A frequency of double the fundamental is called the second harmonic, a frequency of three times the fundamental being the third harmonic, and so on. As an example, a blood pressure waveform with a heart rate of 120 beats per minute would have a fundamental frequency of 2 Hz. To reproduce this signal faithfully, the recording system should have a frequency response which is linear out to at least the tenth harmonic, that is, to 20 Hz. This is a working rule, but for faithful reproduction of fine detail, a linear response out to the 20th harmonic is desirable (Shirer, 1962).

As has been previously mentioned, it is the harmonic frequencies which provide the quality of a musical note. Thus it is essential that the frequency response of a high-fidelity audio amplifier should be sufficient to handle even the high harmonic frequencies, for two frequencies, each above the upper frequency limit of audibility, can beat together to produce an audible frequency.

BEATS

If two electrical signals of nearly equal frequency are added together, a periodic rise and fall in the amplitude of the combined signal can be observed. This is the phenomenon of beats, and the rate of variation is the beat frequency. It can be shown that if the two beating frequencies are f_1 and f_2, the resulting beat frequency will be (f_2-f_1). Beats can easily be observed with the help of a cathode ray tube oscilloscope.

When two sound waves of nearly equal frequency are sounded together, a periodic variation of intensity occurs at the beat frequencies. As the frequencies of the notes are brought together, the

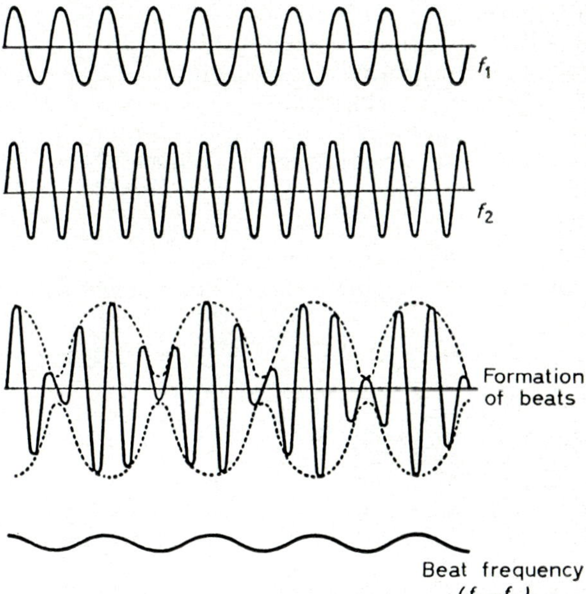

Figure 5.6. The formation of a beat frequency

frequency of the beats falls. When it has fallen to zero, the two frequencies will be exactly equal. In a beat frequency oscillator, an audio frequency output is generated by beating together two ultrasonic frequency oscillators. The formation of a beat frequency is shown in *Figure 5.6* by the addition of two nearly equal frequencies.

FOURIER'S SERIES

The French mathematician Jean Baptiste Joseph Fourier (1768–1830) showed that a periodic waveform can be represented by a trigonometric series of the form

$$y=F(\omega t)=a_0+a_1\cos\omega t+a_2\cos 2\omega t+a_3\cos 3\omega t+\ldots$$
$$+b_1\sin\omega t+b_2\sin 2\omega t+b_3\sin 3\omega t+\ldots$$

ω is the angular frequency of the fundamental where $\omega=2\pi f=2\pi 1/T$, f is the fundamental frequency in Hz and T is the period in seconds of the periodic wave. $F(\omega t)=y$ is the function concerned of ωt and represents the amplitude.

From this series it is seen that any periodic wave can be decomposed into a constant term a_0 and a sum of cosine and sine waves, the angular frequencies of which are $(n\omega)$, where n is an integer having the values 1, 2, 3 . . . etc. $n=1$ gives the fundamental frequency and $n+1, 2, 3$ . . . gives the harmonic frequencies. $a_0, a_1, a_2, a_3 \ldots b_1, b_2, b_3 \ldots$ are the Fourier coefficients. They correspond to the maximum amplitudes of the sine and cosine waves. Many periodic functions encountered in engineering can be represented by only a few terms of a series (Thompson, 1962).

The Frequency Components of a Square Wave

A square wave of amplitude $y=A$ can be represented by the series

$$y=\frac{A}{2}+\frac{2A}{\pi}\left(\sin \omega t+\frac{1}{3}\sin 3\omega t+\frac{1}{5}\sin 5\omega t+\frac{1}{7}\sin 7\omega t+\ldots\ldots\right)$$

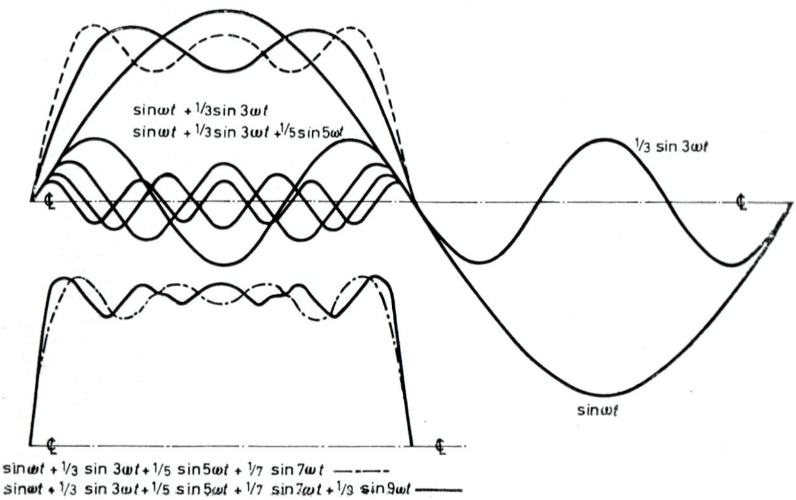

Figure 5.7. The synthesis of a square waveform from the harmonic frequencies

The addition of the fundamental (the repetition frequency) plus odd harmonics up to the ninth is illustrated in *Figure 5.7*. There are no cosine terms. It is evident that the amplitudes of the higher harmonics rapidly decrease. In order to reproduce the fast rise and fall times of a square wave, an amplifier must have a wide frequency response so as to be able to handle a wide range of harmonic frequencies. It is readily possible to form the series which describe the output waveforms from a half or full wave rectifier or a triangular wave.

THE EFFECT OF CAPACITANCE IN AN A.C. CIRCUIT

If either a d.c. or an a.c. voltage is applied to a circuit which contains only pure resistance, then Ohm's law applies. In the a.c. case, r.m.s. values are used, so that $V_{\text{r.m.s.}} = I_{\text{r.m.s.}} \times R$. When a capacitor is connected across a source of direct voltage, a charging current flows at first. This ceases when the capacitor has become fully charged. There is then a potential difference, equal to the source voltage, appearing across the capacitor. No more current flows, and the capacitor 'blocks' the voltage. In contrast, if the capacitor is connected across an a.c. supply, it is found that an a.c. current continues to flow through the capacitor. To find the magnitude of the r.m.s. current passed by the capacitor, the r.m.s. voltage appearing across the capacitor is divided by the 'reactance' of the capacitor. The reactance is given by $X_C = 1/2\pi fC$ where $\pi = 3{\cdot}142$, f is the frequency of the a.c. in Hz, and C is the capacity of the capacitor in farads. X_C is then in ohms. The reactance X_C expresses the opposition offered by the capacitor to the flow of alternating current. A capacitor is a reactive device and it reacts in such a way as to oppose changes produced by the variations of the alternating current. For example, during part of the a.c. cycle, the a.c. supply voltage increases, and this causes the current flowing through the capacitor to increase. This in turn causes the voltage across the capacitor to rise and the current to fall, for it is the difference between the supply voltage and the voltage across the capacitor which causes the current to flow.

From the formula, it can be calculated that the reactance of a 1 μF capacitor at 50 Hz will be 3,185 Ω. If it is connected across a 230 V r.m.s., 50 Hz supply, a current of 72 mA r.m.s. will flow through the capacitor. If it were a pure capacitance, no power would be dissipated. In the case of a 3,185 Ω resistance, passing a 72 mA current would dissipate a power of 16·5 W. The great advantage of using a capacitor to restrict current flow lies in the fact that the power loss is much less than for a resistor having the same ohmic value as the capacitive reactance.

In practice a capacitor can be regarded as a pure capacitance in series with a loss resistance which is normally small. A good quality paper capacitor might have a loss resistance of the order of 5 to 10 Ω, so that little power is dissipated in it. A useful application of capacitive reactance arises in the limiting of the armature current of a servo motor to a safe value when the motor runs slowly (Hill, Hook and Bell, 1961). The half horse-power motor was used to drive a respiratory waveform simulator.

Using an a.c. bridge such as a Schering bridge, it is easy to measure the value of the series resistance associated with a particular capacitor at some particular frequency. Specifications for capacitors quote a maximum value of the power factor for the type at a specified frequency. Thus for a range of miniature bead-type solid tantalum capacitors, the power factor is quoted as 0·24 maximum at 100 Hz. This corresponds to a phase angle of approximately 76 degrees. For a range of polystyrene dielectric capacitors, the power factor is quoted as less than 0·0005 at 1 MHz, corresponding to a phase angle of more than 89 degrees.

PHASE RELATIONSHIPS WITH A CAPACITOR

Using a true double-beam cathode ray tube oscillograph, it is possible to compare the phase relationship existing between the voltage appearing across a capacitor and the current flowing through it. The current waveform is observed by placing a small resistor in series with the capacitor and observing the voltage developed across the resistor. The voltage and current waveforms are both sinusoidal in form, but a quarter of a wave (90 degrees) out of phase. The current leads the voltage by 90 degrees. Physically, it can be visualized that current must flow into the capacitor before the voltage across it can start to rise.

CAPACITIVE COMPENSATION OF A POTENTIAL DIVIDER CIRCUIT

In the case of a d.c. circuit (*Figure 5.8*), the output voltage from an unloaded potential divider is $V_{out} = V_{in}\ R_2/(R_1+R_2)$. If such an arrangement is used to handle a.c. signals, it is found that the output from the divider falls off as the frequency increases. This effect can be overcome by matching the time constants of the divider arms. In *Figure 5.9*, if $R_1C_1 = R_2C_2$, then the divider ratio R_2/R_1+R_2 remains constant at all frequencies (*Figure 5.10*).

Capacity compensation is used on the input attenuators of cathode ray tube oscilloscopes. Pulse waveforms contain significant harmonic frequencies. For each component, a different proportion of the input signal would flow into the stray capacities unless the time constants of the divider arms were matched.

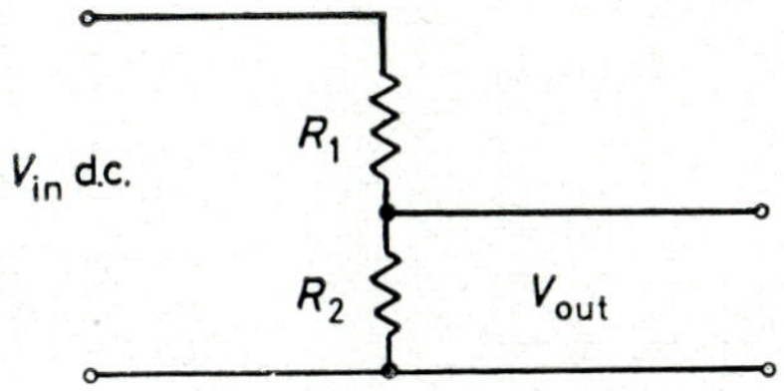

Figure 5 8. A simple voltage-divider circuit

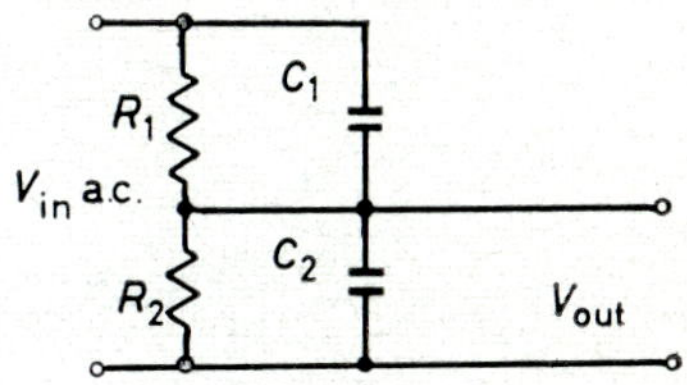

Figure 5.9. Capacitance compensated potential divider

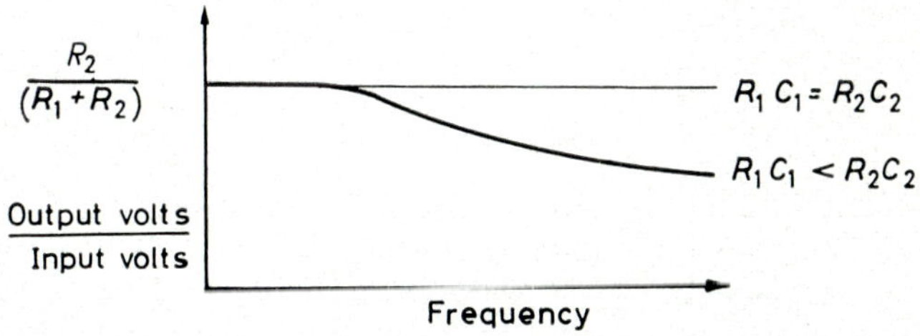

Figure 5.10. The frequency response of a compensated potential-divider circuit

THE EFFECT OF INDUCTANCE IN AN A.C. CIRCUIT

The reactance of a capacitor arises from the capacitor reacting to oppose changes in the circuit conditions. On positive half-cycles, the voltage appearing across the capacitor tends to oppose the flow of charge into the capacitor. On negative half-cycles, the fall in voltage across the capacitor tends to oppose the flow of charge out of the capacitor. A similar opposition effect arises to any change in the flow of current through a coil of wire (an inductor).

When a current flows in a coil of wire, a magnetic field is produced. This is illustrated in *Figure 5.11* for a solenoid coil. If the current is stopped, the collapsing magnetic field gives rise to an electromotive force which acts in such a direction as to try to maintain the current flow. When the coil current is switched on, the direction of the induced e.m.f. will be such as to tend to oppose the build-up of current.

In general, when the coil current is changed, a 'back-e.m.f.' is induced in the coil in such a sense as to try and oppose the current changes.

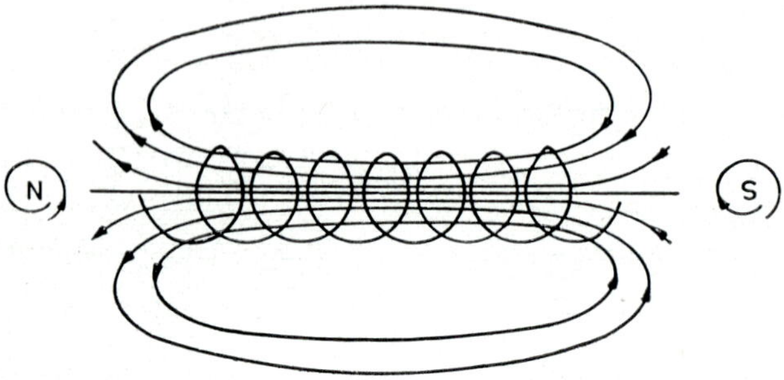

Figure 5.11. The magnetic field generated in a current-carrying solenoid

The action of electromagnetic induction is defined by the following two laws. Faraday's law states that when the magnetic flux through a circuit is changing, an induced e.m.f. is set up and its magnitude is proportional to the time rate of change of the flux. Lenz's law states that the e.m.f. induced in any circuit is always in such a direction as to oppose the motion or change producing it.

SELF-INDUCTANCE

Numerically, the induced voltage V appearing across the coil is related to the time rate of change of current in the coil by the expression $V=-L(\mathrm{d}I/\mathrm{d}t)$ where I is the coil current. The minus sign indicates that the induced voltage is acting to oppose the current change. L is a constant for a particular coil; it is known as the self-inductance of the coil. The inductance of a solenoid coil depends on the number of turns, the winding length, the cross-sectional area of the coil and the permeability of the core material. For an air-cored solenoid, $L=4\pi T^2 A/10^9 l$ where L is in Henries, T is the number of turns, A is the cross-sectional area in cm^2 and l is the winding length in centimetres. The magnetic field produced at the centre of a long air-cored solenoid is given by $H=4\pi \mathrm{n}I/10$ gauss where n is the number of turns and I amperes is the current flowing.

The gauss is the c.g.s. unit of magnetic induction and in any material it is the number of lines of magnetic force passing perpendicularly through the unit area. In the S.I. system of units, the gauss has been replaced by the tesla where 1 tesla$=10^{-4}$ gauss.

The tesla is the unit of magnetic flux density and is equal to 1 weber per square metre of circuit area. The weber is the S.I. unit of magnetic flux. It is equal to the magnetic flux which, linking a circuit of one turn, produces in it an e.m.f. of 1 V as it is reduced to zero at a uniform rate in 1 second.

The henry is the S.I. unit of electrical inductance. It is defined as the inductance of a closed circuit in which an e.m.f. of 1 V is produced when the electric current in the circuit varies uniformly at the rate of 1 ampere per second.

From $V = -L(\mathrm{d}I/\mathrm{d}t)$, if the current is changing uniformly in an inductance of 1 henry at a rate of 1 ampere per second, then the induced voltage will have a magnitude of 1 V. When a switch is used to break an inductive circuit, quite high voltages, sufficient to produce a spark, can appear across the switch contacts. The effect is particularly marked in d.c. circuits and arcing across the contacts can occur. Sparking can rapidly destroy the contacts and a 'spark-quench' circuit is normally wired across them. This consists of a resistor and a capacitor in series, typical values being 0·1 μF and 220 Ω. Sparking must be avoided in operating rooms where explosive agents such as cyclopropane and ether might be used. For this reason, the electrical outlets in operating rooms in the United Kingdom are fitted with sealed mercury switches.

If a sine wave signal is applied to an inductance, and a double beam cathode ray tube oscilloscope used to measure the current and voltage waveforms, it is found that they are both sinusoidal in form. However, the current lags behind the voltage by 90 degrees. The lag arises from the necessity for the applied voltage to overcome the back e.m.f.

The opposition to a.c. current flow of an inductance is expressed in terms of an inductive reactance, X_L. X_L is in ohms when f is in hertz and L is in henrys and $X_L = 2\pi fL$. By Ohm's law $V_{r.m.s.} = I_{r.m.s.} X_L$.

Although the improved performance of modern voltage stabilizer circuits in many cases is doing away with the need for chokes in medium current power supplies, large iron cored inductors are still used to assist in the removal of the residual a.c. ripple component from the output of d.c. power units. Such inductors are known as 'smoothing chokes'. A typical smoothing choke might have an inductance of 20 henrys when carrying a direct current of 100 mA, and an ohmic resistance of 500 Ω. In general, the effect of passing a direct current through a choke is to reduce its effective inductance. Hence when measuring the inductance of a choke, it is desirable to be able to do so whilst passing the value of the direct current through it which will be used in practice. Suitable techniques are the use of Hay's bridge or Turner's method (Scroggie, 1945).

In the case of a d.c. power unit using a full wave rectifier, the ripple current will have a frequency in the United Kingdom of 100 Hz (50 Hz mains supply). At this frequency, the reactance of the 20 H choke will be 12,500 Ω. This is considerably higher than the 500 Ω d.c. resistance of the choke which dissipated 5 W at 100 mA. The 12,500 Ω reactance effectively chokes back the a.c. ripple whilst the only opposition to the direct current flow is the resistance of 500 Ω.

Inductances of the order of millihenrys, having compressed powder cores, are commonly used in audio frequency circuits, often as part of a filter circuit. In radio frequency circuits, inductances of the order of 200 μH at 1 MHz are encountered as chokes to keep signals out of the supply lines and in tuned circuits.

TUNED CIRCUITS

The formulae for the reactance of a capacitor ($X_C=1/(2\pi fC)$) and for the reactance of an inductor ($X_L=2\pi fL$), reveal that the inductive reactance of a coil increases with increasing frequency (*Figure 5.12*), whilst the capacitive reactance of a capacitor falls with

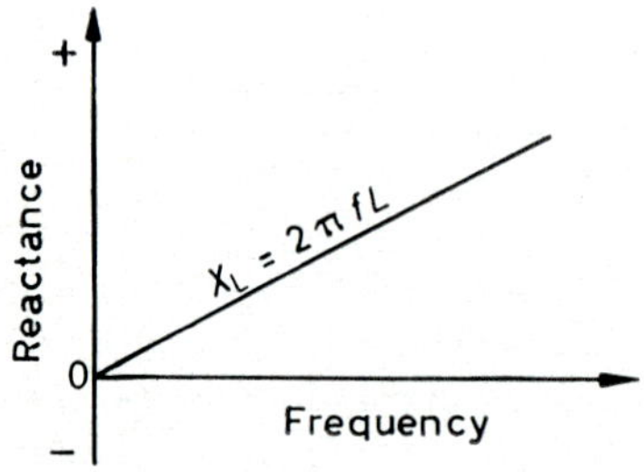

Figure 5.12. The variation of an inductive reactance with frequency

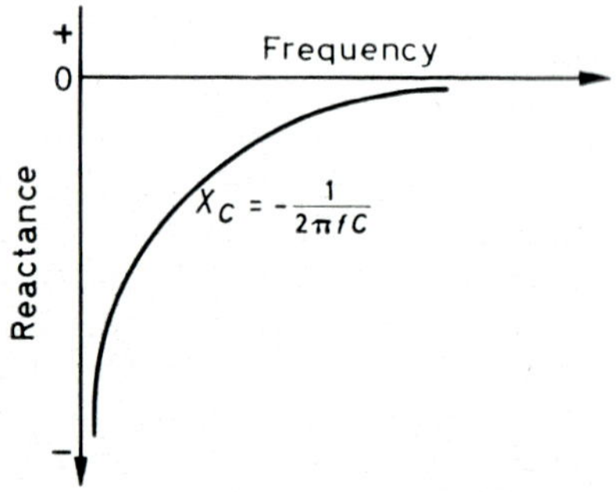

Figure 5.13. The variation of a capacitive reactance with frequency

increasing frequency (*Figure 5.13*). This suggests that cancellation might occur at some particular frequency.

The Series Tuned Circuit

In *Figure 5.14*, a coil L is shown in series with a capacitor C. The ohmic resistance of the circuit is mainly concentrated in the coil. The effective opposition of the circuit to an a.c. signal is given by the impedance of the coil–capacitor combination. Numerically, the impedance Z in ohms is given by $Z=\sqrt{[R^2+(X_L-X_C)^2]}$, where R is the total ohmic resistance of the circuit. The opposition to current flow between electrodes placed across the thorax or in the brain depends on the impedance of the resistance and capacitance of the intervening tissue. Changes occurring in this impedance,

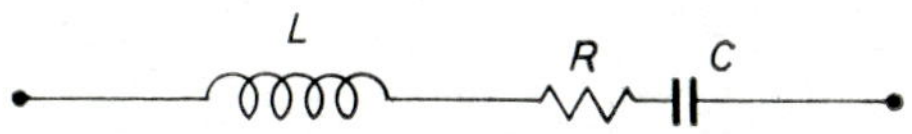

Figure 5.14. The series tuned circuit

for example with respiration, are usually monitored by passing a small current through the electrodes and recording the voltage developed across the electrodes. Impedance techniques have been used to monitor respiration, cardiac output and brain perfusion. Relevant references are Geddes and Hoff (1964) and McCally *et al.* (1963).

Although inductive and capacitive reactances and resistances are all expressed in ohms, it is not possible simply to add them numerically in order to determine the impedance. This is because of the phase differences existing between the voltages and currents in the circuit. In a capacitance, the current leads the voltage by 90 degrees, whilst in an inductance the current lags the voltage by 90 degrees. Thus at any instant, the currents due to a particular voltage will be 180 degrees out of phase, that is, flowing in opposite directions. For this reason, the reactances should be subtracted. It is possible to find a frequency, for a given combination of inductance and capacitance, at which the inductive and capacitive reactances are equal and cancel. At this frequency, the impedance of the combination simply equals the resistance of the circuit. This frequency is called the Resonant Frequency of the circuit. The use of a variable capacitor enables the circuit to be 'tuned' to resonance at a specified frequency. Alternatively, the inductance may be changed by moving a core in or out of the coil in order to tune the circuit.

A series combination of inductance and capacitance is called an Acceptor Circuit, because it presents a low impedance at resonance. Such a circuit may be used to pass the fundamental frequency of a signal whilst rejecting the harmonics. For example, if a square wave is put through a series circuit tuned to the fundamental frequency the output will be a sine wave of that frequency.

The Parallel Tuned Circuit

In *Figure 5.15*, an inductor L is shown connected in parallel with a capacitor C. At the resonant frequency, the numerical values of the inductive and capacitive reactances will be equal, and the currents in L and C will be oppositely directed at any instant. If there is no resistance present in the circuit ($R=0$), then no current flows in or out from the circuit. There is simply a large oscillating current surging backwards and forwards between the capacitance and the

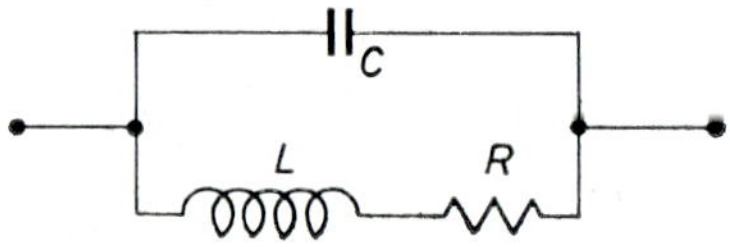

Figure 5.15 The parallel tuned circuit

inductance. In this ideal state, the impedance presented to the signal source by the circuit would be infinite. In practice there is always some resistance associated with the winding of the inductor in particular and to a lesser extent with the capacitor. Hence the signal source has to provide a small make-up current to replenish these losses. Therefore, the circuit impedance, although high, is not infinite. A parallel tuned circuit is known as a Rejector Circuit, because it will not pass (will reject) signals having a frequency equal to the resonant value.

The resonant frequency of either a series or a parallel tuned circuit is given by the formula $f=1/2\pi\sqrt{(LC)}$ where f is in hertz, L is in henrys and C is in farads. As an example, a medium waveband radio coil of 190 μH inductance can be tuned to a frequency of 1 MHz by a variable capacitor of 133 pF capacitance. At resonance, the inductive and capacitive reactances cancel and a large current flows. In the case of a parallel tuned circuit, it is a circulatory current. It is known as a tank circuit, since it provides a reservoir of oscillatory current. The oscillatory current develops a large signal voltage across the circuit. The magnification of the input signal by a parallel tuned circuit enables a radio receiver to be tuned to a particular station. Tuned circuits are used in endo-radiosondes and their receivers and in radio telemetry systems in general. They are also used to pick out the various harmonic frequencies from signal waveforms.

MAGNIFICATION FACTOR

The effectiveness of a coil in producing the magnification of an applied signal is expressed in terms of its magnification factor, or Q. Q is given by the ratio of the reactance of the coil at the resonance frequency to its resistance, i.e. $Q = 2\pi f_0 L/R$ where f_0 is the resonant frequency. The resistance is the a.c. resistance of the coil. This is usually rather higher than its true d.c. resistance. At high frequencies, the current tends to concentrate on the outside of the wire of the coil. The effective cross-sectional area is thus reduced, causing the resistance to be raised. This action is known as the Skin Effect. The 190 μH coil mentioned previously had a Q of 50 and an a.c. resistance of 24 Ω at 1 MHz. The d.c. resistance was 4·5 Ω. To reduce the skin effect, which lowers the Q, radio frequency coils are wound with multi-strand Litz wire in which each individual strand is insulated.

FILTERS

The resistance of a pure resistor is independent of frequency, but the reactance of a capacitor is proportional to $1/f$ and thus falls with increasing frequency. This fact allows simple low and high pass filters to be constructed. These are basically voltage-dividing networks (attenuators) arranged to possess frequency-discriminating properties.

Low Pass R–C Filter

The arrangement shown in *Figure 5.16* favours the lower frequencies. At the higher frequencies, the reactance of C decreases and

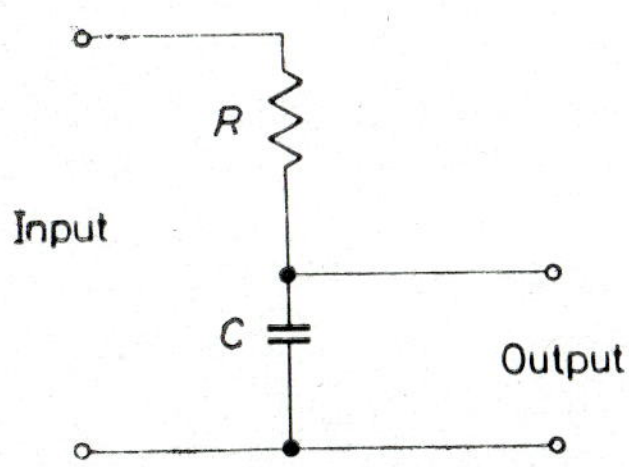

Figure 5.16. A simple low pass R–C filter

the output falls. Referring to the concept of decibels in Chapter 6, the output of the filter is reduced to 0·707 (3 db down) of the input at the frequency which makes the reactance of the capacitor ($1/2\pi fC$) numerically equal to R (*Figure 5.17*). This is known as the cut-off frequency of the filter (f_0), and $f_0 = 1/2\pi RC$ Hz. In an EEG amplifier, different filter capacitors can be switched in to limit the high frequency response of the amplifier. Typically, a 1·2 db loss can be introduced at frequencies of 15, 25 or 75 Hz. In each case the slope of the amplifier's response curve falls off at a rate of 6 db per octave. With a single stage R–C filter of this type, the output falls by 6 db each time the frequency is doubled, that is, at a rate of 6 db per octave. The attenuation produced is negligible at frequencies up to one half of f_0, and is 3 db at f_0, 6 db at $2f_0$ and 12 db at $4f_0$. The shape of the attenuation curve depends only on the product RC and not on the individual values of R and C. For the unwanted signal frequency to be attenuated by a factor of ten compared with

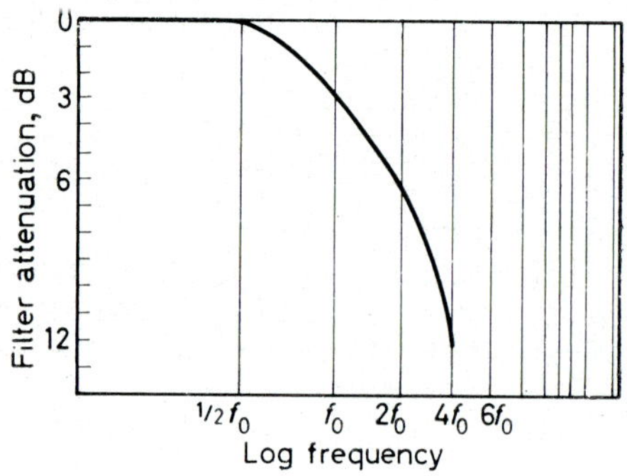

Figure 5.17. The attenuation produced by a simple low pass R–C filter as a function of the signal frequency

the wanted frequency, the ratio of the frequencies must be at least ten to one. Other applications for a low pass filter lie in the removal of electromyographic muscle activity from an electrocardiogram, the extraction of the respiratory modulation from a central venous pressure recording or the removal of cardiac pulsations from an oesophageal pressure recording. For a greater attenuation efficiency, two or more filters may be inserted at different points in an amplifier circuit. Two filters will give a roll-off in the frequency response curve of 12 db per octave, whilst three filters will give 18 db per octave. The roll-off introduced by R–C couplings becomes important when considering the frequency compensation of operational amplifiers. Filters can be connected directly in series if the RC value is kept constant but R is progressively increased.

For the three-stage filter shown in *Figure 5.18*, the cut-off frequency is 50 Hz. Above this frequency the attenuation will be 19 db per octave. Low pass filters will also change the phase of the higher

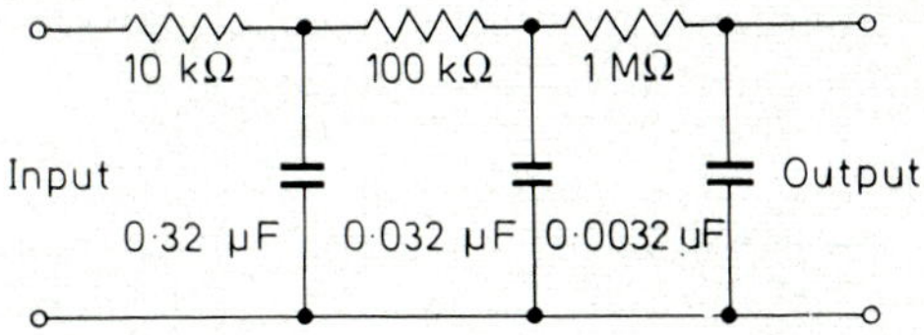

Figure 5.18. Three-stage R–C low pass filter

frequency signal components, and this may introduce serious distortion if a sharply rising signal is applied to the filter.

High Pass R–C Filter

Figure 5.19 shows a simple high pass R–C filter. At the higher frequencies, the capacitive reactance of C falls and the output is

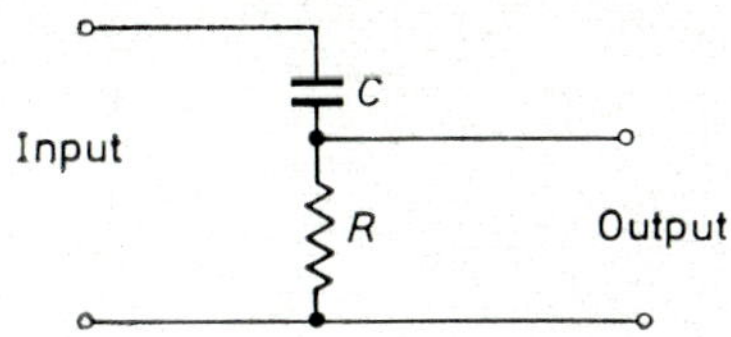

Figure 5.19. A simple high pass R–C filter

increased. The cut-off frequency $f_0 = 1/2\pi RC$ again occurs at such a value that the capacitive reactance is numerically equal to R. At signal frequencies lower than f_0, an attenuation is introduced of 6 db

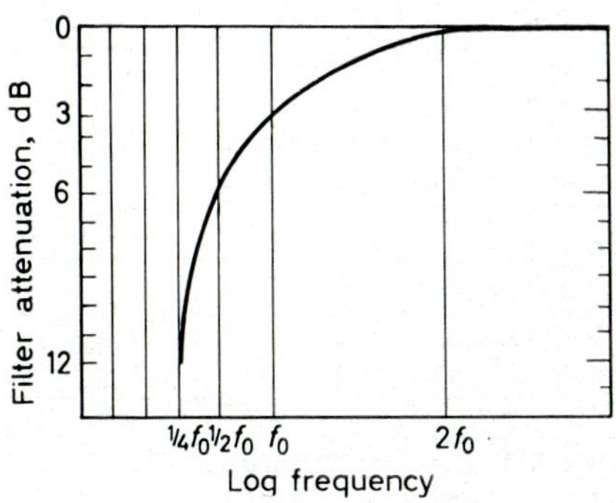

Figure 5.20. The attenuation of a simple high pass R–C filter as a function of frequency

per octave. Signal frequencies higher than $2f_0$ are not significantly affected. This is shown in *Figure 5.20*.

High pass filters are used to discriminate against low frequency signals such as those due to skin electrode contact potential changes occurring when recording an ECG, or for the attenuation of 50 and 100 Hz mains interference in an audio amplifier.

Notch Filter

A requirement exists for a filter which will attenuate a relatively narrow band of frequencies. A typical application occurs in the reduction of 50 Hz 'hum' present in a physiological signal such as an ECG. The usual arrangement is to use a two-stage amplifier having

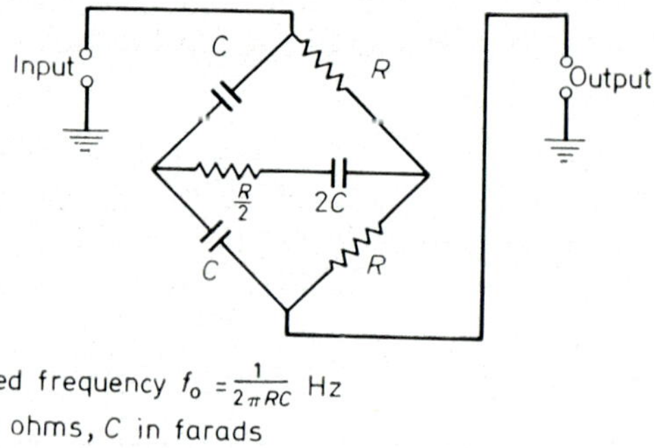

Figure 5.21. A twin-T R–C notch filter

a twin-T network as part of the interstage coupling. The network is designed to present a high impedance at the required frequency. Hence, the gain of the amplifier is a minimum for this frequency.

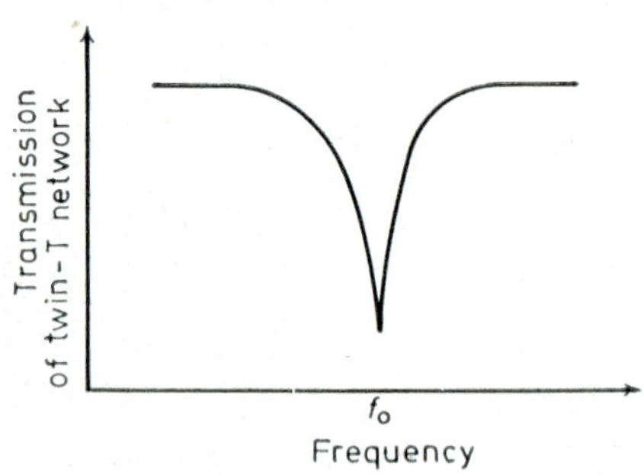

Figure 5.22. The notch characteristic of a twin-T filter

Figure 5.21 shows a parallel-T (or twin-T) network (Wolf, 1946), and *Figure 5.22* shows a typical response for a 50 Hz rejection filter.

To obtain the sharpest possible notch, the values of the components should be carefully matched and good quality capacitors used.

Although a notch filter is simple to construct and effective, it should be used only as a last resort, since it will also remove signal components lying within the pass band and can distort transient signals. Gibson, Gibson and Hirsch (1970) make the point that a parallel-T filter can seriously distort neural data such as 'spikes'.

Low Pass Filters

Another requirement is for variable low pass filters to remove high frequency noise from a signal. A useful paper on the subject is that of Mundl (1968).

Mundl points out that in EEG applications there is a requirement for band pass filters of two types, one having a bandwidth of approximately $\frac{1}{4}$ to $\frac{1}{2}$ octave and the other a bandwidth of $\frac{3}{4}$ to 1 octave. These requirements can be met by the use of three and five stagger tuned stages respectively. Each stage uses a twin-T network in the feedback path of its amplifier, the combination of the stages providing a flat top across the pass band and steep sides. At the tuned frequency, the twin-T network presents a high impedance. Hence the negative feedback is minimal and the gain a maximum, giving a peaked response for that stage. Mundl gives curves for predicting the tuned frequencies and the magnification factors (Qs) of the individual responses for a given centre frequency and Q of the composite filter.

A.C. BRIDGES

The simple type of Wheatstone bridge described in Chapter 4, and energized from a d.c. supply such as a battery, is useful only for measuring resistances. It is usual to employ an a.c. bridge to measure components possessing reactance, such as capacitors or inductors. It may also be desirable to use an a.c. bridge in order to avoid the polarization effects associated with d.c., for example when measuring the conductivity of a solution.

Figure 5.23a shows a d.c. bridge arranged to measure the resistance R_4 of a solution contained in a conductivity cell. *Figure 5.23b* shows the corresponding a.c. arrangement. The bridge is energized from an R–C oscillator, usually at a frequency of 1,000 Hz. The balance detector is now a pair of headphones or a cathode ray tube oscilloscope instead of the galvanometer used in the d.c. bridge. R_3 is adjusted for a minimum sound in the headphones or a minimum amplitude trace on the oscilloscope. There is usually some residual output at balance due to the presence of harmonics. At balance, points *a* and *b* will be at the same potential. Then the voltages developed across the bridge components are such that $V_2 = V_3$ and $V_1 = V_4$, giving $I_2Z_2/I_1Z_1 = I_3Z_3/I_4Z_4$ where Z_1, Z_2, Z_3 and Z_4 are the impedances of the bridge arms. This relationship holds only if the following two conditions are fulfilled: $R_2/R_1 = R_3/R_4$ and $X_2/X_1 = X_3/X_4$ where X_1, X_2, X_3 and X_4 represent any reactances present in the arms. In general, to balance an a.c. bridge, two balance conditions must be fulfilled compared with the one condition for a d.c. bridge.

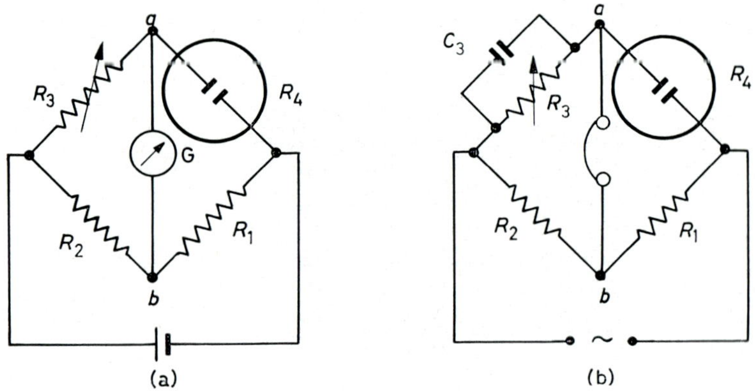

Figure 5.23. D.C. and a.c. bridge circuits

A.C. bridges are widely used to measure both capacitance and inductance (Owen, 1962). Commercial component bridges are available in most electronics laboratories. A typical arrangement would use a d.c. bridge for resistance measurements and an a.c. bridge at 1 kHz or 10 kHz for the measurement of inductance and capacitance. An indication is usually available of the power factor. A valve voltmeter feeding a centre zero meter with flat pole pieces makes a convenient detector. This type of meter has a response which is approximately logarithmic, so that the sensitivity is a maximum around the balance point and falls off rapidly on either side. The use of an oscilloscope in parallel will enable the operator to check on the presence of residual harmonics if their amplitude appears to be excessive.

A most useful bridge for comparing impedances is the transformer bridge shown in *Figure 5.24.* It differs from the conventional Wheatstone bridge network, and offers the advantage of being able to measure an impedance which is still connected in a circuit.

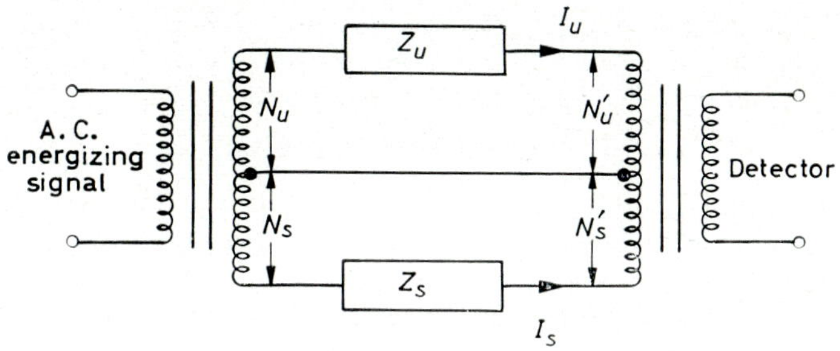

Figure 5.24. Transformer bridge

Z_u is the unknown impedance, and Z_s is a standard impedance Let the transformers be tapped to give N_u, N_s and N'_u, N'_s turns respectively. It can be shown that

$$Z_u = Z_s \cdot \frac{(N_u)}{(N_s)} \times \frac{(N'_u)}{(N'_s)}$$

In order to express the unknown impedance Z_u in terms of the standard impedance Z_s it is only necessary to know the transformer turns ratios accurately. Each ratio may be of the order of 1,000 to 1. A good account of the transformer bridge is given by Griffiths and Lee (1962).

THE MEASUREMENT OF ELECTROLYTIC CONDUCTIVITY

An interesting example of the use of an a.c. bridge in medical practice occurs in the measurement of electrolytic conductivity. Basically conductance is the reciprocal of resistance and is a measure of the ease with which electrical current can flow in a substance. Thus the higher the resistance of the substance, the lower its conductance. The basic unit of conductance is the reciprocal ohm (ohm^{-1}) or mho. In the S.I. system of units the mho is now known as the siemens. When dealing with the conductance of solutions it is usual to use millimhos. The resistance of a substance is a function of its geometry, and this leads to the concept of specific resistance.

Similarly in the case of conductance a specific conductance or conductivity can be defined with units of mhos per cm^3.

The conductivity of solutions arises from the fact that ionic dissociation occurs in solutions of acids and alkalis and in pure water (Miller, 1967). The dissociation process results in the formation of positive and negative ions; in equilibrium, the number of new ions being formed is balanced by ions recombining. As an example, sulphuric acid dissociates as follows:

$$(H_2SO_4) \rightleftharpoons 2(H)^{+} + (SO_4)^{--},$$

and for caustic soda $(NaOH) \rightleftharpoons (Na)^{+} + (OH)^{-}$. The presence of free charge carriers suggests that a current will flow if positive and negative electrodes are placed in the solution. When the positive ions reach the negative electrode they acquire electrons, and similarly the negative ions give up electrons at the positive electrode, so that the ions are neutralized at the electrodes. The current flowing will depend not only upon the concentration of the solution but upon the charge carried by the ions and their velocity or mobility in travelling to the electrodes. Where several species of ions are present, there is a general relationship $E.K = \Sigma q.u.C$ where K is the conductivity of the solution, q is the charge on the ion concerned, C is the concentration of those ions, u is the mobility of the ion, and E is the potential gradient across the solution. The summation sign indicates that the equation takes into account all the species of ion present. In practice, it applies strictly only for dilute solutions where there is a linear relationship between conductivity and concentration. At higher strengths of solution the conductivity is affected by changes in mobility due to attractive forces existing between ions. The relationship between concentration and conductivity for dilute solutions simplifies to $E.K = \alpha C$ where α is a constant. Thus a measurement of the conductivity of the solution should be linearly related to the concentration.

In practice a d.c. potential difference is not applied across the solution and the current flowing taken as a measure of the conductivity. With a d.c. system a marked degree of polarization may be present. When the potential difference applied across the cell is less than a certain value, known as the decomposition potential, the current increases only slightly with increasing voltage and not according to Ohm's law. At voltages higher than the decomposition potential, Ohm's law is obeyed and continuous electrolysis takes place. When gaseous ions are produced, these tend to congregate around the electrodes when they have been neutralized. The action is similar to that of polarization in a primary cell, the neutral layer tending to reduce the effective size of the electrodes and their attraction for ions. The effects of polarization at the electrodes can be minimized by applying an a.c. voltage across the cell. The polarization produced by each half cycle is relatively small and is neutralized with each reversal of the cycle. Typically, a frequency of 1,000 Hz is widely used.

A second form of polarization effect arises when the electrodes are made from the same metal as the metallic salt in solution, for example, silver electrodes in a silver salt solution. Metal passing into solution may give rise to an increase in the conductivity in the region of the anode and a decrease around the cathode due to the deposition of metal. As a result, a concentration cell is formed whose e.m.f. opposes that applied to produce conduction. Conductivity cell electrodes are usually made from carbon, platinum or gold, so that this situation does not normally apply.

As would be expected, the conductance of a solution is directly proportional to the area of the electrodes and inversely proportional to their distance apart. The specific conductivity of a solution is defined as the conductivity of the solution between electrodes 1 cm^2 in area and 1 cm apart. The cell constant of a conductivity cell is defined as the ratio of the specific conductivity of the solution in the cell to the conductance of the solution as measured by the cell. By analogy with the formula for specific resistance, it can be seen that $K = k.(A/L)$ where A is the area of the electrodes and L their separation. Hence the cell constant $\beta = (L/A)$. The value of β may not stay constant in practice due to variations occurring in the effective area of the electrodes. It is best determined by placing a solution of known specific conductivity in the cell and measuring its conductance, rather than by relying on the geometry of the cell. Typical values of cell constants are 0·1, 1 and 10. The conductivity of a solution is temperature dependent, typically varying by 1·5 to 3·5 per cent per degree Centigrade. For this reason, either the temperature of the conductivity cell is stabilized at a known value, or else a thermistor is incorporated into the cell in order suitably to adjust the measuring circuitry in respect of the temperature changes. A cell designed to measure the conductivity of the dialysate used in an artificial kidney might have a pair of carbon ring electrodes and operate with a temperature compensation thermistor. The porous surface fo the carbon gives rise to a large effective surface area, and by reducing the current density it thus reduces the degree of polarization.

The conductivity cell can be placed in one arm of a Wheatstone bridge circuit with the thermistor in the opposite arm (Simpson *et al.*, 1967). The conductivity cell also possesses capacitance. This can be balanced out by adjusting a variable capacitor placed across the opposite arm of the bridge. Basically, the bridge measures the resistance of the solution contained in the cell. A linear calibration in terms of conductance can be obtained if a constant voltage is applied across the cell and the current through the cell is measured. In at least one type of artificial kidney, a pair of conductivity cells is employed, placed in opposite arms of the a.c. bridge. One cell has the dialysing fluid flowing through it, whilst the other (at the same temperature) contains a standard solution of known conductivity. If the conductivity of the dialysing fluid should move outside specified limits, the degree of unbalance of the bridge would be sufficient to close a relay and sound an alarm. The conductivity of a typical dialysate solution of 130 mEq/litre sodium concentration is approximately 13·8 millimhos/cm at 25° C, so that a conductivity meter for use with dialysate solutions might cover the range 11–15 millimhos/cm. Sproule (1967) describes the use of a conductivity meter to control the concentration of the dialysate solution in an artificial kidney.

It is also possible to use an a.c. bridge to estimate blood loss during surgery (LeVeen and Rubricius, 1958). The addition of blood to water will produce changes in the electrical conductivity of the mixture and this is measured with the bridge. Provided other electrolytes are not present, this is an accurate method capable of giving a continuous reading. An alternative method which is simpler and may be more reliable in practice is that of Roe, Gardiner and Dudley (1962). This is a photoelectric estimation of the optical density of the blood solution.

A.C. METERS

With the ordinary moving coil meter as used in d.c. circuits, the deflection of the pointer is proportional to the current I. With very low frequency a.c. currents (approximately 1 Hz), the meter pointer will swing from side to side about the zero mark of the scale with each cycle. At higher frequencies, the inertia of the meter movement will prevent the pointer from following the signal and thus the meter will read the average value of the signal. For a sine wave this is zero.

Rectifier Meters

By feeding the moving coil meter from a full-wave bridge rectifier, the input a.c. is converted to d.c. and can now be measured by the meter. Frequencies up to about 20 kHz can be handled. The arrangement is shown in *Figure 5.25.* This type of rectifier meter reads the mean value of the full-wave rectified waveform, and this is

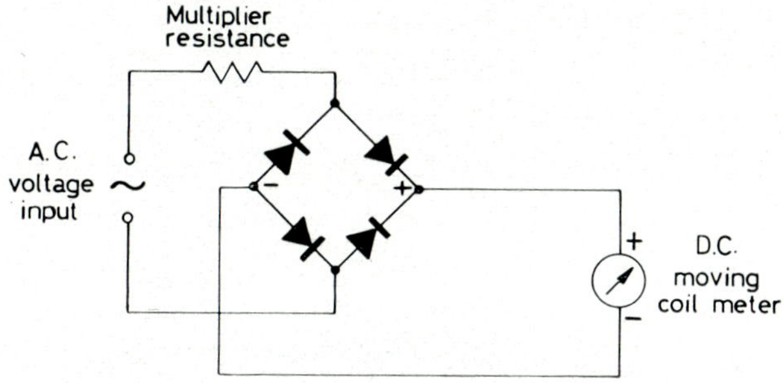

Figure 5.25. A rectifier-type a.c. meter

equal to 0·91 of the r.m.s. value of the a.c. waveform. Multiplier resistances can be used to extend the range of rectifier-type a.c. meters as is the case with d.c. meters. For the a.c. current ranges, however, it is usual to employ current transformers (*Figure 5.26*).

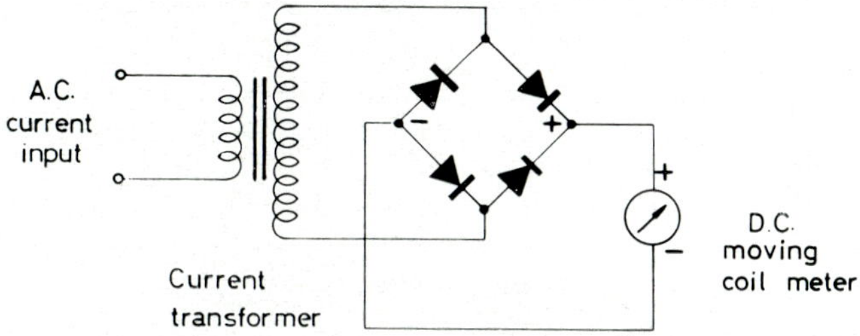

Figure 5.26. The use of a current transformer

For a typical range, the secondary must produce 1 mA d.c. (1·11 mA a.c. r.m.s.) when the primary current is 1,000 mA r.m.s. The turns ratio is thus $T_1/T_2 = 1{\cdot}11/1{,}000 = 1:900$.

Moving Iron Meters

Here the current to be measured is passed through the coil (*Figure 5.27*) and creates a magnetic field. The iron becomes magnetized and is drawn into the coil. The force experienced by the iron depends on the magnetism of the iron and the field of the coil.

Hence the deflection is now proportional to the square of the current. Thus a moving iron meter can be used to measure either d.c. or r.m.s. a.c. This type of meter is employed only at power line frequencies. It is commonly encountered on heavy current hospital

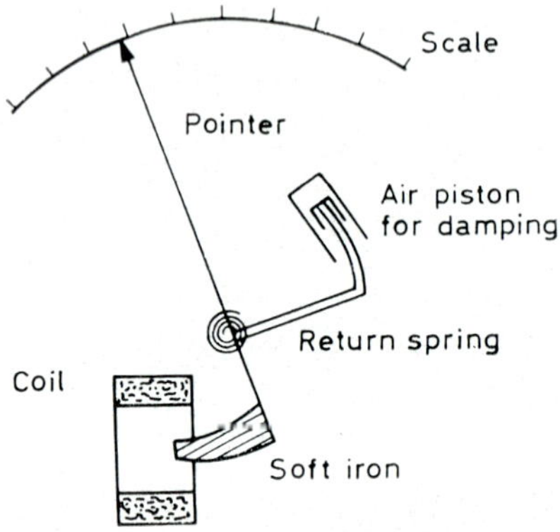

Figure 5.27. A moving iron meter

switchboards where its robust construction is an asset. The scale is made approximately linear by careful shaping of the iron in order to minimize cramping at the top end of the scale.

Thermocouple Meters

In this case the current to be measured is passed through the heater wire of the meter (*Figure 5.28*). The temperature of the heater is sensed by a thermocouple, the output of which is read by a d.c.

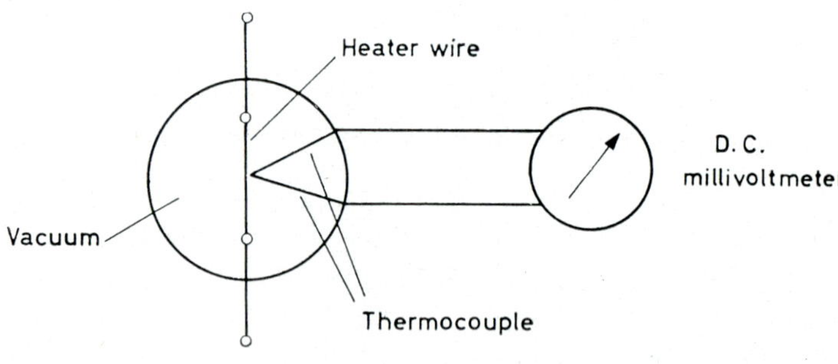

Figure 5.28. A thermocouple meter

millivoltmeter. Since the heating effect is proportional to the square of the heating current, the meter can be scaled in terms of d.c. or r.m.s. a.c. The scale is non-linear. Thermocouple meters are encountered on surgical diathermy units, where they are used to indicate the magnitude of the radio frequency output current.

REFERENCES

Geddes, L. A. and Hoff, H. E. (1964). 'The measurement of physiologic events by electrical impedance.' *Am. J. med. Electron.* **3,** 16.

Gibson, J. M., Gibson, M. M. and Hirsch, H. R. (1970). 'Distortion of neural data by "notch" filters.' *Med. biol. Engng* **8,** 95.

Griffiths, V. S. and Lee, W. H. (1962). *The Electronics of Laboratory and Process Instruments.* London: Chatto & Windus.

Hill, D. W., Hook, J. R. and Bell, E. G. (1961). 'Servo-operated respiratory waveform simulator.' *J. scient. Instrum.* **38,** 100.

LeVeen, H. H. and Rubricius, J. L. (1958). 'Continuous, automatic, electronic determinations of operative blood loss.' *Surgery Gynec. Obstet.* **106,** 368.

McCally, M., Barnard, G. W., Robins, K. E. and Marko, A. R. (1963). 'Observations with an electrical impedance respirometer.' *Am. J. med. Electron.* **2,** 322.

Miller, J. T. (1967). 'Electrolytic conductivity.' *Biomed. Engng* **2,** 490.

Mundl, W. J. (1968). 'Practical design of low-frequency bandpass filters.' *Med. biol. Engng* **6,** 203.

Owen, D. (1962). *A.C. Measurements,* 3rd edn. London: Methuen.

Roe, C. F., Gardiner, A. J. S. and Dudley, H. A. F. (1962). 'A simple method for the continuous accurate measurement of operative blood loss.' *Lancet* **1,** 672.

Scroggie, M. G. (1945). *Radio Laboratory Handbook,* 3rd edn. London: Iliffe.

Shirer, H. (1962). 'Blood pressure measuring methods.' *Trans. Inst Radio Engrs* **BME-9,** 116.

Simpson, K. M., Blainey, J. D., Dawson-Edwards, P., Hilton, D. D., Williams, B. T., Sutherland, A. C. and Cantrill, K. I. (1967). 'A single-patient haemodialysis-monitoring and dialysate-proportionating machine.' *Lancet* **1,** 1247.

Sproule, R. A. (1967). 'Artificial kidney dialysate control by electrolytic conductivity measurement.' *Biomed. Engng* **2,** 172.

Thompson, N. P. (1962). 'Fourier analysis of the electrocardiographic function.' *Am. J. med. Electron.* **1,** 299.

Wolf, A. (1946). 'Note on a parallel-T resistance–capacitance network.' *Proc. Inst. Radio Engrs* **34,** 659.

Chapter 6

Semiconductor Devices

ELECTRON ENERGY LEVELS

In free atoms, the orbital electrons are distributed amongst so-called stationary states which are characterized by each electron having a discrete energy. The electrons which are most strongly bound in the atom are those which are situated close to the nucleus, whilst those in the outermost orbits are the most weakly bound. The electron energy states in an atom are grouped into shells known as K, L, M, etc., the K shell being occupied by the innermost electrons. The energy possessed by any electron is mainly determined by the particular shell to which it belongs. The average energy difference between shells is very much greater than that existing between electrons in the same shell. The Pauli exclusion principle limits the number of electrons which can occupy each shell to the number of discrete energy states available in that shell. The chemical properties of an element are determined by the arrangement of the outermost or valency electrons in its atoms.

ELECTRONS IN SOLIDS

Important modifications to the arrangements of the electron energy levels occur when the atoms concerned are separated by distances of the same order of magnitude as the atomic diameters. In the case of a crystalline solid, the atoms are bound together in the form of a rigid, regular array or lattice and the valence electrons may no longer be associated with a particular atom. They constitute a group of 'free' electrons which are associated with energy levels belonging to the whole lattice. In the simplest case, if two atoms each having one orbital electron are brought sufficiently close together, interaction occurs and the motion of each valence electron is influenced by both atoms. As a result the energy level of one electron becomes slightly higher and that of the other slightly lower than the levels they would have had in the free atomic state. The change from the free state levels increases as the atoms come closer together. When a large number of atoms each having one valency electron are brought together, the individual energy levels spread out into a narrow band. The difference in energy between the top and the bottom of the band depends upon the spacing between atoms and the extent to which adjacent atoms overlap.

The conduction of electricity in solids is believed to be due to the movement of electrons through the solid under the influence of an applied electric field. When this happens, the electron will be accelerated by the field and will receive energy. For the resulting motion to be possible, there must exist a higher energy level into which the electron may move. Electrons which are able to attain these higher energy levels are able to move about reasonably freely without being tied to nuclei and are known as conduction electrons. When the nuclei are separated so that a wide forbidden energy gap exists between the valence and conduction bands, electrons cannot easily move from the former to the latter. A material of this nature is an electrical insulator. If the separation of the nuclei is such that the conduction and valence bands overlap, then conduction can occur provided that some of the upper energy levels in the conduction band are not occupied by electrons. When the width of the forbidden gap between the valence and conduction bands is relatively small, the material is classified as an insulator. As the name implies, a semiconductor has a specified resistance or resistivity lying between that of a conductor and that of an insulator. The resistance R in ohms of a substance of cross-sectional area A and length l is given by $R=ls/A$ where s is the specific resistance of the substance. A general classification might be that conductors have specific resistances of less than about 0·1 ohm-metres, semiconductors have specific resistances in the range 0·1 to 10^{12} Ω–m, and insulators have specific resistances greater than about 10^{12} Ω–m.

Semiconductors have the property that their electrical resistance decreases with increasing temperature. This property is widely used to measure temperature in clinical applications by means of a semiconductor 'thermistor' probe. In contrast, metallic conductors exhibit an increase in resistance with increasing temperature. Some materials, such as germanium, exhibit semiconducting properties only when they contain a small proportion of another element as an impurity. In its pure state germanium, although it looks like a metal, is in fact an insulator. On the controlled addition of a small amount (approximately one part in 10^7) of another element such as arsenic or indium, the resistivity of the material decreases and it acquires semiconducting properties. Such forms of both germanium and, increasingly, silicon 'doped' with controlled amounts of impurity are used in the fabrication of diodes and transistors.

THE STRUCTURE OF PURE GERMANIUM AND SILICON

Both germanium and silicon are tetravalent, that is, they have four valency electrons to each atom. They can be made to exist in a regular crystalline form in which the four valency electrons of each atom are linked with those of four adjacent atoms to form covalent bonds. For a valence electron to cross the forbidden gap between the valence and conduction bands, it must acquire a minimum energy of 0·72 electron volts in the case of germanium and 1·03 electron volts in the case of silicon. The addition of energy in the form of heat or light should help valence electrons to cross the gap and reach the conduction band. Because of this, the conductivity of the crystal should depend both on the ambient temperature and on the strength of the incident light. Germanium is more affected than silicon because of the smaller energy gap.

An atom of germanium consists of a central positively charged nucleus surrounded by 32 orbital electrons arranged in shells (or orbits), the valency electrons being in the outermost shell. The arrangement of the covalent bonds is shown in *Figure 6.1*. Diamond, which is a form of carbon, is also tetravalent and the structure of a semiconductor crystal is often referred to as a 'diamond lattice'.

If the valence electrons were free to move in the conduction band under the influence of a potential difference applied across the germanium, the material would be a good conductor of electricity. The poor conduction of pure germanium arises from the forming of the covalent bonds. As a result, each valence electron is shared between two adjacent atoms. The only electrons available for conduction are those liberated by the action of light or heat. The additional energy imparted breaks up some of the covalent bonds. At normal room temperatures the effect is small, but the higher the temperature, the greater becomes the conductivity. The release of the charge-carrying electrons and holes is known as 'ionization'.

THE ADDITION OF IMPURITY TO PURE GERMANIUM

Pure single crystal germanium, with a resistivity of approximately 0·5 Ω–m at room temperature, is known as an Intrinsic Semiconductor. The word 'intrinsic' indicates that the germanium would conduct significantly at a higher temperature even if it were in an absolutely pure state and possessed a perfect crystal structure.

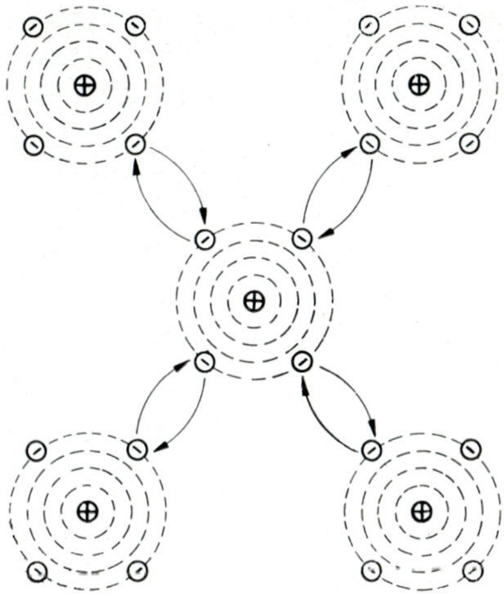

Figure 6.1. Covalent bonds in germanium

THE ADDITION OF A CONTROLLED AMOUNT OF IMPURITY TO PURE GERMANIUM

The addition of a pentavalent atom, such as antimony or arsenic, to pure germanium makes available a free electron to act as a carrier of electric charge. This follows since only four valency electrons of the impurity atom form covalent bonds with germanium atoms. When the impurity atom loses an electron to the current flow, it has a net positive charge and is called a Donor, since it has donated one electron. In practice, the germanium is first purified and then doped with a controlled amount (1 part in 10^7) of the desired impurity. With a pentavalent impurity, the charge carriers are negatively charged electrons and the material is known as *n*-type germanium (*n* for negative). The doped material is an Extrinsic or Impurity Semiconductor. It has a resistivity approximately 200 times greater than that of the pure single crystal material.

On the other hand, if a trivalent impurity such as gallium or indium is added, the impurity atoms each borrow an electron from a neighbouring germanium atom to make up the number of covalent bonds to four. The removal of the electron leaves a 'hole' in the crystal lattice. This hole now exerts an attractive force on any electron which is liberated from a germanium atom by thermal energy and passes near the hole. As a result, a new hole is formed, and this in turn can be filled by the capture of another electron. The effective movement of holes throughout the germanium constitutes a flow of positive charge carriers. In this situation, an impurity atom will gain an electron and is called an Acceptor. Germanium with this type of tetravalent impurity added is called *p*-type germanium (*p* for positive).

THE ADDITION OF A CONTROLLED AMOUNT OF IMPURITY TO PURE SILICON

Pure silicon, like pure germanium, has four valency electrons and is an intrinsic semiconductor. It has a diamond lattice and a resistivity of approximately 2,500 Ω–m at room temperature. The melting point of silicon is 1,420° C compared with 936° C for germanium. This fact has made the purification processes and hence the fabrication of silicon devices considerably more difficult than is the case with germanium. The evolution of suitable manufacturing technology, such as the silicon planar construction, has led to the almost universal use of silicon devices and the emergence of a large family of integrated circuits based on silicon. The energy gap for silicon is higher than that for germanium, which means that since leakage currents are lower, devices are capable of operating at higher temperatures and higher reverse voltages when fabricated in silicon.

THE *p–n* JUNCTION DIODE

Consider a junction formed between two pieces of germanium or silicon, one *p*-type and the other *n*-type, as shown in *Figure 6.2.* At first sight it might be expected that electrons would simply flow from the *n*-type to the *p*-type material and there neutralize the holes, while at the same time there would be a flow of holes from the *p*-type to the *n*-type material. However, the result of electrons flowing from the *n*-type material is to leave it positively charged. Similarly, the result of holes flowing from the *p*-type material is to leave it negatively charged. This process results in the build-up of a 'potential barrier' which prevents any further flow of charge carriers across the junction. The barrier produces the same effect as would a battery connected with the polarity as shown in *Figure 6.2*. The tendency is for the electrons and holes to move in opposite directions away from the junction.

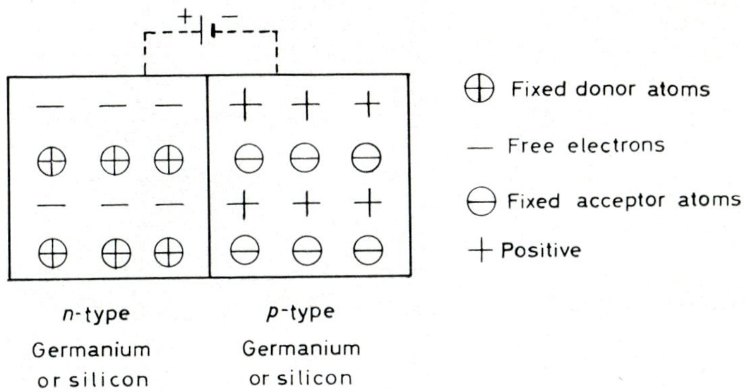

Figure 6.2. Fixed and mobile charges in the region of an n–p or p–n junction

Suppose that a real (external) battery is connected across the junction so that its polarity is the same as that of the internal potential barrier (fictitious) battery. The action of the external battery is to increase the magnitude of the effective potential barrier and to separate the holes and electrons more effectively. Under these conditions, no current flows across the junction from the battery and the junction is said to be reverse biased. This is an ideal case. In practice there is usually a small current flowing, arising from the thermal dissociation of the covalent bonds of germanium or silicon atoms. This leakage current is very small at room temperatures and is practically independent of the voltage.

However, if the polarity of the real external battery is reversed, it will act to neutralize the potential barrier which appears across the junction. Electrons are now attracted into the *p*-region, and holes into the *n*-region. The junction is said to be forward biased. Electrons and holes meet and neutralize each other at the junction. Each time this happens, a covalent bond breaks near the positive terminal, an electron joins the terminal and a hole proceeds to the junction. Simultaneously, an electron leaves the negative terminal and also proceeds to the junction. The resulting effect is that of a substantial electron stream flowing through the junction.

It is apparent that the junction acts as a rectifying or one-way device (a diode). The graph of current flow against applied voltage for a *p–n* junction is illustrated in *Figure 6.3a* for the ideal case and in *Figure 6.3b* for a practical diode.

For a practical diode, a small forward voltage must be applied in order that the flow of current may start. The forward voltage drop is about 0·5 V for germanium and 0·8 V for silicon. The power dissipated by the diode is equal to the product of the forward voltage drop multiplied by the forward current. The small size of

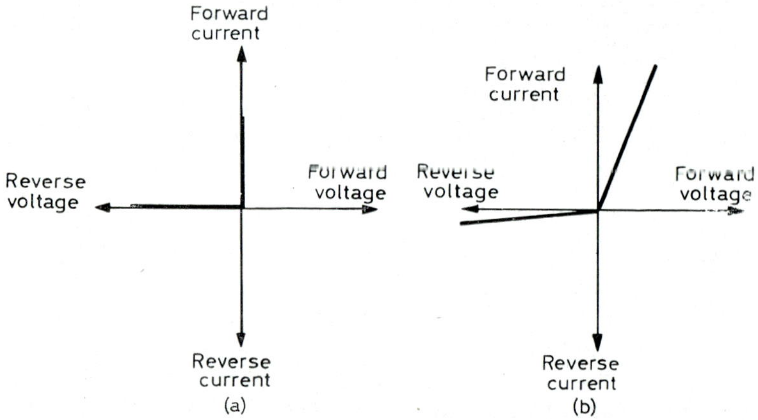

Figure 6.3. Characteristics of ideal and practical junction diodes

semiconductor diodes limits the amount of heat that can be safely dissipated. For the larger diodes this can be increased by mounting the diode in a heat sink. The forward impedance of a junction diode is only a few tens of ohms, whilst the reverse impedance is of the order of megohms. Junction diodes are efficient, and hence can pass large currents in spite of their small size. They are frequently used as power and signal rectifiers. The maximum reverse voltage specified for a diode must not be exceeded even by transients, since this will damage the device.

THE POINT-CONTACT DIODE

A point-contact diode consists of a piece of *p*-type or *n*-type semiconductor and a fine wire making a springy contact with it (*Figure 6.4*). A very small zone around the point is converted to the opposite type of material, producing a miniature *p–n* junction. The point-contact diode has similar rectifying properties to the junction diode, but its self-capacitance is much smaller because of the relatively small junction area and its current-carrying capacity is less. A

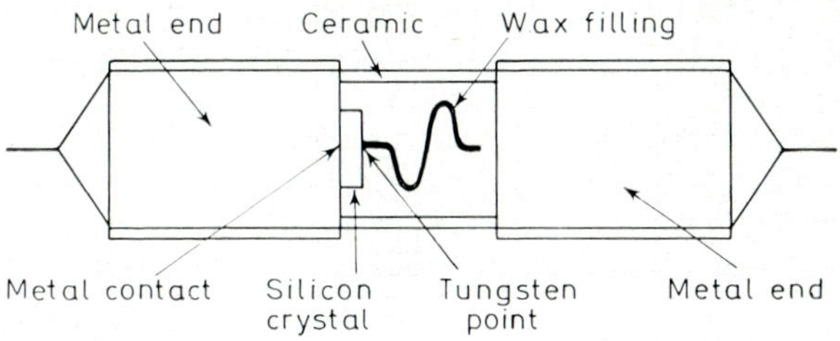

Figure 6.4. Construction of a point-contact diode

typical application arises as a demodulation diode in a radio frequency circuit.

LEAKAGE CURRENT

The charge carriers produced by the addition of controlled amounts of impurity in *p*-type and *n*-type semiconductors are known as majority carriers. Charge carriers can also be liberated by thermal effects and these are known as minority carriers. Thus for example, although the majority carriers are electrons in *n*-type material, there will also be a small number of holes and electrons present as minority carriers. These minority carriers give rise to the leakage current which is associated with all semiconductor devices and which increases with increasing ambient temperature.

THE VOLTAGE BREAKDOWN OF SEMICONDUCTOR DIODES

Under normal circumstances, the reverse current of a semiconductor diode is small. However, if the reverse voltage applied to the diode is made sufficiently large, a critical voltage is reached at which the diode breaks down. When this occurs a large reverse current starts to flow. The effect is normally due to the electric field strength rising to such a magnitude that the charge carriers are accelerated and attain sufficient energy to be able to ionize the fixed atoms in the crystal lattice by collision, generating further hole–electron pairs. This process is known as the Avalanche Effect. It is utilized in the Silicon Avalanche Rectifier (Duddridge, 1964), which is able to absorb reverse voltage transients of such a magnitude that they would damage a conventional rectifier. Because of this facility, a voltage surge suppression network may not be required.

Junction diodes which have a relatively high concentration of impurity added may break down at a lower reverse voltage than would be required to give rise to an avalanche effect. This other breakdown mechanism is internal field emission and is called the Zener Effect. It depends on the fact that an electron can pass through a high-potential barrier if the barrier is sufficiently thin. This action contrasts with the view of classical mechanics, where the only way in which an electron could cross the barrier is by gaining sufficient energy to surmount it. The effect is also known as the Tunnel Effect and will be mentioned again in describing the Tunnel Diode.

Whichever of the mechanisms operates, the breakdown voltage is fairly constant. If it is arranged that the current shall be limited by an external series resistance to a value which will not overload the junction, then the original high-resistance reverse biased condition will be resumed when the applied voltage is reduced below

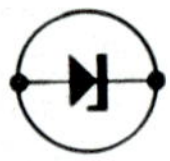

Figure 6.5. Circuit symbol for a Zener diode

the breakdown level. Once the diode has broken down, the voltage drop developed across it will remain almost constant over a wide range of currents. For this reason, a diode operated under these conditions finds many applications as a voltage reference element. Silicon diodes made specially for this purpose are known as Zener diodes (Rigg, 1962; Miles and Tumber, 1964) whether or not the breakdown is specifically due to the Zener effect. *Figure 6.5* shows the circuit symbol for a Zener diode. Apart from their use as voltage reference elements in stabilized power supply circuits, Zener diodes are widely used as voltage-limiting devices in protective circuits. Typical applications include the protection of the input and output of integrated circuit operational amplifiers, and the protection of the input circuitry of electrocardiograph amplifiers against accidental damage when a d.c. defibrillator is used on the patient.

VARACTOR DIODES

On either side of a *p–n* junction there is a transition region. In the *p*-type material this consists of ionized acceptor atoms and in the *n*-type region it consists of ionized donor atoms. These two facing regions of opposite charges constitute a dipole layer. If the potential difference across this region is altered by the application of an external potential difference, the width of the transition region and hence the charge on the dipole will be altered. Since the charge depends on the voltage, the dipole layer acts as a voltage-dependent capacitance across the junction (Straub, 1958). For a 1 mm^2 junction area, a typical capacitance would be of the order of 10^3 pF. The change in capacity with variation of the reverse voltage applied to a diode can be used to swing the carrier frequency of a frequency modulation circuit. Gregory and Lewin (1962) used this technique in a radio frequency arrangement for the measurement of small currents in a mass spectrometer and flame ionization gas chromatograph. The use of overall current feedback resulted in a stable gain and day-to-day drifts of less than 10^{-11} A. A similar technique has also been used in the input circuits of multi-channel electroencephalographs, but

Figure 6.6. Circuit symbol for a variable capacitance diode

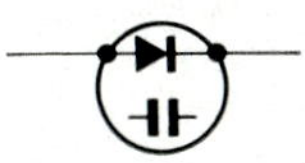

current (1972) practice is to use field effect transistors. *Figure 6.6* shows the circuit symbol for a variable capacitance diode, known as a varicap.

THE TUNNEL DIODE

The operation of amplifying devices such as transistors depends upon the emission of charge carriers into a region where their motion can be influenced by a control electrode. The charge carriers are subsequently collected at the output electrode of the device. The response time of the device depends on the time it takes for the charge carriers to move from the emitter to the collector. The basic mode of conduction in tunnel diodes has a theoretical frequency limit of 10^7 MHz. This is several orders of magnitude

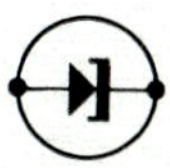

Figure 6.7. Circuit symbol for a tunnel diode

higher than the drift and diffusion processes occurring in conventional semiconductor diodes and transistors (Lowry *et al.*, 1961; Adler and Selikson, 1962; Rigg, 1962; Chang, 1964; Chow, 1964). *Figure 6.7* shows the circuit symbol for a tunnel diode and *Figure 6.8* illustrates the forward and reverse voltage–current characteristics of a tunnel diode and a conventional diode. Between the points marked 1 and 2, the current through the tunnel diode decreases whilst the voltage across it is increased. For a conventional resistor obeying Ohm's

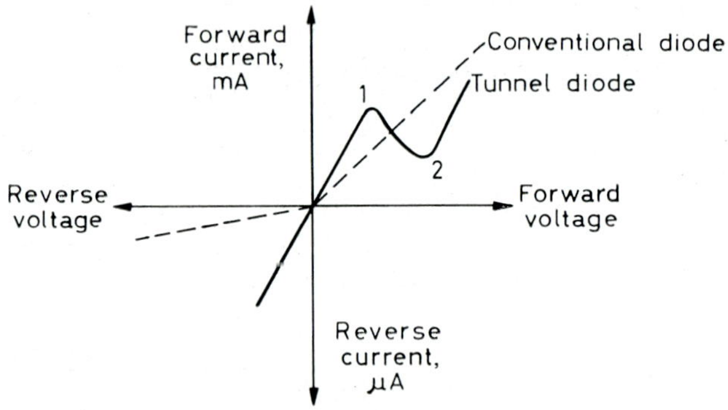

Figure 6.8. Forward and reverse voltage–current characteristics of a tunnel diode and a conventional diode

law, the current through it will increase in proportion to the voltage applied across it, and this applies to an ordinary diode. Between points 1 and 2, the tunnel diode is said to possess the property of a negative resistance.

The tunnel diode takes its name from the Tunnel Effect. This is a mechanism whereby a particle, which obeys the quantum theory, can disappear from one side of a potential barrier and appear instantaneously on the other side although it does not have sufficient energy to surmount the barrier. The barrier in the case of a tunnel diode is the transition or space charge depletion region of a *p–n* junction. This is the barrier which prevents current flowing in a reverse biased conventional semiconductor diode. The barrier of a tunnel diode is made extremely narrow—less than one millionth of an inch. Thus tunnelling becomes possible. This action produces an additional component of current at very small forward bias voltages. The additional current diminishes as the value of the forward bias is increased.

This negative resistance property enables the tunnel diode to maintain a tuned circuit in operation at frequencies as high as 2,000 MHz. Crystal-controlled tunnel diode radio transmitters have been made to operate in the United Kingdom medical telemetry band at 102 MHz. In one form, due to L. Kavannah at the Royal College of Surgeons, an integrated circuit amplifier was used to apply the ECG waveform to the tunnel diode oscillator. The complete transmitter was powered by two mercury cells and was small enough to be implanted in a rabbit. Tunnel diodes have also been employed in high speed switching circuits for digital computers.

THE SILICON-CONTROLLED RECTIFIER

The silicon-controlled rectifier, or Thyristor, consists of four alternate layers of *n*-type and *p*-type silicon (*n–p–n–p*) brazed between substantial plates of molybdenum or tungsten. These plates have the same coefficient of expansion as silicon. The device functions as a very efficient rectifier, and as a switch which can operate in microseconds and only requires a triggering power of a few microwatts, but can control powers of up to 400 W. When handling a.c. loads, an SCR can act both to control and to rectify (Butler, 1963).

An SCR can be turned ON in about 1–4 μs and OFF in 10–20 μs. It acts as a 'latching' switch, since it can be turned ON by the momentary application of control current to the gate electrode (the gate signal can be as short as a fraction of a microsecond). This contrasts with thermionic valves and transistors, where a continuous ON signal must be applied to the device. The circuit symbol for a silicon-controlled rectifier is illustrated in *Figure 6.9.*

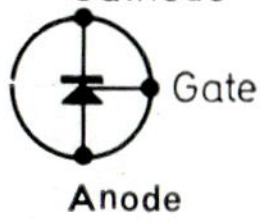

Figure 6.9. Circuit symbol for a silicon-controlled rectifier

The mode of operation of the device can be explained by considering it as consisting of a *p–n–p* and an *n–p–n* transistor with a common collector junction as shown in *Figure 6.10.* The *p–n–p* portion has an α_1 which defines the fraction of the hole current injected at the *p*-type emitter which reaches the *p*-type collector. The *n–p–n* portion has an α_2 which defines the fraction of the electron current injected at the *n*-type emitter which reaches the *n*-type collector. The total current flowing across junction J is $I\alpha_1+I\alpha_2+I_{CO}$ where I_{CO} is the leakage current, $I\alpha_1$ is the hole current from the *p*-end region and $I\alpha_2$ is the electron current from the *n*-end region.

However, since the total current at junction J must be equal to the external current I, then $I = I\alpha_1 + I\alpha_2 + I_{CO}$, thus $I = I_{CO}/(1-\alpha_1-\alpha_2) = I_{CO}/(1-(\alpha_1+\alpha_2))$. If $(\alpha_1+\alpha_2)$ is equal to 0·9, then the current flowing through the device will be equal to ten times the leakage current. Since the leakage current in a silicon *p–n* junction is only of the order of milli-microamps, the total current through the SCR will be small. This is the OFF state of the SCR. If $(\alpha_1+\alpha_2)$ is nearly unity, then I becomes large and is limited only by the external circuit resistance R. This is the ON state of the SCR. In this state the two centre regions of the SCR are saturated with carriers, making all the three junctions biased in the forward direction.

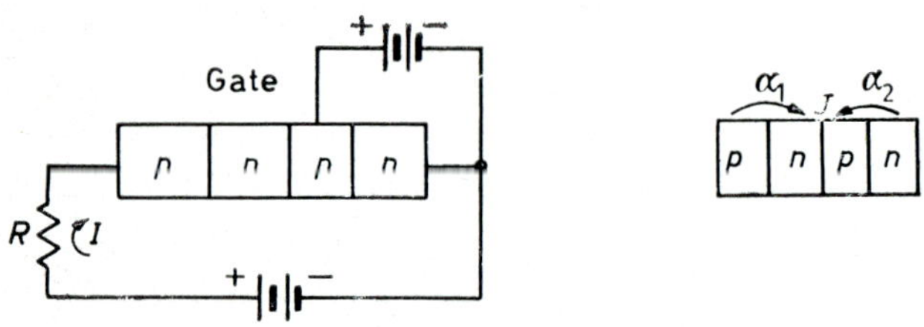

Figure 6.10. Schematic diagram of a silicon-controlled rectifier

The SCR can be turned ON by injecting current at one of the bases. The turn-on occurs because for most silicon transistors, α is quite low at low emitter currents but increases fairly rapidly with increasing emitter current. The SCR can also be made to conduct by placing a fairly high forward voltage across it. Breakdown then occurs by avalanche action. The SCR is usually operated well below this forward 'break-over' voltage and is triggered ON by injecting current into the GATE lead. Conduction will continue unless the value of the forward current is reduced below a minimum 'holding current' value, when conduction will cease. Once the gate has triggered the SCR ON, it no longer has any control over the current. The only method for turning the SCR OFF is to reduce the main current to below the holding current level.

In practice, an SCR may be used to feed current from a full wave unsmoothed supply to a load such as the heater of an oven or water bath or the armature of a motor. The SCR is arranged to conduct for a predetermined fraction of each half cycle. The SCR is automatically extinguished towards the end of each half cycle as the voltage falls and the current drops below the holding level. Adjustment of the fraction of each cycle for which the SCR is firing provides a smooth control of the power delivered to the apparatus connected in series with the SCR. The action of the trigger pulses in initiating the firing of the SCR at a certain portion of the mains cycle is shown in *Figure 6.11*. By incorporating a variable phase circuit, the portion

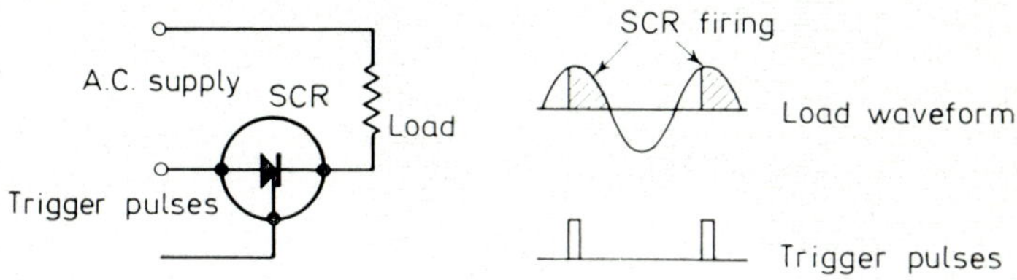

Figure 6.11. The action of the trigger pulses in firing an SCR

of the cycle during which the SCR fires can be adjusted. *Figure 6.12* shows an R–C network in the secondary of a mains transformer for providing a variable phase shift. The saturable transformer is employed to square off the a.c. waveform in order to provide triggering pulses every cycle for the SCR.

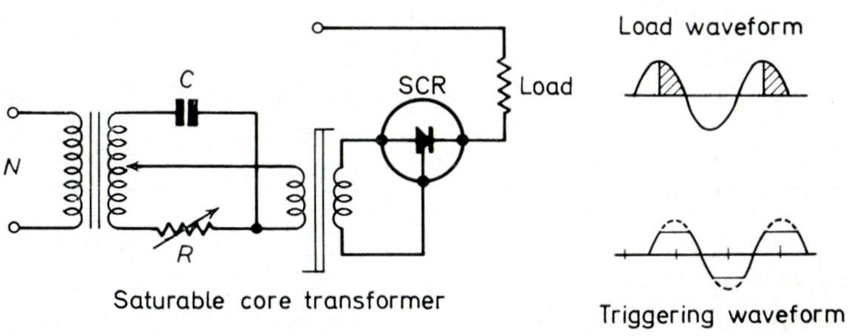

Figure 6.12. The use of a phase-shifting network to control the firing of an SCR

SCRs are being increasingly used for this type of load control in medical equipment. An example occurs in the proportional temperature controller developed for use with an incubator for neonates. A thermistor temperature probe is attached to the baby's abdomen and the temperature at which the baby is to be maintained is set on the controller. As the temperature of the baby approaches the preset value the firing time of the SCR is progressively reduced, so giving a proportional temperature control.

Bidirectional SCRs or triacs are available consisting of two

SCRs connected back-to-back and having a common trigger (*Figure 6.13*) for full wave rectifier applications.

Figure 6.13. Circuit symbol for a bidirectional SCR (triacl)

p–n–p JUNCTION TRANSISTORS

The Common Base Circuit

A *p–n–p* type transistor in germanium or silicon consists of a layer of *n*-type material, a few thousandths of an inch thick, sandwiched between two regions of *p*-type material. The two outer regions are known as the emitter and the collector, the middle region being the base. The polarity of the voltage applied to the various electrodes is important. If it is incorrect, damage to the transistor may result. *Figure 6.14a* depicts the circuit symbol for a *p–n–p* transistor. The fact that it is a *p–n–p* transistor is indicated by the arrow pointing from the emitter towards the base. It is also possible to have an *n–p–n* transistor, and in the circuit symbol the arrow is drawn pointing away from the base towards the emitter to indicate that it is an *n–p–n* device (*Figure 6.14b*).

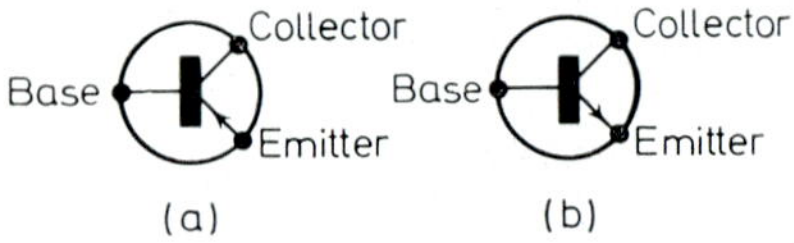

Figure 6.14. Circuit symbol for (a) a p–n–p transistor and (b) an n–p–n transistor

Figure 6.15 shows a *p–n–p* transistor connected in a common base configuration. This is so called because the base electrode is common to both the input and the output circuits. The emitter is biased positive with respect to the base and hence the emitter–base junction functions as a junction diode connected in the forward direction. Positive holes from the *p*-type emitter are attracted into the base region by the forward bias. The current through the diode can be measured with the 0–5 mA meter, and the 1·5 k Ω resistor serves to limit the current to a safe value. A small proportion of the holes will be neutralized by collision with electrons in the *n*-type base. Since the base is narrow, many holes will diffuse across the base–collector junction. The base–collector diode is reverse biased, and the holes are attracted across the junction to the collector. There they can be neutralized by recombination with electrons flowing into the collector from the battery.

Electrons which are removed by recombination in the base region are replaced by an electron current drawn from the bias battery. By making the base region as narrow as possible, and ensuring that it contains only a small number of free electrons compared with the number of holes in both the emitter and collector regions, it is arranged that the collector current becomes very nearly as large as the emitter current. Typically, each 1 mA change of current in the base–emitter circuit will produce a 0·98 mA current change in the base-collector circuit. The current that flows

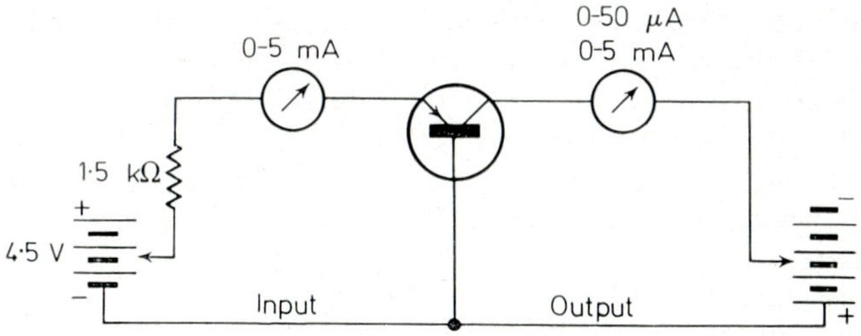

Figure 6.15. A transistor in the common base configuration

in the base lead is small and is equal to the difference between the emitter and collector currents. The impedance of the forward biased base–emitter diode is about 50 Ω, whilst that of the reverse biased base–collector diode can be as high as 1 M Ω. The ratio of the corresponding current change in the collector circuit to the change in the emitter circuit is known as 'alpha' (α), the current gain. In the common base circuit, α is less than unity (0·98) but since the output impedance is much higher than the input impedance, large power and voltage gains are possible.

In *Figure 6.15*, the meter in the collector circuit is provided with a low and a high sensitivity range. The high sensitivity range is used to measure the leakage current which flows in the reverse biased base–collector circuit when the base–emitter circuit is open.

Let the emitter current be I_E, the base current I_B and the collector current I_C. Then $I_B=(I_E-I_C)$. For small signals, the current gain α can be taken as $\alpha=I_C/I_E$. Substituting $I_C=\alpha I_E$ gives $I_B=(1-\alpha)I_E$. In addition to the portion of the emitter current which passes through the base to the collector, there is also a component of the collector current which arises from leakage. This leakage current

I_{CO} adds to the collector current, but is in the opposite direction to the base current. I_{CO} corresponds to the collector current when the emitter circuit is open. When the emitter circuit is closed, the collector current increases due to the addition of the useful current I_E from the emitter circuit. Taking into account the leakage current gives $I_B=(1-\alpha)I_E-I_{CO}$ and $I_C=\alpha I_E+I_{CO}$.

For a small germanium transistor, the leakage current is small, of the order of 5 μA at 25° C. It increases in an approximately linear fashion, reaching about 50 μA at 55° C. However, it is still small compared with the useful collector current I_E, which might be 1 mA. Changes in the leakage current will not affect the collector current significantly, so that the common base amplifier configuration possesses good thermal stability. Because of the higher energy gap involved, silicon transistors will exhibit a lower leakage current for comparable transistor types. At 25° C, for a silicon transistor, the leakage current might be one thousandth of a micro-ampere, and this makes it feasible to operate silicon transistors with collector currents of only a few micro-amperes when it is necessary to minimize transistor noise.

The Common Emitter Circuit

In this configuration, the emitter is common to both the emitter–base (input) circuit and the emitter–collector (output) circuit (*Figure 6.16*). The positive hole current flowing from emitter to collector forms the output current. The input current consists of

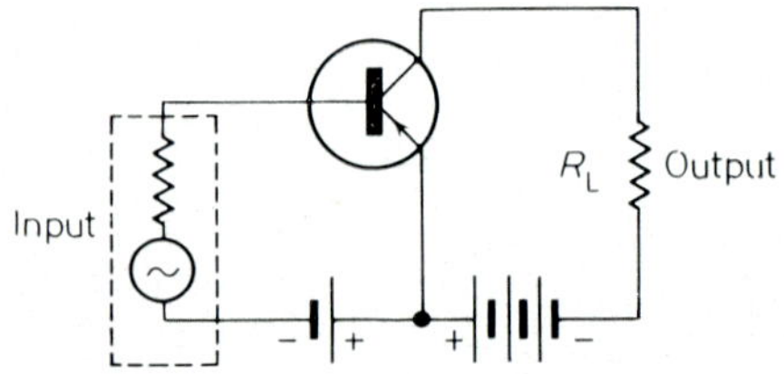

Figure 6.16. The common emitter configuration

electrons flowing into the base to replace the base electrons which have been lost as a result of recombination with the positive hole current. Maximum emitter-to-collector current can flow when the base can be supplied with all the electrons it needs. If the input current to the base is reduced, the base becomes positively charged as it loses, without complete replacement, electrons by recombination. Thus the relatively large collector current is controlled by the relatively small base current. The transistor essentially functions as a current amplifier. The current amplification factor is defined as the ratio of the change in output current to the corresponding change in input current. For the common emitter circuit this is denoted by β or h_{fe}. Strictly this value β holds for d.c. changes, but it is usually taken as being the same as h_{fe} for low frequency signals. The collector-to-emitter voltage V_{CE} is assumed to remain constant. h_{fe} is one of a set of so-called *h* parameters which can be used to characterize the behaviour of a transistor. A typical value for h_{fe} would be of the order of 50 to 60. The characteristics of common emitter circuits are high current gains (20–100), a low input impedance (400–2,000 Ω), and a leakage current I'_{CO} which can be high in the case of germanium transistors.

If the emitter–base circuit is opened, then only the leakage current flows in the collector–base diode. This is small since the collector–base diode is reversed. Since there is no external base current, the base–emitter circuit being open, the leakage current in the collector–base diode is matched by an equal and opposite current flowing to the base from the emitter. This emitter–base current acts as an effective input current and becomes magnified by transistor action, appearing as a current approximately h_{fe} times greater at the collector. For a useful collector current of 1 mA,

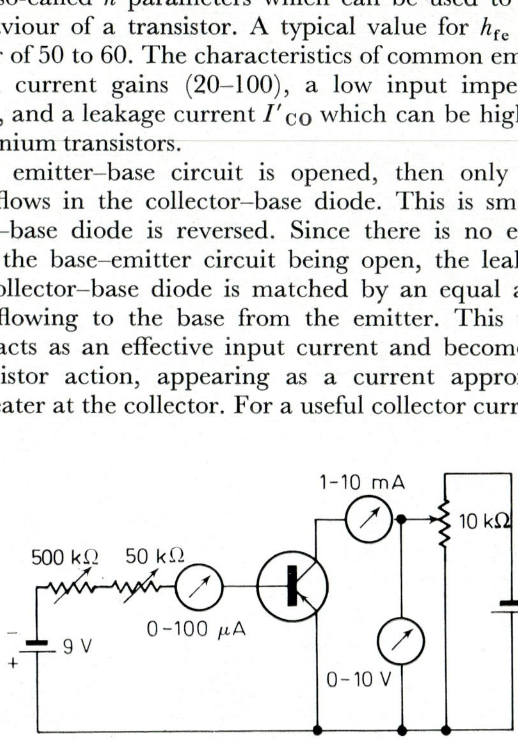

Figure 6.17. Measurement circuit for the common emitter configuration

the leakage current of a germanium common base amplifier might be 50 μA at 55° C, whereas for a common emitter amplifier at 55° C it might be 2·5 mA. For a silicon transistor in a common emitter configuration it might be of the order of $\frac{1}{20}$th of a micro-ampere. With germanium transistors, it is important to provide circuit protection against the possible production of large leakage currents. These could seriously limit the amplification available, and possibly damage the transistor if 'thermal runaway' occurred.

For a common emitter configuration, the relationship obtaining between base current, collector current and collector voltage can be found from the circuit of *Figure 6.17*. A typical family of curves for a small audio frequency transistor is shown in *Figure 6.18*.

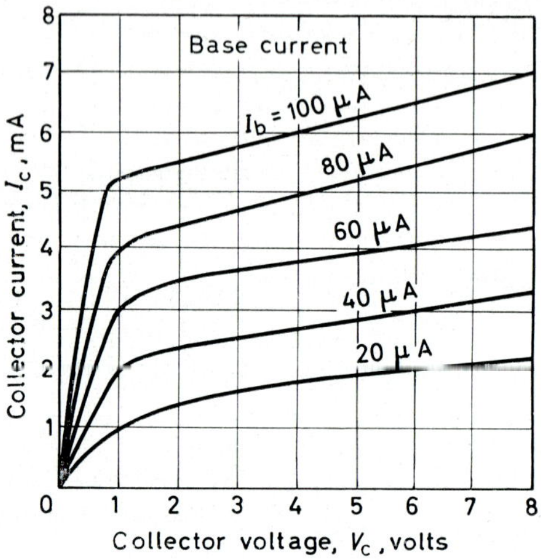

Figure 6.18. The relationship between collector current and voltage for various base currents in the common emitter configuration

The forward current gain in the common emitter connection h_{fe} can be determined from the curves by considering small increments. The current gain h_{fe} is given by

$$\frac{\text{the change in collector current}}{\text{the corresponding increment in base current}}$$

and it can be shown that h_{fe} falls slightly with increasing collector current. It is also dependent on the voltage across the transistor V_{CE} at the junction temperature. The collector incremental output resistance can also be found from the curves since this is given by

$$\frac{\text{the increment in collector voltage}}{\text{the corresponding change in collector current}}$$

It is evident that the curves each possess a well-defined 'knee' followed by a region in which the slope is relatively small, corresponding to a high value of the incremental output resistance. A similar situation arises in the case of a pentode thermionic valve when anode current is plotted against anode voltage for various values of grid–cathode voltage.

The Common Collector Circuit

Figure 6.19 gives the basic circuit of a common collector amplifier. It can be seen that the collector is common to both the input and the output circuit. The input is applied between the base and the collector and the output taken from between the collector and the emitter. The output voltage is in phase with the input voltage and the circuit is usually known as an 'emitter follower' since signal changes at the emitter follow those at the base. The voltage gain of the emitter follower is less than unity, but current and power gains are possible. Compared with the common emitter and common

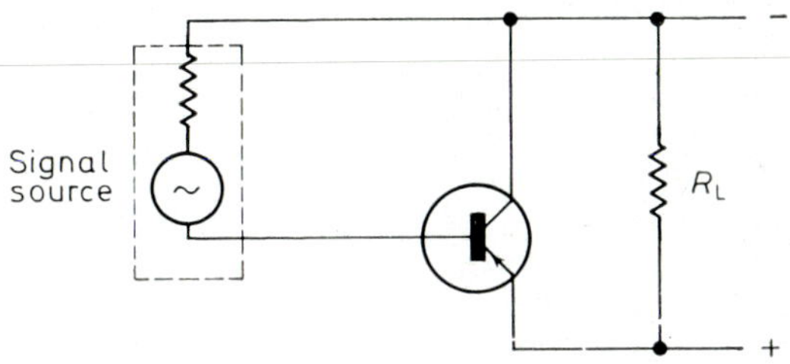

Figure 6.19. The common collector configuration

base circuits, the input impedance is high and the output impedance is low, but these values depend markedly upon the magnitude of the input (source) impedance and the load impedance. A more detailed analysis of the emitter follower stage will be given later. A common collector amplifier might have an output impedance of the order of 50 Ω and an input impedance as high as 2 MΩ. For this reason it is often employed as a 'buffer' stage in an amplifier to isolate a stage in the amplifier from the one preceding it and thus minimize interaction between them.

A COMPARISON BETWEEN VALVE AND TRANSISTOR CIRCUITS

Thermionic valves are rapidly disappearing from scientific apparatus, but they are still encountered where high voltages have to be handled, for example, in stabilized high voltage power supplies and in the deflection circuits of large screen cathode ray tube systems. Although the transistor is best considered in its own right as a semiconductor device, it is possible to compare transistor and valve configurations, as in *Figure 6.20.* It is evident that the collector, base and emitter of a transistor can be considered as analogues of the anode, grid and cathode of a thermionic triode. The characteristics of a pentode

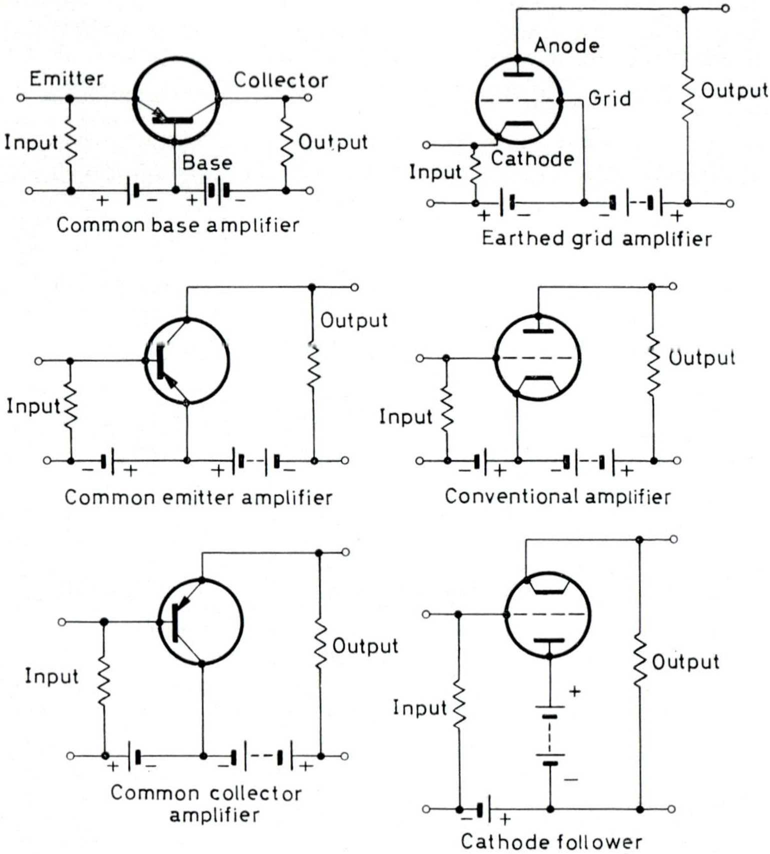

Figure 6.20. A comparison between valve and transistor circuits

valve have much in common with those of a field effect transistor and this has revived an interest in the circuit techniques developed for use with pentodes.

BIAS AND STABILIZATION

The collector current of a bipolar junction transistor consists of two components, one of which is under the control of the base current, the other being independent of it. The first component enables the transistor to function basically as a current amplifier, but the second component is useless in this respect and is known as the leakage current. The magnitude of the leakage current is markedly temperature dependent. If the leakage current becomes excessive, it gives rise to a significant self-heating of the transistor. This in turn generates a further increase in leakage current. This may result in a 'thermal runaway' and the destruction of the transistor. When stability of the transistor characteristics is important, it may be necessary to thermostat the transistor (Belsey and Gabriel, 1963).

It is necessary to supply a steady bias current to the base of a transistor when it has to operate as a linear amplifier. The changing signal current can then be superimposed on this steady forward bias current and the transistor is arranged to operate with a relatively linear relationship between base and collector currents. Without this bias, the transistor would be cut off and inoperative for part of the input signal cycle.

Figure 6.21 shows a common emitter amplifier stage. The base of the transistor is connected to the junction of two resistors R_1 and R_2 which form a potential divider circuit across the supply voltage. If the base current is considerably smaller than the current flowing

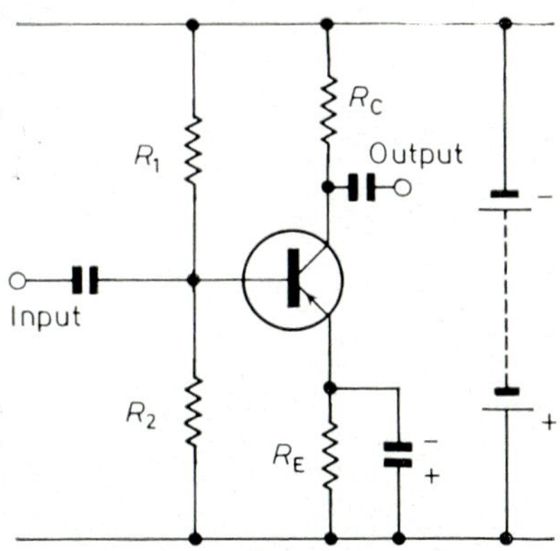

Figure 6.21. A common emitter amplifier stage

through the divider circuit, then the voltage applied to the base can be taken as sensibly constant. Suppose that the ambient temperature rises, causing an increase in the leakage current; this will produce an increase in the total collector current. As a result there will be an increased voltage drop across R_E, the external resistance in series with the emitter, and the emitter and base voltages will tend to approach each other. The collector current is thus diminished and, when an equilibrium is attained, the collector current will be greater than it was initially but less than it would have been in an unstabilized circuit. Typically, such an arrangement might reduce variations in collector current to about one-fifteenth of their value in an unstabilized circuit.

Stability Factor

Referring to *Figure 6.22*, a fixed bias current is fed to the transistor via R_B. Then $I_C = \alpha I_E + I_{CO}$, so that $I_E = I_C/\alpha - I_{CO}/\alpha$ and $I_E = I_C + I_B$, $I_B = I_E - I_C$.

$$I_B = I_C/\alpha - I_{CO}/\alpha - I_C = I_C(1-\alpha)/\alpha - I_{CO}.$$

Now
$$V_I = I_E R_E + V_{BE} + I_B R_B,$$

giving
$$V_I = \frac{I_C R_E}{\alpha} - \frac{I_{CO} R_E}{\alpha} + V_{BE} + \frac{I_C(1-\alpha)R_B}{\alpha} - \frac{I_{CO} R_B}{\alpha},$$

and
$$I_C = \frac{(V_I - V_{BE})}{R_E + (1-\alpha)R_B} + \frac{I_{CO}(R_E + R_B)}{R_E + (1-\alpha)R_B}$$

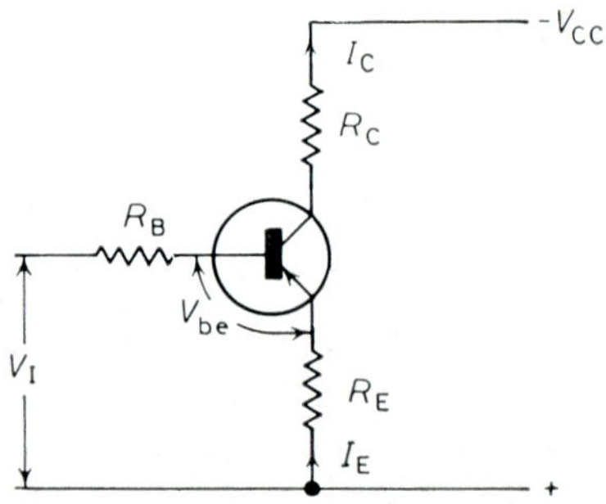

Figure 6.22. The application of a steady bias current to a transistor

This relationship shows how the collector current I_C depends on the values of the input voltage, the base-to-emitter voltage and the leakage current. The factor

$$\frac{(R_E + R_B)}{R_E + (1-\alpha)R_B}$$

equals the rate of change of collector current with leakage current and is known as the stability factor of the circuit. If $\alpha=0{\cdot}98$ and $R_B/R_E=10$, rearranging the stability factor gives

$$\frac{1+R_B/R_E}{1+(1-\alpha)R_B/R_E}=9{\cdot}2.$$

Clearly it is desirable to make the stability factor as small as possible, and it increases with an increase in the ratio R_B/R_E. The total external resistance between the base and collector terminals should be made as small as possible and the total external resistance between the emitter and collector should be made as large as possible in order to minimize the effect of temperature upon the collector current.

A COMMON EMITTER AMPLIFIER STAGE

The circuit of *Figure 6.23* is due to Watson (1966). It uses a Texas Instruments 2S 302 silicon *p–n–p* transistor. This has an h_{fe} at 1 mA of 15. Taking a supply voltage $-V_{CC}$ of -24 V and allowing 9 V for the voltage V_{CE} across the transistor and 9 V across the collector load resistor, R_C, then 6 V must be dropped across the emitter resistor R_E. Using Ohm's law, $R_C=9$ kΩ and $R_E=6$ kΩ. When

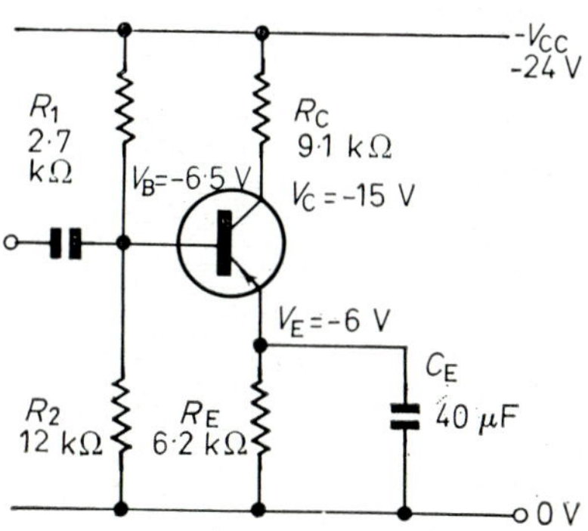

Figure 6.23. Common emitter amplifier circuit

(Reproduced from Watson, 1966, by courtesy of Rank Precision Industries Ltd.)

the transistor is hard ON, the maximum current through it will be $24/(9\text{ k}\Omega+16\text{ k}\Omega)=1{\cdot}6$ mA. For $h_{fe}=15$, the corresponding maximum base current will be $1{\cdot}6/15=0{\cdot}108$ mA. It is desirable that the current flowing through the potential divider R_1R_2 should not be less than about five times the maximum base current, i.e. 0·54 mA. For normal operation of the transistor, the base–emitter voltage V_{BE} is about 0·5 V, so the voltage developed across R_2 must be −6·5 V, and for a current of 0·54 mA this gives R_2=12 kΩ. The voltage to be dropped across R_1 is −(24−6·5)=−17·5 V, and at 0·54 mA this gives R_1=28·7 kΩ. The nearest preferred values employed were R_E=6·2 kΩ, R_C=9·1 kΩ, R_1=27 kΩ and R_2= 12 kΩ. With a particular transistor, Watson found the measured gain of the single stage was a voltage gain of about 200. The emitter resistor R_E is bypassed with a 500 μF capacitor in order effectively to short-out signal variations appearing across R_E which would constitute a series negative feedback. Taking into account the production spread of the transistor parameters, the calculated voltage gain for the stage could vary from 200 to 350. If a second identical stage is added to the first, the gain range is extended and becomes 2,000 to 15,000. The problem is that the large range of gain for the stages depends both on the particular transistor used and on the variation of its parameters with temperature. For this reason, it is usual to sacrifice a considerable amount of the gain available in order to achieve gain stability. The gain available is then largely determined by the stable characteristics of the feedback network rather than by those of the active elements.

THE SIMPLIFIED ANALYSIS OF TRANSISTOR AMPLIFIERS

A number of equivalent circuits have been introduced to represent the operation of a transistor in a circuit. Basically $I_C = \alpha I_E + I_{CO}$, but the situation is complicated by the fact that the collector current depends upon the value of the collector-to-emitter voltage as well

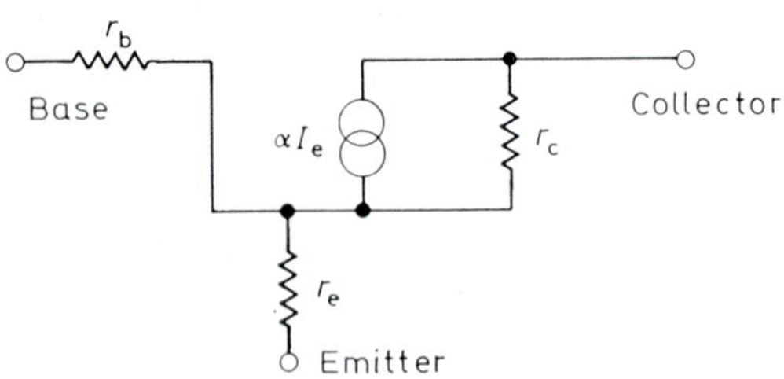

Figure 6.24. T-equivalent circuit of a transistor

as on the magnitude of the base current and the temperature-dependent leakage current. Also the base-to-emitter voltage is not independent of the base current. One method of specifying the performance of a transistor is in terms of a set of hybrid or h parameters; another is by means of a T-equivalent circuit (*Figure 6.24*) where r_e, r_b and r_c are the intrinsic emitter, base and collector resistances of the particular transistor. Typical values for a transistor would be $\alpha=0{\cdot}98$, $r_c=1$ MΩ, $r_e=10\Omega$, and $r_b=750\Omega$. Using this low frequency T-equivalent circuit, Yarker (1962) gives the voltage gain of the single stage amplifier of *Figure 6.21* as

$$\frac{R_C(r_e+R_E-\alpha r_c)}{(r_b+r_e+R_E)R_C+(r_b+r_c)\,(r_e+R_E)+(1-\alpha)r_b r_c}$$

and the output impedance as

$$R_0=r_c+\frac{(R'_S+r_b)\,.\,(R_E+r_e-\alpha r_c)}{(R'_S+r_b+r_e+R_E)}$$

where R'_S is the effective source impedance and the effective output impedance R'_0 is the parallel combination of R_0 and R_C, i.e. $R'_0=R_0R_C/(R_0+R_C)$. From *Figure 6.21*, the effective input impedance R'_S is the parallel combination of the base bias resistors R_1 and R_2, together with the input impedance looking into the base. The input impedance looking into the base alone is given by

$$R_{in}=r_b+\frac{(r_e+R_E)\,(r_c+R_C)}{R_C+r_e+R_E+(1-\alpha)r_c}$$

Referring to the two-stage amplifier of *Figure 6.25*, any load resistance connected to the output will appear in parallel with

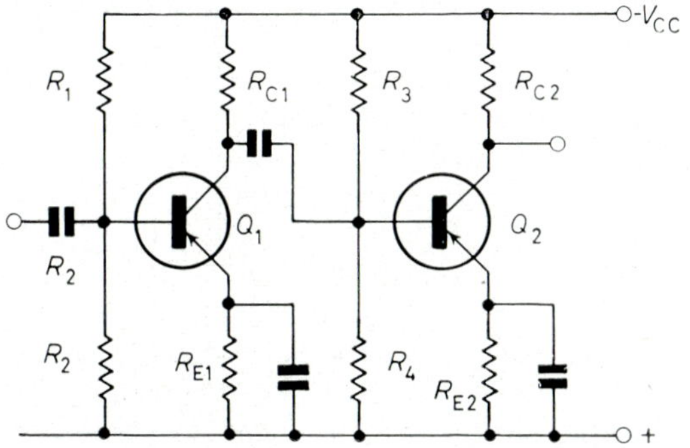

Figure 6.25. Two-stage R–C coupled amplifier

R_{C_2}, giving a resultant load of R'_2. Using the value of R'_2, the input impedance R_{in_2} of the base of Q_2 can be calculated. The bias resistors R_3, R_4 are in parallel with R_{C_1} to give R'_{C_1}. The input impedance at the base of $Q_1=R_{in_1}$ can be found in a similar fashion since the effective load for Q_1 is R'_{C_1} in parallel with R_1 and R_2.

The output impedance of the first stage can be calculated by first calculating the effective source impedance, which consists of R_1 and R_2 in parallel with R_S to give R'_S. Using this value, the output impedance R_{01} of the first stage can be found. This in parallel with R'_{C1} gives the source input impedance for Q_2 and allows the output impedance R_{02} to be calculated. R_{02} in parallel with R'_{C2} gives the amplifier output impedance. The voltage gains A_{v1} and A_{v2} can now be found, and thus the overall gain $A_{v1} \times A_{v2}$.

THE LOAD LINE

A typical set of characteristic curves for a transistor is given in *Figure 6.26.* When the transistor is switched OFF, the voltage between the collector and the emitter is the supply voltage V_{CC} since the device is not drawing current. On the other hand, when the transistor is hard ON, the maximum current which can flow is given by V_{CC}/R_L. These two points can be plotted on the characteristics and joined together by a Load Line. For any value of base current I_B the values of the collector current and collector–emitter voltage will be defined by the line. The instantaneous operating

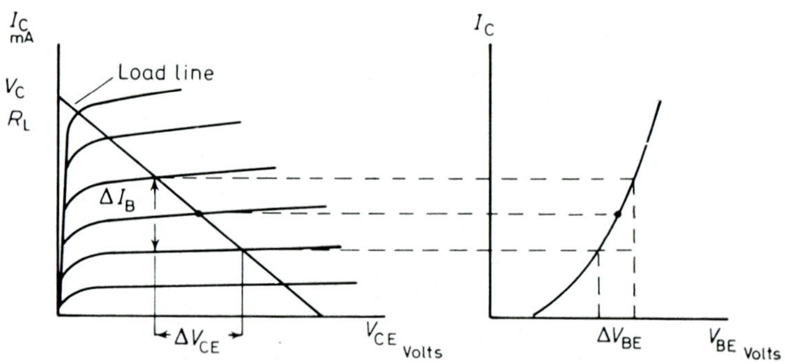

Figure 6.26. The superimposition of a load line on a set of transistor characteristics

point of the transistor will be where the characteristic corresponding to the particular input voltage intersects the load line. In a practical device the curves corresponding to the various values of V_{BE} will not be equally spaced, so that the load voltage swing will not faithfully follow the input voltage swing to the base. As a compromise, a steady value of bias voltage is applied to the base in order to bias it so that the transistor operates where the characteristic curves are most evenly spaced. This defines the working point, and the application of a varying input signal superimposed on the bias sweeps the device around the operating point. A Load Line is shown in *Figure 6.52* for a field effect transistor.

The right-hand curve of *Figure 6.26* relates load current to the control voltage under actual operating conditions and is known as a dynamic mutual characteristic. The voltage gain of the circuit can be found by measuring V_{CE} and V_{BE} from the load line, and then $A_v = \triangle V_{CE}/\triangle V_{BE}$.

CUT-OFF DISTORTION

If the value of the bias plus signal voltage applied to the gate of an FET or the base of a transistor is sufficiently large to cause the output

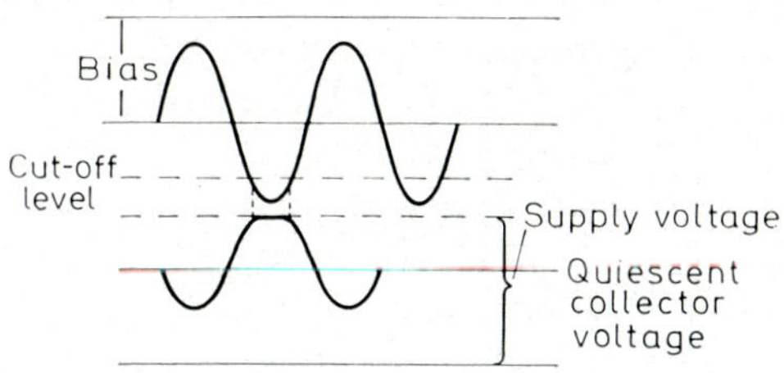

Figure 6.27. Cut-off distortion of a sine wave signal

current to be limited or cut off, then gross distortion of the output waveform results. The effect with a sinewave input is illustrated in *Figure 6.27.*

THE USE OF DECIBELS

The gain of amplifiers, or the loss introduced by an attenuator network or filter or a telephone line, is usually expressed in terms of decibels. Basically, the decibel is used to express power ratios. Consider a network connecting a generator of power to a load. Let the input power supplied to the network be P_1 and the output power delivered to the load be P_2. The ratio of output to input power is P_2/P_1. If the network contains active elements and produces a power gain, then P_2/P_1 is greater than unity. If the network introduces a loss, then P_2/P_1 is less than unity.

For n networks connected in series, the overall power ratio is obtained by multiplying together the various individual power ratios. Thus

$$P_n/P_1 = P_2/P_1 \times P_3/P_2 \times P_4/P_3 \times \ldots P_n/P_{n-1}.$$

Logarithmic Units

In a complicated system containing a large number of amplifiers, filters and attenuators, the continued multiplication makes the overall gain calculation tedious. Hence the individual power ratios can be conveniently expressed in terms of a logarithmic unit, enabling simple additions to be used instead of multiplications. The logarithmic unit is the decibel (db), and a power ratio of 10:1 is defined as one bel (after Alexander Graham Bell). The bel is too large for most purposes and so is subdivided into decibels, and the power loss or gain of a network in db is given by $D=10\ \log_{10}(P_2/P_1)$. If P_2/P_1 is less than unity, then $10\ \log_{10}(P_2/P_1)$ becomes negative. A negative sign indicates a power loss and a positive sign a power gain. Since $10\ \log_{10}(P_2/P_1)=-10\ \log_{10}(P_1/P_2)$, the numerical value will be the same whether P_2/P_1 or P_1/P_2 is used, but in order to obtain the correct sign, P_2/P_1 must be considered. A power gain of 10 will be equivalent to a gain of 10 db, a gain of 100 will equal 20 db, and so on.

Absolute Power Levels Using the Decibel Notation

The decibel is a unit of power ratio and not of absolute power. If some standard level of power is taken as a reference, any other power level can be expressed in terms of decibels relative to this standard level. For audio and telephone work, this power level reference is often one milliwatt (1 mW). Decibels referred to 1 mW are written as dbm. Thus an audio amplifier having a gain of 30 dbm would produce a power output of one watt.

Voltage and Current Ratios

The powers developed in two equal resistors can be compared by considering the voltage drops produced or the two currents. The power ratio in decibels (db) is now equal to 20 times the common logarithm of the voltage or current ratio. Let two equal resistors of $R\Omega$ each, carrying r.m.s. currents I_1 and I_2, have voltage drops of V_1 and V_2 developed across them respectively. The powers developed are $P_1=V_1I_1=I_1^2R=V_1^2/R$ and $P_2=V_2I_2=I_2^2R_2=V_2^2/R$, so that the power ratio is

$$P_2/P_1=(V_2/V_1).(I_2/I_1)=(I_2/I_1)^2=(V_2/V_1)^2.$$

In decibels the power gain is

$$\mathrm{D}=10\ \log_{10}\ (V_2/V_1)^2=20\ \log_{10}\ (V_2/V_1).$$

The power ratio in decibels is strictly equal to $20\times\log_{10}$ (current ratio) or $20\ \log_{10}$ (voltage ratio) provided that the two resistances, across which the voltages or through which the currents are measured, are equal. A voltage gain of 10 is equivalent to a gain of 20 db, whilst a voltage gain of 1,000 is equivalent to a gain of 60 db.

In electronic engineering practice it is conventional to express the voltage gain of an amplifier in db in terms of the ratio of its output to input voltages even if the input and output impedances are not the same. In practice it is unlikely that they will be the same.

Amplifier Bandwidth Expressed in Terms of Decibels

The gain of a well-designed a.c. amplifier is relatively flat over a wide range of frequencies, but falls off at the upper and lower ends of the frequency band. Conventionally, the voltage gain of an amplifier is expressed in db. The bandwidth of the amplifier is usually quoted in terms of the frequency interval between the upper and lower 3 db points. For a constant input voltage, these frequencies represent the points at which the output voltage will have fallen to 0·707 of the maximum value obtaining over the flat mid-band portion of the frequency response curve. A voltage ratio of 0·707 represents a power ratio of one half, so that the 3 db points are also the half power points. As an example, the gain of the Y amplifier of a good general purpose oscilloscope is quoted as being 3 db down at 2 Hz and 15 MHz when used in the a.c. coupled mode. Table 6.1 gives some voltage and power ratios expressed in decibels.

Table 6.1

Decibels	*Voltage ratio*	*Current ratio*
0	1·0	1·0
0·5	1·059	1·122
1·0	1·122	1·259
2·0	1·259	1·585
3·0	1·413	1·995
5·0	1·778	3·162
10	3·162	10·0
20	10·0	100
30	31·6	1,000
40	100	10,000
50	316	100,000
60	1,000	1,000,000

A logarithmic scale allows a wide range of gain to be encompassed within a limited scale length, and this is advantageous when plotting frequency responses. The advantages of a linear plot are also obtained, since if the gain of an amplifier is expressed in db it can be plotted on a linear graph of db against frequency.

Decibels occur frequently in medical electronics. The slope of the frequency response curve of filters is expressed in db per octave; the output voltage attenuator of an audio oscillator is often calibrated in db, as is the gain control of some types of electroencephalograph amplifier. Decibels are also used to compare sound levels and to plot the response of microphones. Taking the threshold of hearing as 0 db, the noise level in an average office is about 40 db and that of heavy traffic 80 db (Fogel, 1963). The intensity of a sound depends on the audio power involved, and since the sensation of hearing produced by the ear follows a law which is approximately logarithmic, equal increments of audio power correspond to equal increments of loudness. For this reason logarithmic law potentiometers are used as volume controls for the audio section of radio receivers.

Amplifiers constructed so as to have a logarithmic response are useful when a wide range of input signal amplitudes has to be handled without overloading. An example occurs with one type of liquid scintillation counting system for use with beta particle emitting radio-isotopes. The small flashes of light produced in the scintillant by the incident beta particles are detected by photomultipliers and the resulting pulses are amplified by pulse amplifiers which have a logarithmic response curve. The output pulses from the amplifiers are fed to pulse height analysers in order to be able to select those originating from a particular isotope for counting. The logarithmic response simplifies the controls, since the range of isotope beta particle energies of interest can be handled without the need for changing the amplifier gains.

THE FREQUENCY RESPONSE OF AN R–C COUPLED STAGE

Referring to *Figure 6.28*, the fall-off in gain observed at the higher

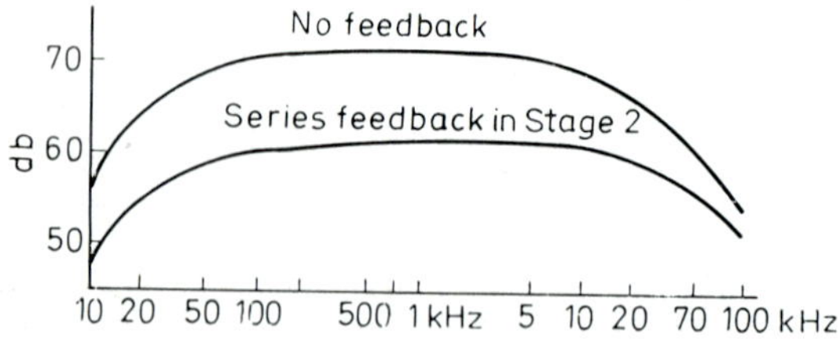

Figure 6.28. The frequency response curves of a two-stage R–C coupled amplifier with and without negative feedback

(Reproduced from Watson, 1966, by courtesy of Rank Precision Industries Ltd.)

frequencies is due to the shunting effect of stray capacitances, and that at the low frequencies is due to the fact that the reactance of the coupling capacitors can no longer be neglected at the lower frequencies. Resistance–capacitance coupling is widely used in multi-stage a.c. transistor amplifiers.

In *Figure 6.29* the output signal swing from the first stage is developed across R_{C_1} and fed via coupling capacitor C_{C_1} to the base of the second transistor. C_{C_1} also serves to block the d.c. collector voltage of Q_1 from reaching the base of Q_2. If it is assumed that the internal impedance of the supply voltage is very small at the signal frequencies considered, i.e. it can be considered as a short

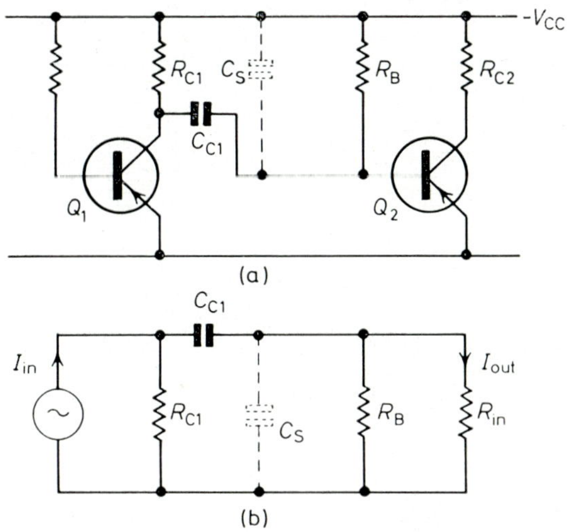

Figure 6.29.(a) The shunting effect of stray capacitance in a two-stage R–C coupled amplifier. (b) Equivalent circuit of a two-stage R–C coupled amplifier

circuit at signal frequencies, then the equivalent circuit of *Figure 6.29a* is given in *Figure 6.29b*. The shunt capacitance C_S is the stray capacitance consisting of the input capacitance of the second stage (this includes Miller effect capacitance) and the capacitance to the supply lines of components and wiring. I_{out} is the output current of the first stage which flows into the input resistance of the second stage. The transistor is basically a current amplifying device, so that if I_{in} is the input current supplied from the signal source to the first stage, and neglecting the effect of C_S at low frequencies, the current transferred between the stages is

$$I_{out}/I_{in} = \frac{R_{B_2}}{R_{B_2}+R_{in}} \times \frac{R_{C_1}}{R_{C_1}+R} \times \frac{X_{C,C_1}\ (R_{C_1}+R)}{1+X_{C,C_1}\ (R_{C_1}+R)}$$

where X_{C,C_1} is the reactance of the coupling capacitor at the frequency concerned and R is the equivalent resistance of R_B and R_{in} in parallel, i.e. $R = R_B R_{in}/(R_B+R_{in})$. The low-frequency cut-off point occurs approximately at the frequency where $f = \frac{1}{2}\pi\, C_{C_1}(R_{C_1}+R)$. At mid-band the effects of C_{C_1} and C_S can be ignored and approximately

$$I_{out}/I_{in} = \frac{R_{C_1}R_B}{R_{C_1}R_B + R_{C_1}R_{in} + R_B R_{in}}.$$

At high frequencies C_{C_1} can be ignored, but C_S must be considered; then

$$I_{out}/I_{in} = \frac{R_B}{R_B+R_{in}} \times \frac{R_{C_1}}{R_{C_1}+R} \times \frac{1}{1+X_{C,C_S} R_{C_1}R/(R_{C_1}+R)}.$$

The high frequency cut-off occurs approximately at

$$f = \frac{1}{2\pi C_S R_{C_1}R/(R_{C_1}+R)}.$$

THE USE OF NEGATIVE FEEDBACK

Suppose that a fraction β of the output voltage of an amplifier is fed back and applied in series opposition to the existing input voltage, that is to say, the phase of the voltage fed back is 180 degrees out of phase with the input signal. Let the voltage gain of the amplifier without the application of negative feedback be A_v; then a 1 V signal change applied to the input would produce an output voltage swing of A_v volts if there was no distortion. By means of a suitable network, a voltage of $-\beta A_v$ is fed back and this subtracts from the original input signal. In order to maintain an effective input signal change of 1 V, the input to the amplifier must be increased to $(1+\beta A_v)$ volts to compensate for the subtraction of βA_v volts. The gain of the amplifier with negative feedback is then

$$\frac{\text{output voltage change}}{\text{input voltage change}} = A_v/(1+\beta A_v) = 1/(\frac{1}{A_v}+\beta) = \frac{\text{forward gain}}{1+\text{loop gain}}.$$

β is the transfer function of the feedback loop and $A_v\beta$ is the loop gain. Normally A_v is high, several hundred, so that $1/A_v$ is small compared with β. β is possibly of the order of 0·1, so that the gain with negative feedback applied approximates to $1/\beta$.

The fraction β depends only on the components of the feedback path. If these are resistive and capacitive they can be made stable. Hence, under these conditions the value of the voltage gain is almost independent of the transistor characteristics and the supply voltages over reasonable ranges. If the feedback path is purely resistive, the fraction of the output voltage fed back will be independent of frequency. The effect of the negative feedback is now to maintain the gain constant over a wider frequency range than is possible with the higher gain obtainable without feedback. The fact that the gain becomes almost constant with negative feedback relies on the gain in the absence of negative feedback being high. In an a.c. amplifier this will not be so at the upper and lower ends of the frequency range due to stray capacitances and the reactance of the coupling capacitors respectively (*Figure 6.29*). Thus the use of negative feedback will not extend the frequency response of an amplifier which is not directly coupled down to d.c.

The effect on the frequency response of applying series negative feedback to the second stage of a two-stage amplifier (*Figure 6.30*)

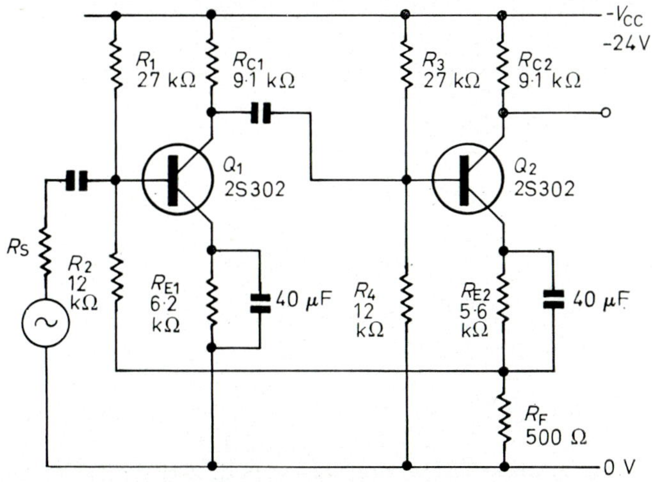

Figure 6.30. Two-stage R–C coupled amplifier with negative feedback
(Reproduced from Watson, 1966, by courtesy of Rank Precision Industries Ltd.)

is shown in *Figure 6.28*. By leaving 500 Ω of the 6·1 kΩ emitter resistor of the second stage un-bypassed, the voltage gain at mid-band was reduced from 3,900 to 1,020.

A simple way of providing voltage-derived series negative feedback is to leave part of the emitter resistance un-bypassed. The voltage swing developed across the un-bypassed resistor will be in phase with the input voltage, so that the effective input voltage swing will be the original input—the signal appearing across the un-bypassed resistor. *Figure 6.30*, also due to Watson (1966), shows the addition of a second stage to the amplifier of *Figure 6.23*. The un-bypassed feedback resistor R_F has reduced the gain from 3,900 to 1,020, but the fact that there is no negative feedback applied to the first stage means that the input impedance of the amplifier will be very dependent on the transistor parameters. The measured value quoted was 1,800 Ω. By further sacrificing gain, it may be stabilized at a lower value by the application of shunt-injected negative feedback. A suitable anti-phase signal is available by connecting R_2 to R_F. This will not significantly affect the bias conditions of Q_1 since $R_2 \gg R_F$. With the feedback loop connected, the gain of the amplifier was reduced from 1,020 to 770. The measured values for the voltage gain of the first stage and the input impedance were 64 and 200 Ω.

The Use of Negative Feedback in Impedance Matching

An important use of negative feedback lies in its ability to alter the input and output impedances of an amplifier. The effect produced depends on the particular feedback connections employed. *Figure 6.31* shows how the feedback signal can be derived from either a

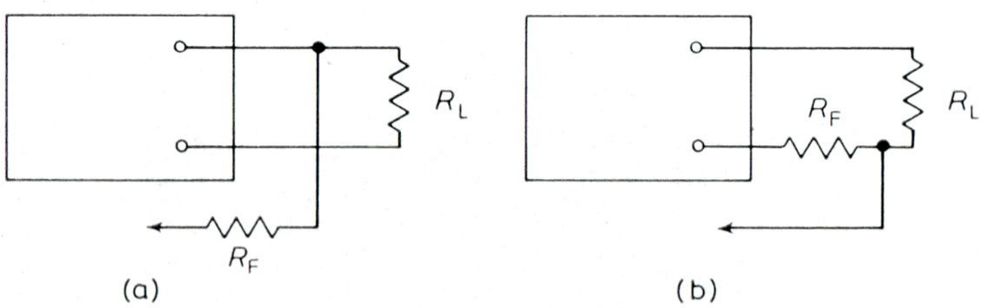

Figure 6.31. (a) Shunt-derived and (b) series-derived negative feedback

parallel or a series connection to the output and then taken to an attenuator network. In the parallel case, the feedback signal is proportional to the output voltage. Any increase in the load resistance tends to increase the output voltage and hence the feedback signal. Thus the gain of the amplifier is diminished and the output voltage tends to be constant. The effect of shunt-derived voltage negative feedback is to reduce the value of the output impedance. When a feedback signal is derived from a resistor in series with the load, the feedback signal is proportional to the output current. An increase in negative feedback acts to reduce the output current and thus effectively to raise the output impedance.

Similarly, the feedback voltage can be either placed in parallel with the input to the amplifier or injected in series with it (*Figure 6.32*). In the parallel injection case, the input signal has to offset

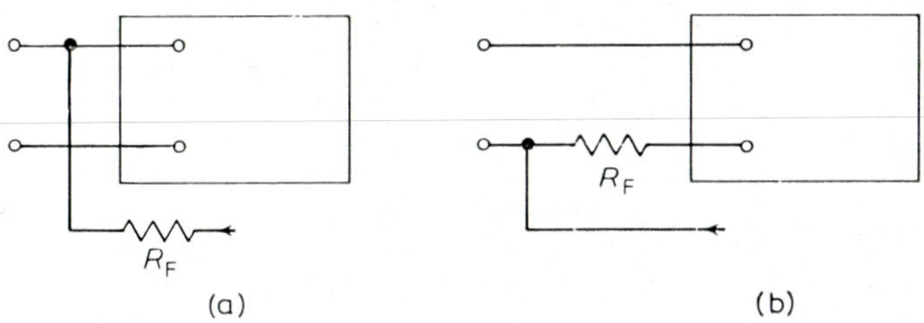

Figure 6.32. (a) Shunt-injected and (b) series-injected negative feedback

the current from the feedback network and also to supply the amplifier's input current. For a given input voltage, a larger input current is now required, so that the effect of the feedback is to reduce the effective input impedance. Finally, when series-injected feedback is employed, the input signal has to offset the feedback voltage and also to supply the amplifier's input voltage. For a given amplifier input current, a greater input voltage is required, so that the negative feedback has effectively raised the input impedance.

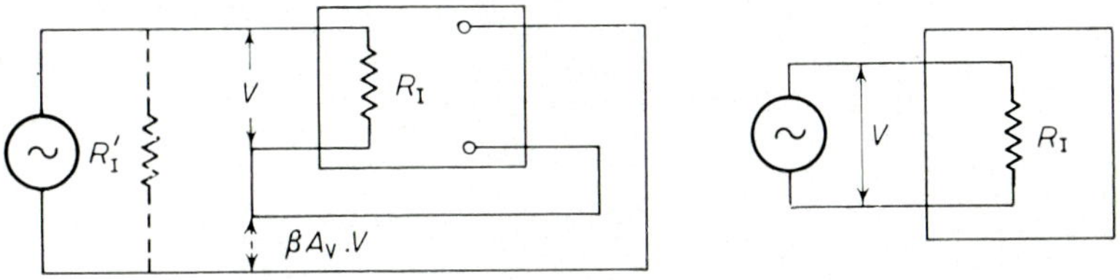

Figure 6.33. Effect of negative feedback on the input impedance of an amplifier

In *Figure 6.33*, let the input impedance of the amplifier be R_I. If an input voltage V is applied across R_I, then a current $I = V/R_I$ will be drawn from the signal source. To maintain the same effective value of the input voltage in the presence of the negative feedback, the source voltage must be raised to $V(1+|\beta A_v|)$. However, the voltage across R_I remains at V and the current drawn as I. Thus the effective value of the input impedance has been raised to $R'_I=V(1+|\beta A_v|)/I$, so that the effective input impedance has now been multiplied by a factor $(1+|\beta A_v|)$. In earlier models of transistor electrocardiographs, the use of negative feedback was employed in order to raise the input impedance. Currently, matched field effect transistors are used in the input stage.

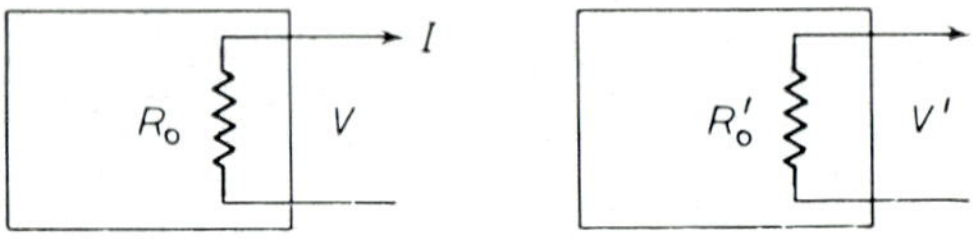

Figure 6.34. Effect of negative feedback on the output impedance of an amplifier

Suppose that the output impedance of the amplifier without negative feedback is R_o (*Figure 6.34*). If the input signal voltage is V, the output voltage without negative feedback will be $V.A_v$. The application of shunt-derived voltage negative feedback will reduce the output voltage to $V'=V(1-|\beta A_v|)A_v$. If the same load current is drawn, the effective value of the output impedance becomes $R'_o=V'/I$, so that the application of the feedback has lowered the output impedance (Table 6.2).

Table 6.2

Type of feedback	*Effect on input impedance*	*Effect on output impedance*
Series-derived		Increase
Shunt-derived		Decrease
Series-injected	Increase	
Shunt-injected	Decrease	

Cascaded Feedback Stages

The design of a multi-stage transistor amplifier is complicated by the fact that the input impedance of each stage is partly dependent on the input impedance of the following stage. If a series feedback stage is followed by a shunt feedback stage (*Figure 6.35*), the output impedance of the first stage will have a much greater value than the input impedance of the second stage. This ensures that the input impedance of the second stage has little effect on that of the first stage. The output impedance of the second stage is low, whilst the input impedance of the third stage is high, so that there is little interaction between the second and third stages. This

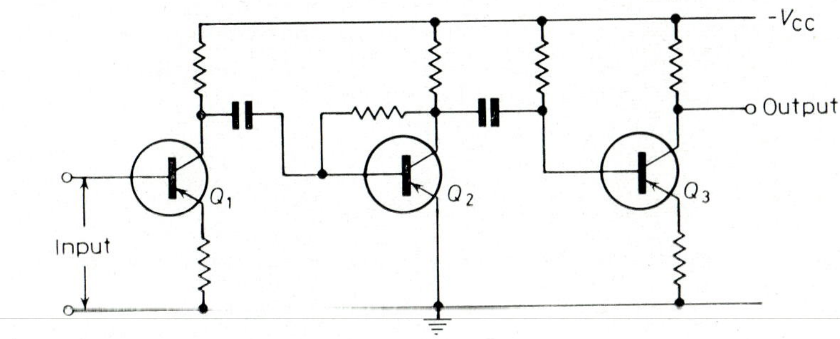

Figure 6.35. The cascading of series and shunt feedback stages in an amplifier

approach allows low frequency amplifier stages to be designed almost independently of one another.

DECOUPLING

Feedback in amplifiers is not always intentional, and the fact that alternative feedback pathways exist can give rise to unwanted oscillation. For example, if the common power supply to several stages of an amplifier does not have a negligible internal impedance,

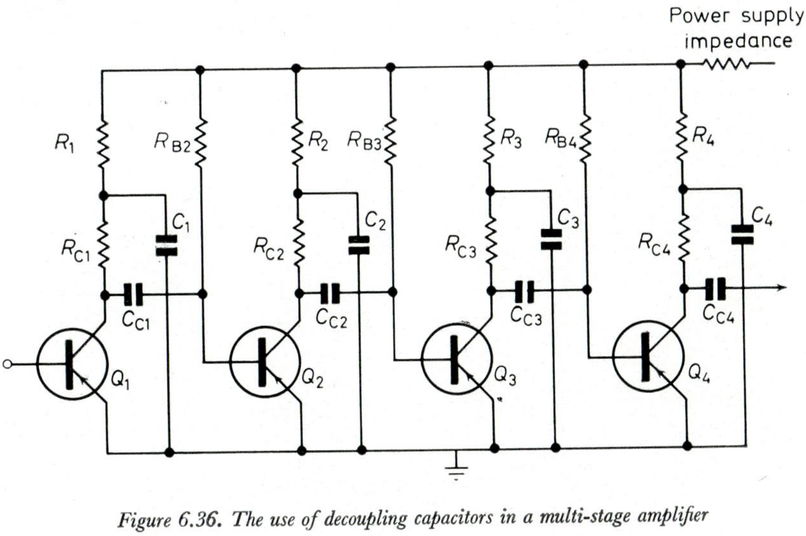

Figure 6.36. The use of decoupling capacitors in a multi-stage amplifier

it is possible for a signal to be developed across this and fed back to an earlier stage in the correct phase to cause a positive feedback. To guard against this happening, it is usual to arrange to 'decouple' each stage as shown in *Figure 6.36*. The components R_1C_1, R_2C_2 and R_3C_3 form low pass filters between the supply line and the inputs to the stages. They also help to reduce the effects of any residual ripple left on the supply line.

THE EMITTER FOLLOWER

A simplified equivalent circuit for a transistor in an emitter follower is shown in *Figure 6.37*. It is seen that the output is taken from the emitter resistor rather than from a collector load. This is a case of an

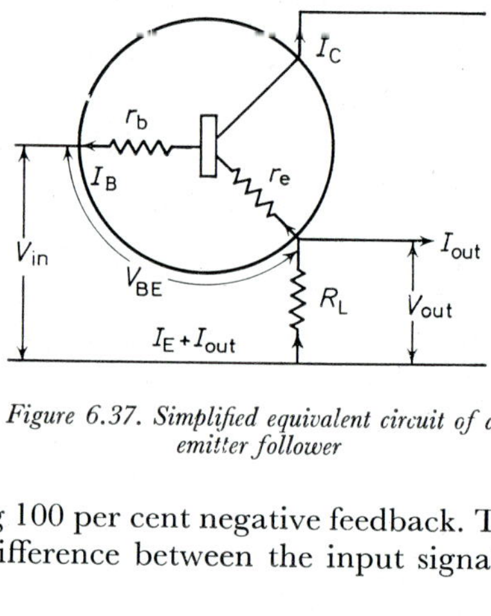

Figure 6.37. Simplified equivalent circuit of an emitter follower

amplifier having 100 per cent negative feedback. The effective input voltage is the difference between the input signal voltage and the output voltage.

Basically, $I_C = \alpha I_E + I_{CO}$. $I_B = I_E - I_C = I_E(1-\alpha) - I_{CO}$. $V_{BE} = I_E r_e + I_B r_b$ and is assumed not to vary with temperature. $V_{in} = I_B r_b + I_E r_e + (I_E + I_{out}) R_L$.
Substituting for I_B,

$$V_{in} = I_E[r_b(1-\alpha) + r_e + R_L] - I_{CO} r_b + I_{out} R_L,$$

so that

$$I_E = \frac{V_{in} + I_{CO} r_b - I_{out} R_L}{r_b(1-\alpha) + r_e + R_L}.$$

Now,

$$V_{out} = (I_E + I_{out}) R_L = \frac{V_{in} R_L + I_{CO} r_b R_L + I_{out} R_L (r_b(1-\alpha) + r_e)}{r_b(1-\alpha) + r_e + R_L}.$$

The open-circuit voltage gain is $V_{out}/V_{in}=R_L/(r_b(1-\alpha)+r_e+R_L)$. If R_L is much greater than $r_b(1-\alpha)+r_e$, the voltage gain approaches unity. The output resistance is

$$V_{out}/I_{out}=\frac{R_L(r_b(1-\alpha)+r_e)}{R_L+r_b(1-\alpha)+r_e}.$$

By inspection this is seen to be equal to R_L in parallel with $r_b(1-\alpha)+r_e$, and this is small if r_b and r_e are small, perhaps of the order of 50 Ω.

The effect on the output voltage of the temperature-dependent reverse leakage current I_{CO} is given by

$$V_{out}/I_{CO}=\frac{r_b R_L}{r_b(1-\alpha)+r_e+R_L}.$$

When R_L is large, the effect is approximately proportional to r_b, the base resistance, which can include any external series base resistance.

$$I_B=I_E(1-\alpha)-I_{CO},$$

and substituting for I_E,

$$I_B=\frac{V_{in}(1-\alpha)-I_{out}R_L(1-\alpha)-I_{CO}(r_e+R_L)}{r_b(1-\alpha)+r_e+R_L}.$$

The input resistance

$$R_{in}=V_{in}/I_B=r_b+\frac{r_e+R_L}{(1-\alpha)}.$$

If $R_L=10$ k Ω and $\alpha=0{\cdot}98$, then R_{in} is approximately 500 k Ω.

The Use of an Emitter Follower as an Impedance Converter

The high input impedance and low output impedance of an emitter follower make it useful as a buffer stage interposed between two amplifier stages to minimize interaction between them. Although the voltage gain of an emitter follower is slightly less than unity, it is also widely used as a buffer amplifier when a high input impedance is required, and an emitter follower might be connected to each electrode of an ECG recording system. The low output impedance is also useful when a capacitive load, such as a long cable, has to be driven. If there were an appreciable output impedance, the time constant formed by it and the cable capacitance could be sufficiently long to distort the signal waveform.

TRANSISTOR D.C. AMPLIFIERS

The main problems in the design of d.c. amplifiers which are required to have a frequency response extending down to d.c. are the minimization of zero (baseline) drift and variations in gain. The application of negative feedback reduces both the gain and the effective zero drift proportionately, so that zero drift has not been eliminated. A good discussion of the design of transistor d.c. amplifiers is that of Grigson (1964). Baseline drift arises from three main causes.

The first cause is variation in the leakage current I_{CO} of the transistors. Typical values for I_{CO} for a germanium transistor might be 3–4 μA at 25° C, whilst for a silicon transistor the corresponding values would be 10–20 nanoamperes. For a germanium transistor the leakage current will double for every 9–10° C rise in temperature. For normal room temperature operation it is possible to neglect changes in the leakage current occurring with silicon transistors. $I_C = I_B . h_{fe} + I_{CO}$ shows how the collector current, and hence the voltage at the collector, will alter if the leakage current changes. Hence d.c. amplifiers make use of silicon transistors.

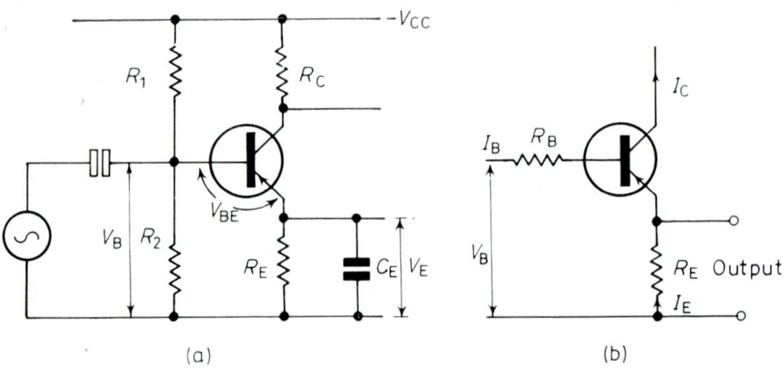

Figure 6.38. Emitter follower circuit

Secondly, drift can arise from changes with temperature of the h_{fe} of the transistors. For a silicon transistor, h_{fe} might change by about 0·4 per cent per degree Centigrade. Temperature variations between transistors can be minimized by mounting them in a common heat sink or even arranging to thermostat the circuit.

Thirdly, the variation with temperature of the base-to-emitter voltage V_{BE} can be very important when the leakage current of silicon transistors is neglected. V_{BE} is in effect the forward voltage drop across the base–emitter diode. Consider the circuit of *Figure 6.38*. In *Figure 6.38b*, the base bias resistors R_1 and R_2 have been combined to give $R_B = (1/R_1) + (1/R_2)$. The voltage V_B drives the base current I_B round the circuit so that $V_B = I_E R_E + V_{BE} + I_B R_B$. Assuming that the base current supplied I_B remains constant, then if V_{BE} decreases with a rise in the temperature, I_E and hence the collector current I_C must increase. For both silicon and germanium transistors, V_{BE} decreases by about 2 mV per degree Centigrade rise. In a simple common emitter stage (*Figure 6.39*),

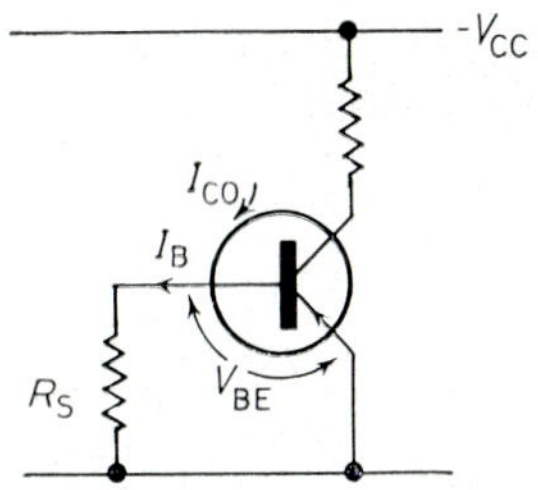

Figure 6.39. Drift in a simple common emitter stage

the equivalent current drift referred to the input consists of the three components

$$\Delta I_{CO} + \frac{\Delta V_{BE}}{{}_{S}R} + I_B \frac{\Delta h_{fe}}{h_{fe}}.$$

The equivalent voltage drift referred to the input is

$$\Delta I_{CO} R_S + \Delta V_{be} + \frac{(I_B . \Delta h_{fe})}{h_{fe}} R_S.$$

The relative importance of voltage or current drift depends not only on their absolute values, but also on the ratio of the signal–source incremental resistance to the amplifier input incremental resistance. If this ratio is high, the source approximates to a current source and the amplifier is 'current operated'. Current drift is then relatively more important. When the ratio is low, the source approximates to a voltage source and the amplifier is 'voltage operated'. The expressions for drift show that if R_S is small, current drift predominates. If R_S is large, voltage drift predominates.

The changes occurring in V_{BE} can be cancelled by using similar pairs of transistors in a long-tailed pair configuration. This is a differential or balanced amplifier. Such an arrangement is described by Mason and Braunwald (1963). By using silicon transistors, the leakage current changes can be neglected up to 35° C.

DIFFERENTIAL AMPLIFIERS

Apart from their employment as components of various scientific instruments, a principal use of amplifiers in medical electronics occurs in the measurement of small signals such as the EEG, EMG and ECG. In a balanced or push–pull stage, the output is taken as the difference between two collector voltages. If two signals identical in amplitude and phase are applied one to each base, and the stage is completely symmetrical, there will be no output voltage change. This assumes that the transistor characteristics are matched and all the resistors are identical. (Vierhout and Vendrik, 1964). Then both collector voltages will change by the same amount, and there will be no voltage difference between the collectors. This balanced arrangement has the useful property that changes in the ambient temperature and supply voltages tend to affect each half of the stage by equal amounts and thus the effect on the output is minimized.

On the other hand, if one of the input signals is 180 degrees out of phase with the other, an output change will result. One collector current will increase by the same amount that the other decreases, and thus there will be a difference between them. The total collector current for the pair of transistors will remain constant. The voltage drop across the resistor in the emitter circuit also remains constant. There is thus no series negative feedback for anti-phase signals. When in-phase signals are applied to the stage, both emitter currents change together and the change in emitter current gives rise to negative feedback across the resistor in the emitter circuit. Thus the gain of the stage is lower for in-phase signals than it is for anti-phase signals. This is helpful, since in practice the stage may not be completely balanced and some output will be produced for in-phase signals. The electrodes from which signals such as the ECG and EEG have to be recorded are usually subjected to the pick-up of mains interference voltages from the wiring and lights in the room. These unwanted signals are in-phase at each electrode, whereas if the electrodes are suitably sited the biological signals will be in anti-phase.

Figure 6.40, due to Towers (1968), illustrates a two-stage balanced d.c. amplifier, using *p–n–p* transistors in the first stage directly coupled to *n–p–n* transistors in the second stage. Negative feedback is provided between the stages. Two balance controls are provided for setting the d.c. level of the output. One is used with the input open-circuited and the other with the input short-circuited. As shown, the output stage drives a moving coil meter, and the adjustable series resistor acts as a sensitivity control. Another d.c. amplifier is that of Oberg *et al.* (1967).

Push–pull biological amplifiers such as those used in electrocardiographs and electroencephalographs contain at least one a.c.

coupled stage in order that baseline shifts of the recording may not occur due to changes in the d.c. potentials present on the recording electrodes. The balance control can be adjusted by applying an in-phase signal to the differential inputs of the amplifier and adjusting the balance to produce a minimum output. The in-phase rejection ratio of the amplifier can be measured by means of a low frequency oscillator which is provided with a push–pull output and a calibrated

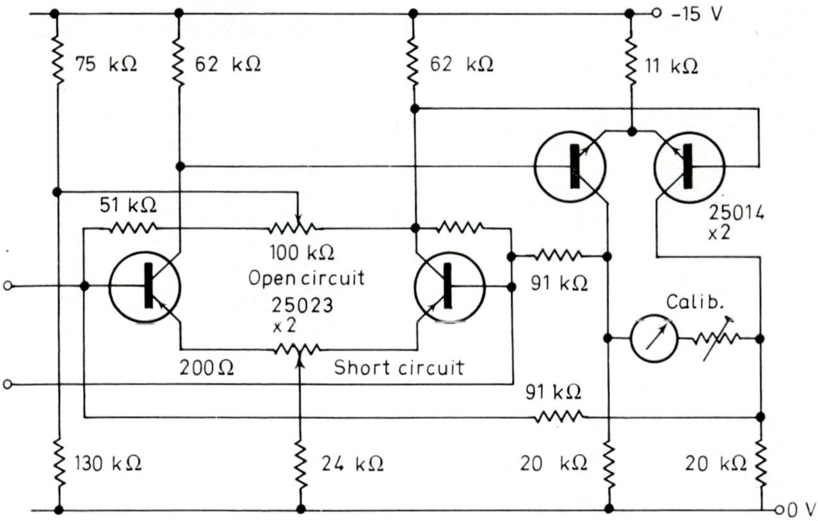

Figure 6.40. Two-stage differential d.c. amplifier

(Reproduced after Towers, 1968, by courtesy of the Editor of *Wireless World*)

attenuator capable of reducing the oscillator output down to tens of microvolts. The common (earth) terminals of the amplifier and oscillator are joined together. Initially, the two active input terminals of the amplifier are joined together and connected to one output terminal of the oscillator. The oscillator output is gradually increased from zero until a small output is produced from the amplifier. It is necessary to keep the amplitude of the output small, since the large in-phase signals which would otherwise be produced in the final stages of the amplifier could cause overloading and distortion. The link joining the two inputs of the amplifier is now opened and they are connected to the output of the oscillator.

Now that the input to the amplifier is push–pull, a smaller signal will be required to produce the same output amplitude as before. The ratio of the amplitude of the in-phase to that of the out-of-phase input signals gives the required rejection ratio. With a modern electrocardiograph this will be at least 1,000. However, it should be remembered that it is the overall rejection ratio of the complete recording system which is important, rather than that for the amplifier alone.

THE COMPOUND OR DARLINGTON CONNECTION

The connection of two transistors in a Darlington connection is shown in *Figure 6.41.* The power rating of Q_2 is usually greater than

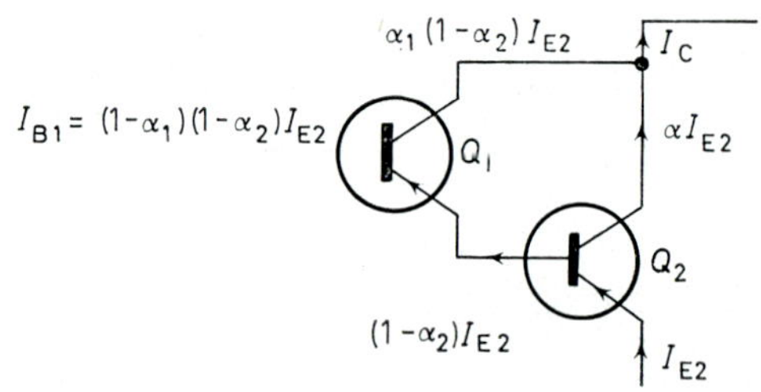

Figure 6.41. Currents in the Darlington compound connection

that of Q_1 since the base current of Q_2 is the collector current of Q_1. If the emitter current of Q_2 is I_{E_2}, then the collector current is $\alpha_2 I_{E_2}$ and the base current is $(1-\alpha_2 I_{E_2})$. This base current is the emitter current of Q_1, so that the collector current of Q_1 is $\alpha_1(1-\alpha_2)I_{E_2}$, while the base current of Q_1 is $(1-\alpha_1)\ (1-\alpha_2)I_{E_2}$. Treating the compound pair as a single transistor,

$$I_C/I_E=\alpha_1\ \frac{(1-\alpha_2)I_{E_2}+\alpha_2 I_{E_2}}{I_{E_2}}=1-(1-\alpha_1)\ (1-\alpha_2)\simeq 1.$$

$$h_{fe}=I_C/I_b=\frac{\alpha_1(1-\alpha_2)I_{E_2}+\alpha_2 I_E}{(1-\alpha_1)\ (1-\alpha_2)I_E}\simeq\frac{1}{(1-\alpha_1)\ (1-\alpha_2)}.$$

If the transistors each had an alpha of 0·98, then for the compound pair $\alpha=0{\cdot}9996$ and $h_{fe}=2{,}500$. When the compound connection is used in the form of an emitter follower (*Figure 6.42*), a high input resistance is obtained over a limited range of working since $R_{in}=h_{fe}R_L$.

Figure 6.43 shows a two-stage circuit which employs two 'compound transistors', each of which is made up of one *n–p–n* and one *p–n–p* transistor. A resistor in each emitter lead provided feedback. The circuit produces drifts of 7–12 μV per degree Centigrade using unselected components, provided that the input transistors are maintained at equal temperatures to within a few millidegrees.

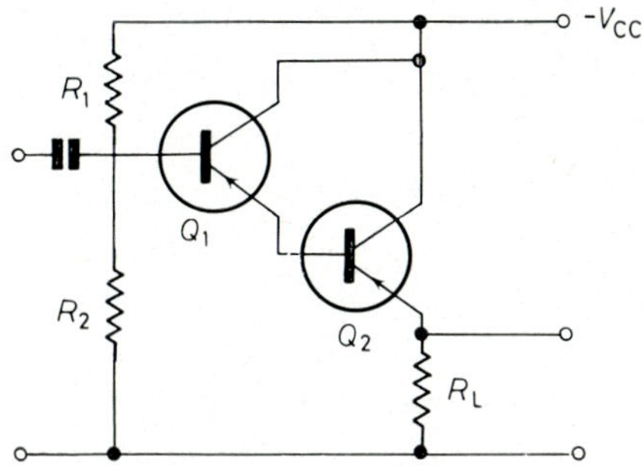

Figure 6.42. The Darlington connection

This amplifier configuration due to Beneteau, together with an improved version, are described by Jones (1963).

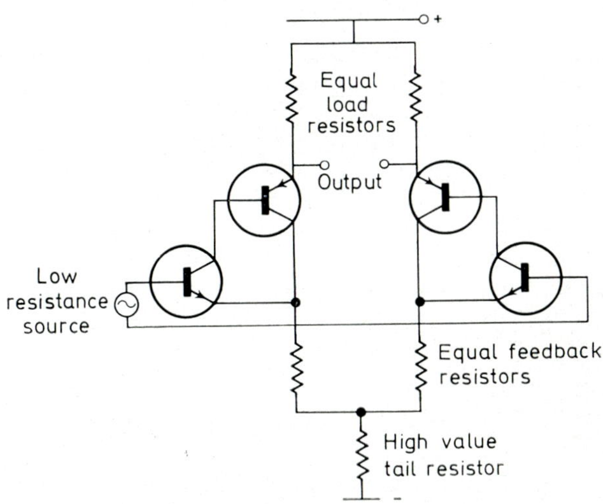

Figure 6.43. Two-stage amplifier using p–n–p and n–p–n transistors
(Reproduced from Jones, 1963, by courtesy of I.T.T. Components)

BOOTSTRAPPING

Bootstrapping is a technique used for raising the input impedance of an amplifier. Positive feedback is connected to the supply end of the input resistor of a stage so that the input current is reduced and the apparent value of the input resistance is increased. In the circuit of *Figure 6.44*, the base biasing resistor has been split into two and the junction is coupled to the output of the emitter follower via the capacitor C_F. The output signal will be in phase with the input

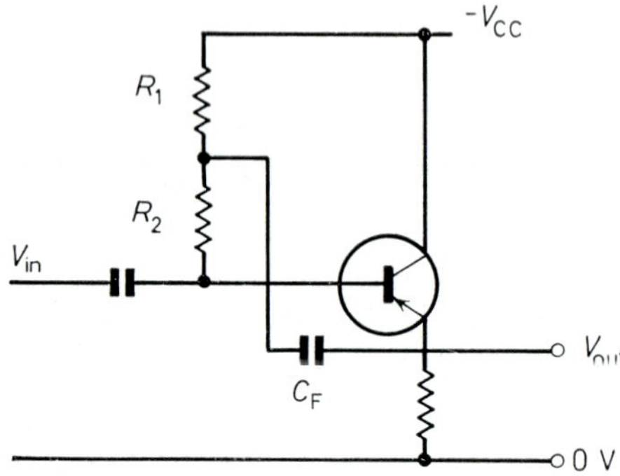

Figure 6.44. Bootstrapping of the base bias resistor

and slightly less in amplitude. Let the input signal to the stage be V_{in}, so that the voltage developed across R_2 will be $V_{in} - V_{out}$, and the signal current shunted off by this resistor will be $(V_{in} - V_{out})/R_2$, whereas without bootstrapping it would have been $V_{in}/(R_1+R_2)$. If the gain of the emitter follower is 0·95, then bootstrapping reduces the current into the biasing resistor by a factor of 20. The collector a.c. resistance r_c shunts the equipment output current generator of the transistor and is in parallel with the load resistor. A bootstrapping technique can also be used to raise the apparent value of r_c.

A PRE-AMPLIFIER FOR ECG OR EEG RECORDING

In biological amplifiers it is necessary to maintain a high value of the rejection ratio for common mode signals in the presence of a d.c. imbalance at the input terminals, usually due to the presence of varying d.c. potentials on the various recording electrodes. Using a dual transistor with both active elements mounted in the same can, it is possible to produce a common mode rejection of between 80 and 90 db without negative feedback being used. However, a d.c. imbalance at the input of only a few millivolts will give rise to an appreciable reduction in the ratio. The effect is not so apparent in valve circuits, but in transistor differential amplifiers it requires the application of a considerable amount of negative feedback in order to stabilize the bias currents of the first stage and thus to preserve the rejection of in-phase signals. Although more stages of amplification will be required than is the case with valve circuitry, advantages accrue in respect of stability and gain linearity (Murari, 1967).

Electrocardiograph amplifiers use interstage coupling time constants of the order of 2 seconds in order to be able to pass the low frequency components of ECGs. This necessitates the use of capacitors which may be several microfarads in capacity. When the lead selector switch at the input of the amplifier is operated, voltage transients charge and discharge the amplifier coupling capacitors and 'block' the amplifier. No recording is possible until the amplifier recovers its balance.

The approach adopted by Murari (1967) to the design of a pre-amplifier which could be adapted to either ECG or EEG requirements was to settle for a low-noise d.c. coupled differential amplifier

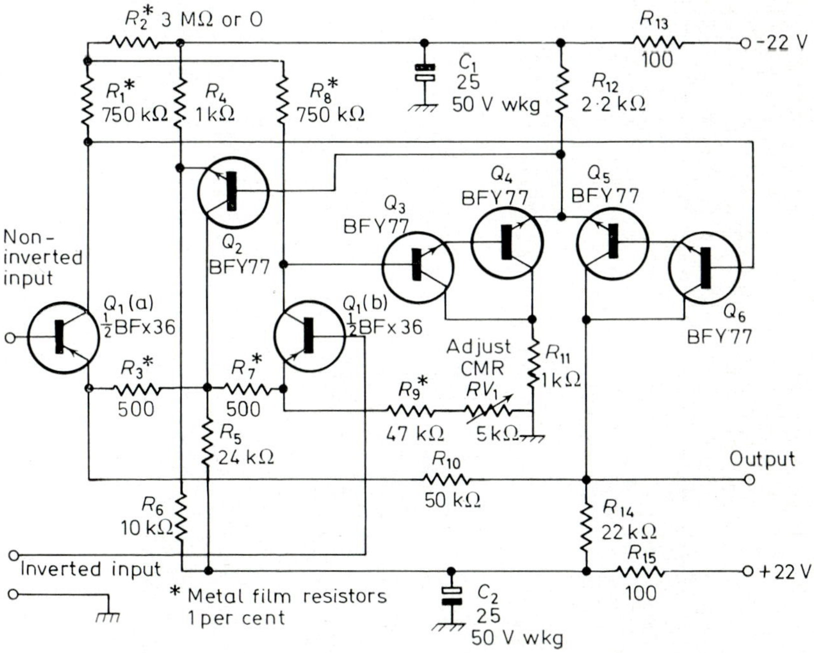

Figure 6.45. A pre-amplifier for ECG or EEG signals. For ECG applications $R_2 = 3$ MΩ. For EEG applications $R_2 = 0$

(Reproduced from Murari, 1967, by courtesy of Pergamon Press)

with a gain of about 100. Its output signal could then be fed from a single-ended output via a single coupling time constant into a power amplifier for driving a recording pen.

With a supply voltage of approximately 22 V, a d.c. input signal of as large as ± 150 mV can be accepted without causing distortion. This, ± 150 mV, is a d.c. differential (anti-phase) signal. The maximum unwanted common mode (in-phase) signal that can be applied to the inputs is ± 10 V. When differential signals of ± 150 mV are applied, a current as large as ± 15 V/50 k $\Omega = 300$ μA flows through R_{10}, and for common mode signals of ± 10 V a current as large as 10 V/50 k $\Omega = \pm 200$ μA flows through R_9 and R_{10} (*Figure 6.45*). To provide these substantial currents, a transistor Q_2 functions as a current source for the first stage. Q_2 draws approximately 1 mA through R_5 and provides the currents for R_9 and R_{10}, thus maintaining the current handling capacity for both differential and

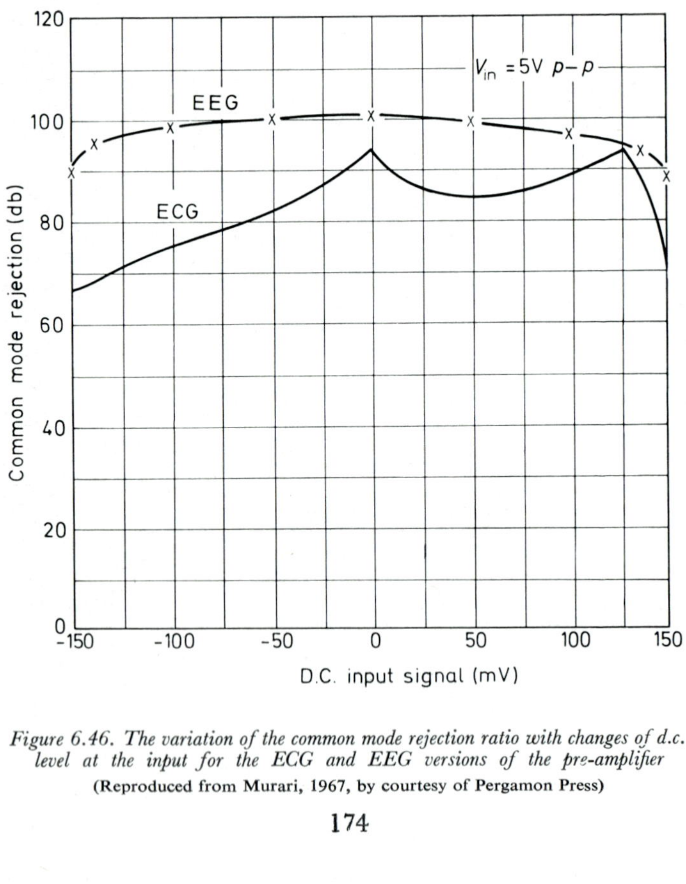

Figure 6.46. The variation of the common mode rejection ratio with changes of d.c. level at the input for the ECG and EEG versions of the pre-amplifier

(Reproduced from Murari, 1967, by courtesy of Pergamon Press)

common mode signals. Q_2 also stabilizes the mean collector current of the first stage and increases the common mode rejection. *Figure 6.46* gives the variation of the common mode rejection ratio, with changes of d.c. level at the input, for both ECG and EEG configurations. The difference is due to the application of only 20 db of differential feedback in the ECG version as compared with

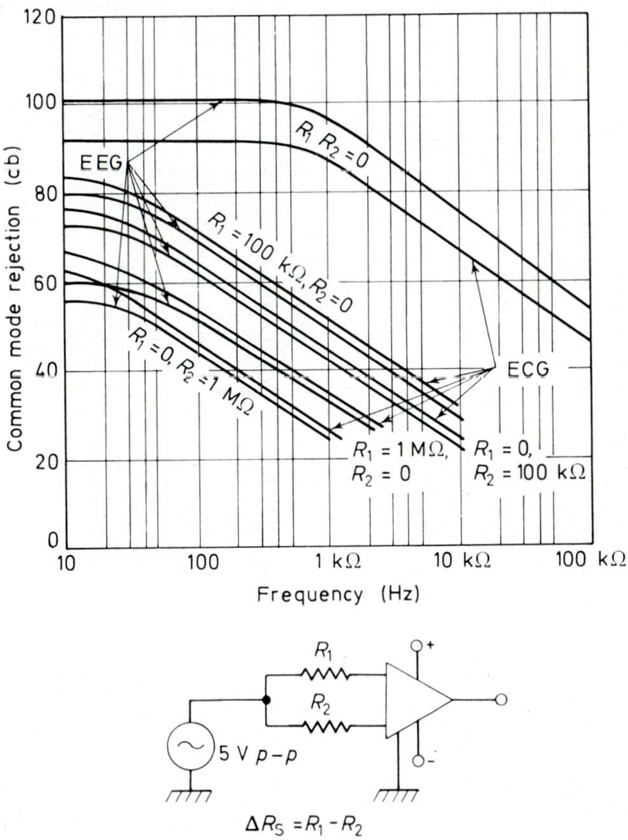

Figure 6.47. The variation of the common mode rejection ratio with the difference in the input source resistances for the ECG and EEG versions of the pre-amplifier

(Reproduced from Murari, 1967, by courtesy of Pergamon Press)

40 db in the EEG version. The common mode rejection ratio is decreased when the source resistances of the two inputs are unequal, but in *Figure 6.47* it can be seen that for both versions a rejection ratio of better than 40 db is available at 100 Hz.

The circuit for the pre-amplifier is given in *Figure 6.45.* There are two differential stages, the second using 'compound' transistors. The circuit has a high current gain with phase inversion in both stages. Hence the differential negative feedback through R_9, R_7 and R_{10}, R_3 is also negative for the common mode signals. RV_1 is used to maximize the common mode rejection ratio. The variation with frequency of the differential and common mode input impedances is shown in *Figure 6.48.* The ECG version has a lower differential

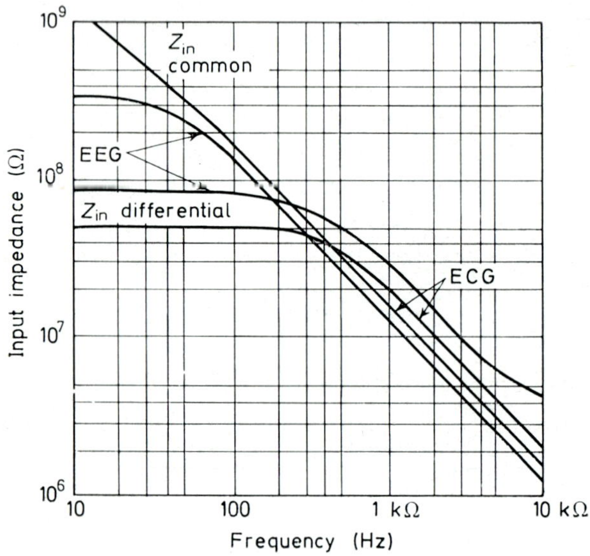

Figure 6.48. The variation with frequency of the differential and common mode input impedances for the ECG and EEG versions of the pre-amplifier

(Reproduced from Murari, 1967, by courtesy of Pergamon Press)

input impedance than the EEG version. This is because of the reduction in the h_{fe} of Q_1 arising from the reduction in collector current when R_2 is made 3 M Ω. However, the presence of this resistor raises the voltage gain in the common mode signal loop and results in an increase in the common mode input impedance.

The performance quoted by Murari for the two versions is given in Table 6.3.

The *p–n–p* transistor type BFX36 was chosen for the first stage because of its low noise level. For the ECG version the collector current of Q_1 is set at 8 μA, and for the EEG version at 1 μA in order to keep the noise level down. The ECG version has a typical noise level of lower than 10 μV pk-to-pk when used with source resistances of up to 300 k Ω. For the EEG version, the noise level is optimized at below 2·5 μV pk-to-pk for source resistances in the range 20–30 k Ω. This represents the limit which could be attained with direct coupled transistor stages.

Table 6.3

	ECG version	EEG version
Open loop gain	60 db	80 db
Closed loop gain	39 db	40 db
Bandwidth (−3 db)	10 kHz	100 kHz
Differential input impedance	50 MΩ+7 pF	80 MΩ+5 pF
Common mode input impedance	1,000 MΩ+10 pF	300 MΩ+12 pF
Output resistance (0–1,000 Hz)	2 kΩ	200 Ω
Common mode rejection ratio (5 V pk-to-pk; 0–500 Hz, V_{in}=±150 mV)	60 db	80 db
Max. common mode input signal	±10 V	±10 V
Supply voltage sensitivity	30 μV/V	30 μV/V
Output voltage swing	32 V pk-to-pk	32 V pk-to-pk
Noise (bandwidth 0·08–100 Hz)		
R_S=10 kΩ	6 μV pk-to-pk	1·8 μV pk-to-pk
R_S=100 kΩ	8 μV pk-to-pk	6 μV pk-to-pk

(Reproduced from Murari, 1967, by courtesy of Pergamon Press)

FREQUENCY SELECTIVE AMPLIFIERS

In many applications it is necessary to amplify signals having a wide range of component frequencies, and the amplifier must therefore have as flat a frequency response as possible within stated limits. However, when it is required to amplify only signals lying within a narrow frequency range, recourse must be made to a frequency selective or tuned amplifier. Here the full gain of the amplifier is available over only a limited frequency range.

Figure 6.49 gives the outline circuit of an audio frequency selective amplifier based on the use of a parallel-T (twin-T) frequency selective network. The parallel-T network presents a high impedance at a chosen frequency given by $f_0=\frac{1}{2}\pi\ RC$ Hz where R is in ohms and C in farads. The twin-T network can be connected in the feedback loop of an amplifier as shown in *Figure 6.49*. The load impedance on the network should be higher than the source impedance feeding it. In this case, the impedance at the base of Q_1 is higher than that at the emitter of Q_2. The graph of gain against

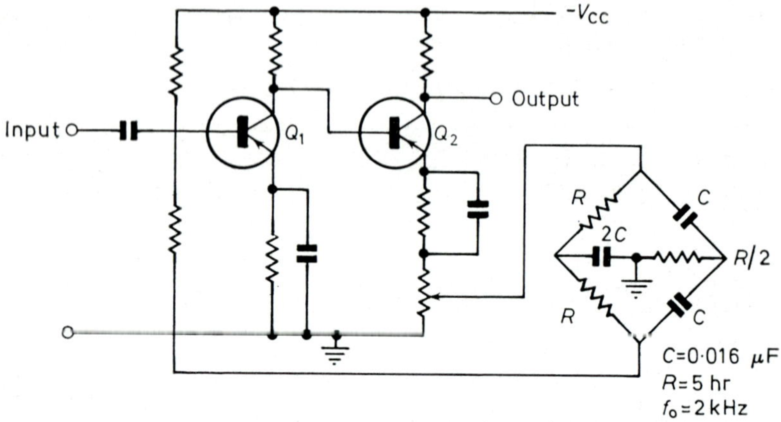

Figure 6.49. Outline circuit of a tuned audio amplifier using a twin-T network in the negative feedback path

frequency is shown in *Figure 6.50*. In order to obtain a sharp (high-Q) curve, the components should be matched to within 2 per cent and good quality (silvered mica) capacitors should be employed. At the desired frequency, minimum negative feedback and hence maximum gain occurs.

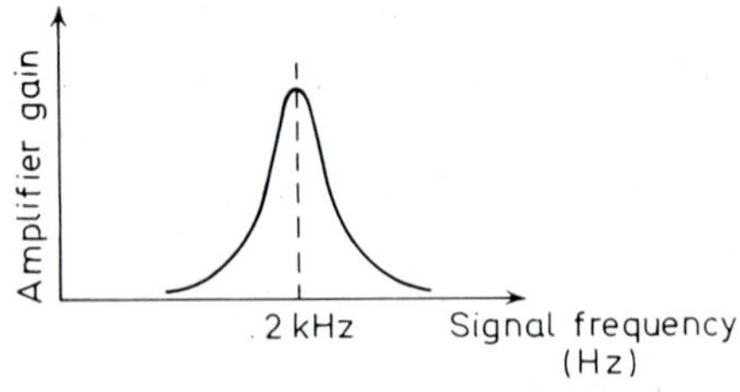

Figure 6.50. The frequency response curve for the amplifier of Figure 6.49

This type of amplifier is invaluable when it is necessary to record a particular frequency in the presence of other frequencies. A popular application is as a selective detector amplifier in an a.c. bridge.

Without its use, the balance point of the bridge would be obscured by residual harmonic frequencies of the excitation signal. Selective amplifiers are also employed in the tuned filters of wave analysers used for estimating the various frequency components of an electro-encephalogram. Twin-T filters on their own are widely used to reject mains hum on biological signals, but care must be taken to guard against distortion which might be introduced in signals such as action potentials (Gibson, Gibson and Hirsch, 1970). A trimmer capacitor is often placed across the capacitor $2C$ in order to adjust the frequency to the exact value required.

The selectivity of the amplifier is adjustable by means of the potentiometer in the feedback circuit. If it is advanced too far it may happen that the amplifier will burst into oscillation. In one particular amplifier tuned to 1,025 Hz, the gain at the centre frequency was 8 and this was 3 db down at 1,020 and 1,030 Hz. An analysis of the twin-T network has been made by Hastings (1946).

FIELD EFFECT TRANSISTORS

In 1928 the American physicist, J. E. Lilienfeld, discovered that the electrical conductivity of a substance could be altered by applying an electric field at right angles to the direction of current flow. Shockley in 1952 described the theory of a device in which the majority carrier current in a resistor made of a semiconductor material was controlled by the reverse voltage applied to a *p–n* junction formed on one side of the resistor. Two main forms of construction have evolved. The first uses one or more *p–n* junctions and is known as an FET. The second operates as a result of an induced depletion or enhancement layer and has an insulating film interposed between the *p–* and *n–* regions. It is known as an IGFET or Insulated Gate Field Effect Transistor.

Figure 6.51 outlines the construction of an *n*–channel FET. The two main electrodes are called the Source and the Drain and are ohmically connected to the ends of the channel. This is shown as *n*–channel material, but it could also be *p*–type material. In an *n*–channel FET the majority carriers are electrons, whilst in a *p*–channel FET they are holes. When connected as shown, a potential gradient is developed along the channel from source to drain. This acts on the majority carriers and a current flows. The gate electrode is formed from *p*–type material placed at one side of the channel. When this diode is reverse biased, an extended depletion region (short of majority carriers) exists on either side of the junction.

Increasing the reverse bias of the junction will increase the depletion region and thus reduce the width of the majority carrier path between the source and the drain. Thus the magnitude of the current between source and drain can be controlled by the reverse bias applied to the gate electrode. Hilbourne and Miles (1965) describe the mode of operation of FETs.

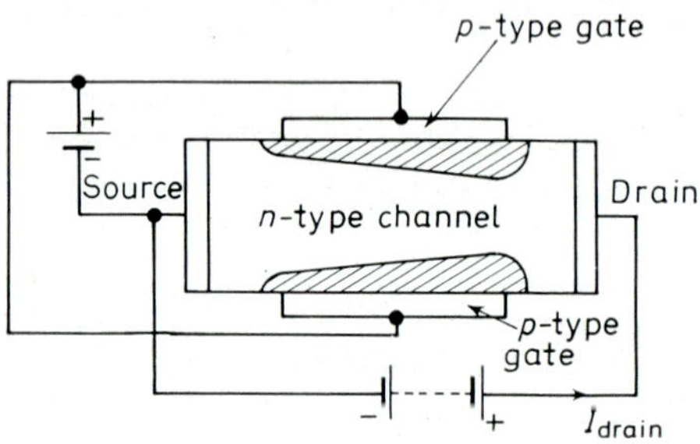

Figure 6.51. Schematic diagram of the construction and biasing of an n-*channel field effect transistor*

Figure 6.52 gives the characteristic curves of an FET connected as in *Figure 6.51*. When the gate electrode is connected to the source electrode, increasing the drain-to-source voltage traces out the curve for $V_{GS}=0$. At first the drain current increases rapidly, and the

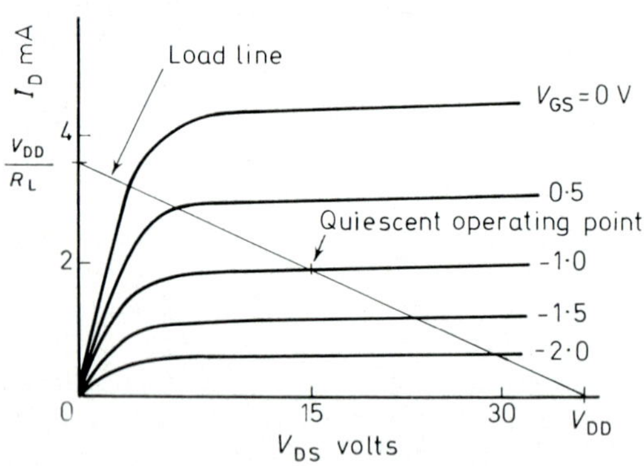

Figure 6.52. The characteristic curves of an n-*channel field effect transistor connected as in Figure 6.51*

increase falls off as the depletion region extends out from the gate electrode and constricts the conduction path available in the channel. Eventually the channel becomes so restricted that the drain current becomes almost constant and independent of the magnitude of the drain voltage. When this occurs, the channel is said to be pinched-off. Here the characteristic curves are almost horizontal. When the gate is made more negative relative to the source, pinch-off arises at lower values of the drain current and drain voltage. Thus for a given drain-to-source voltage, the value of the drain current in the pinch-off region can be controlled by the gate-to-source voltage. Let V_{DS} be the drain–source voltage, V_{GS} the gate–source voltage and V_{PS} the drain–source voltage at which pinch-off occurs, then $V_{DS} = V_{PS} - V_{GS}$.

Parameters of Field Effect Devices

If $\triangle V_{DS}$, $\triangle V_{GS}$ and $\triangle I_D$ represent small changes in these quantities, then the Amplification factor $\mu = \triangle V_{DS}/\triangle V_{GS}$, the Slope Resistance $R_D = \triangle V_{DS}/\triangle I_D$, and the Mutual Conductance $g_m = \triangle I_D/\triangle V_{GS}$.

The amplification factor is measured at a constant drain current, the slope resistance in ohms at a constant gate-to-source voltage, and the mutual conductance in mA/V at a constant drain-to-source voltage. The three parameters are connected by the relationship

$$\frac{\triangle V_{DS}}{\triangle V_{GS}} = \frac{\triangle V_{DS}}{\triangle I_D} \times \frac{\triangle I_D}{\triangle V_{GS}}.$$

Thus $\mu = R_D \times g_m$.

When V_{DS} is fixed and V_{GS} varied, $\triangle I_D = g_m \triangle V_{GS}$. When V_{GS} is fixed and V_{DS} varied, $\triangle I_D = \triangle V_{DS}/R_D$. When both V_{DS} and V_{GS} are altered together, the total change in drain current is given by $\triangle I_D = g_m \triangle V_{GS} + \triangle V_{DS}/R_D$. This equation governs the basic operation of the device. It can be written as $I_D = g_m V_{GS} + V_{DS}/R_D$ where the symbols refer to small changes in the variables, and it holds for low frequency operation.

The Use of an FET as an Amplifier

The drain current can be passed through a load resistor in the usual way in order to obtain an output signal as shown in *Figure 6.53a*. The arrow pointing inwards on the gate electrode shows that this is an n–channel FET. For a p–channel FET it would point outwards (*Figure 6.53b*). V_S represents a constant supply voltage. Increasing I_D will increase the voltage $I_D R_L$ developed across R_L and hence diminish V_{DS}, i.e. $\triangle I_D R_L = -\triangle V_D$. Substituting for $\triangle I_D$ in the equation for FET operation, $-\triangle V_{DS}/R_L = g_m \triangle V_{GS} + \triangle V_{DS}/R_D$, giving $\triangle V_D = -R_L R_D g_m \triangle V_{GS}/(R_L + R_D)$. Since $\mu = g_m R_D$, the voltage gain of the stage $\triangle V_{DS}/\triangle V_{GS} = -\mu R_D/(R_D + R_L)$.

From *Figure 6.54* it is evident that the field effect transistor could be replaced by an equivalent voltage generator producing $-g_m \triangle V_{GS}$ volts with an internal resistance (incremental resistance) of R_D.

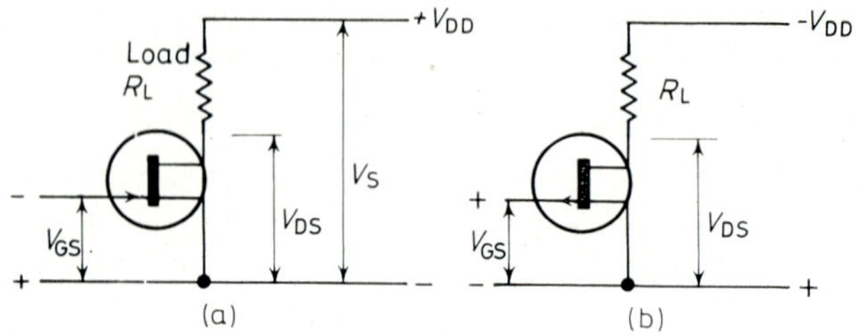

Figure 6.53. The use of a load resistor with (a) an n-channel FET and (b) a p-channel FET

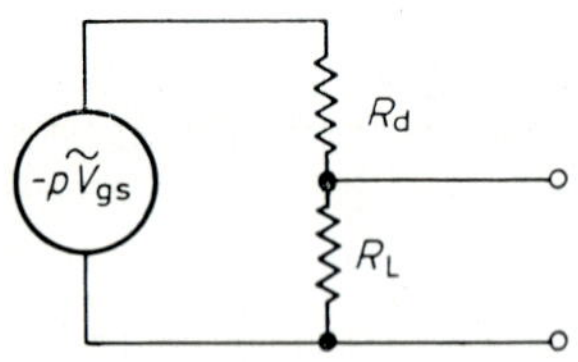

Figure 6.54. Replacement of an FET by an equivalent voltage generator

Since $\mu = g_m R_D$, substituting for μ in the stage gain equation, $\triangle V_{DS} = g_m \triangle V_{GS} R_L R_D / (R_L + R_D)$. From *Figure 6.55* this shows that the FET can also be regarded as a current generator producing

Figure 6.55. Replacement of an FET by an equivalent current generator

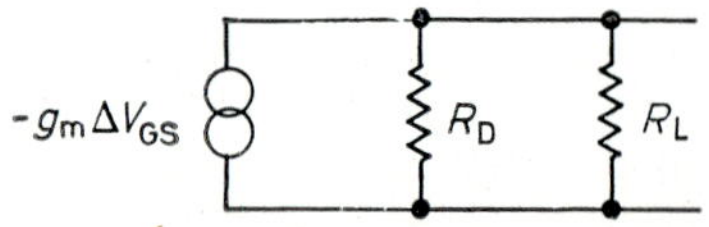

a current of $-g_m \triangle V_G$ and having an internal shunt resistance of R_D.

Output Resistance of the FET

In *Figure 6.53*, when the load resistor R_L is open-circuited, $\triangle V_{DS} = -\mu \triangle V_{GS}$, so that $\mu = -\triangle V_{DS} / \triangle V_{GS}$ under these conditions. In *Figure 6.54*, when the load is now short-circuited, $I_D = -g_m \triangle V_{GS}$. Since $R_D = \mu / g_m$, R_D = open circuit output voltage change/short circuit output current change. From *Figure 6.54* it is evident that the load resistor R_L is always shunted by the drain–source resistance

R_d. This a.c. (incremental) resistance is typically of the order of 1 M Ω.

Bias Stabilization

Unlike a conventional bipolar transistor which is normally OFF and must be turned ON, the FET is normally ON when the gate voltage is zero and the device must be turned OFF. If the gate–source diode is forward biased, the input impedance of the FET rapidly becomes non-linear, eventually limiting the signal at approximately −0·6 V with respect to zero bias. The operating point of an FET is also inherently temperature-sensitive, so that these

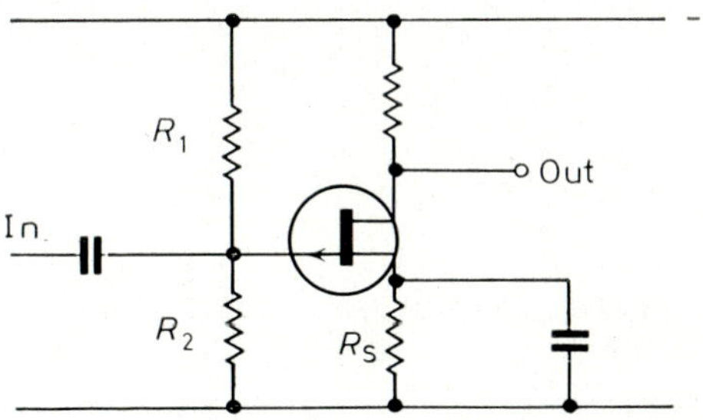

Figure 6.56. Bias network for a field effect transistor

considerations lead to the adoption of a bias stabilization network (*Figure 6.56*) on the lines of that used for a bipolar transistor.

Coupling the FET to Following Stages

Figure 6.57 shows a *p*–channel FET input stage followed by an emitter follower using an *n–p–n* transistor. With R_1=15 M Ω and R_2=3·3 M Ω, the input resistance was 3 M Ω and the overall gain

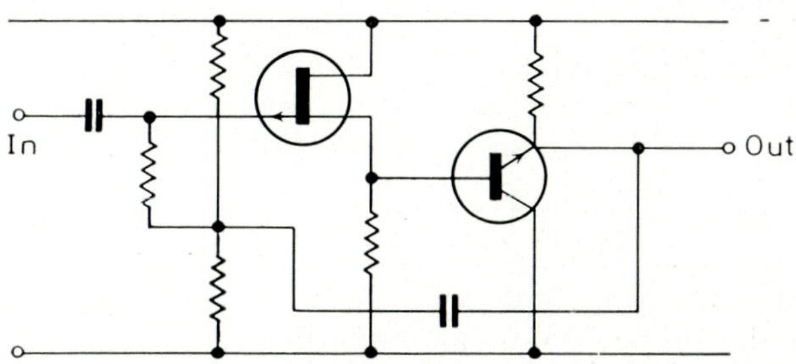

Figure 6.57. The use of a p*-channel FET input stage followed by an emitter follower*

of the amplifier was 10. The input resistance can be raised to approximately 30 M Ω by bootstrapping the input bias resistors as shown in *Figure 6.57*. The overall voltage gain is 18.

Inter-electrode Capacitances

Capacitances exist between the various electrodes of a three-terminal device as shown in *Figure 6.58*. The input impedance of the device consists of the input resistance in parallel with the effective value of the input capacitance. Current flows into or out

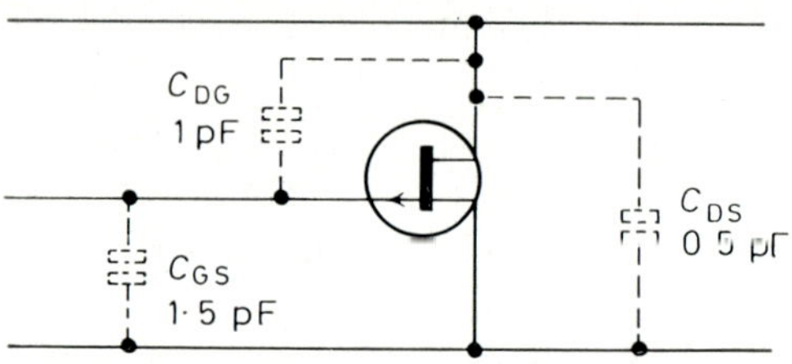

Figure 6.58. Inter-electrode capacitances of a field effect transistor

from the effective input capacitance only when the input voltage is changing. The capacitance C_{GS} between the gate and the source shunts the input signal, but the effect of the drain–gate capacitance C_{DG} is particularly important in its effect on the amplifier performance. Suppose that an a.c. signal of 1 V (superimposed on a suitable d.c. bias) is applied between gate and source. If the voltage gain is A_v, this appears as a signal A_v in amplitude and 180 degrees out of phase as V_{DS} at the drain. Because the input and output voltages are 180 degrees out of phase, the voltage V_{DG} appearing between the gate and the drain must be (A_v+1) V. The voltage across C_{DG} is (A_v+1) V, giving a current through the capacitor C_{DG} which is the same as that which would occur if 1 V were applied across a capacitance equal to (A_v+1) times C_{DG}.

In the case of an FET, the current through C_{DG} cannot flow into the gate which draws almost no current, so that it must flow into the input circuit. The total input current for the device is now the same as though a capacitor of value $C_{GS}+(A+1)C_{DG}$ were connected across the input. The action of the amplifier gain in effectively increasing the value of the input capacitance of the device is known as the Miller effect. Unless steps are taken to neutralize it or reduce it by device construction, the Miller effect acts to limit the high frequency bandwidth of amplifiers. With bipolar transistors when the input current into the base cannot be taken as zero, it must be allowed for in Miller effect calculations.

The Insulated Gate Field Effect Transistor (IGFET)

The construction of an insulated gate field effect transistor is illustrated in *Figure 6.59.* Two islands of *p*–material are diffused close together into a high resistivity *n*–substrate and covered by a thin insulating layer of silicon dioxide. Metal electrodes are evaporated into the oxide layer in contact with *p*–type islands to act as the source and the drain. The gate electrode is evaporated on to the oxide layer and is insulated from both source and drain.

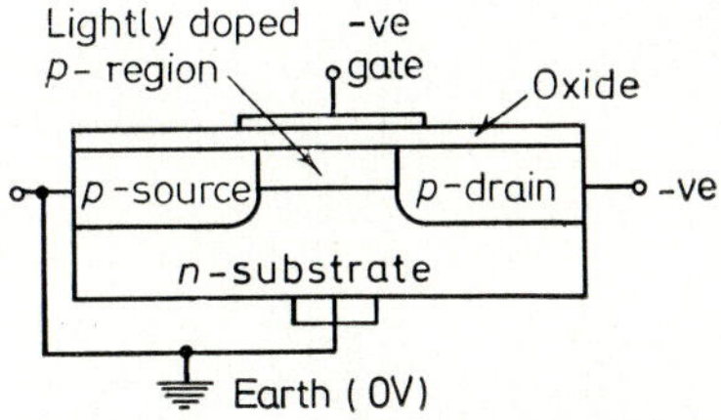

Figure 6.59. Schematic diagram of the construction of a p-*channel insulated gate field effect transistor*

A fourth electrode, known as the base substrate, is connected to the bottom of the *n*-type material. The polarity of the gate and drain supply voltages is as shown for a *p*-channel IGFET. This is also known as a MOSFET (Metal Oxide Silicon Field Effect Transistor). The type shown in *Figure 6.59* is of a silicon planar epitaxial construction.

The MOST is a planar device in which the field generated by the voltage applied between the gate and the channel penetrates into the channel and induces either a depletion or an enhancement region. The induced conducting channel is insulated from the substrate by a reverse biased *p–n* junction, and the substrate acts only as a support. In the *n*-type channel MOST, a positive voltage is applied to the drain. This reverse biases the *p–n* junction at that point. A space charge region forms and little current flows. The gate, oxide layer and substrate form a parallel plate capacitor. The application of a positive voltage to the gate induces a positive charge on the gate electrode and a corresponding negative charge on the surface of the silicon. This induced region extends from the source, which is at zero voltage, to a point in the space charge region around the drain which is approximately at the same potential as the gate. Most of the induced electrons are 'free' and can move under the influence of the transverse electric field which occurs along the length of the layer. Any electrons which reach the end of the induced layer are swept across the space charge region to the drain. Current flow between the drain and the source is determined by the resistance of the induced layer. As the current is not markedly dependent upon the drain voltage, the output resistance is high. When the drain voltage is less than the gate voltage, the induced layer stretches completely from the source to the drain and the output resistance becomes low, producing a 'knee' in the output characteristics (*Figure 6.60*).

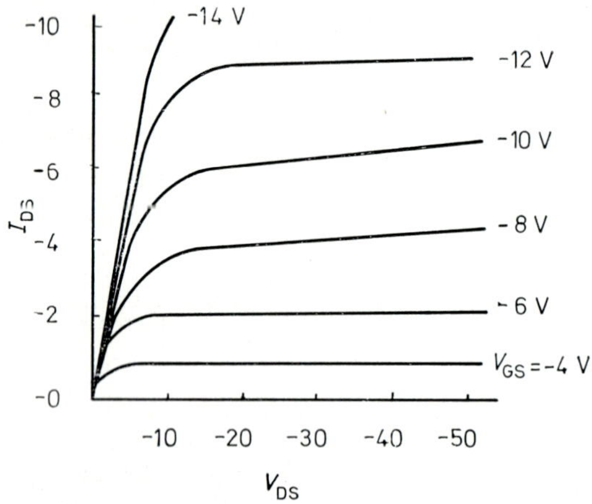

Figure 6.60. Output characteristics of a p*-channel insulated gate field effect transistor*

As has been mentioned previously, it is also possible to make a *p*-type channel MOST by using an *n*-type silicon substrate with *p*-type source and drain electrodes. Conduction is now due to induced positive holes. The resistance of the induced layer of holes is greater than that found with electrons and the hole mobility is lower. Hence, for the same geometry, a *p*-type MOST has a lower g_m (transconductance). Whereas a silicon planar FET might have an input impedance of several thousand megohms, that of a MOST is much higher, typically being in excess of $10^{13}\ \Omega$. The IGFET or MOST compares favourably with an electrometer valve, having better drift characteristics and warm-up time, but its noise level may be higher (Bolic, 1960).

The ordinary FET depends for its operation upon the formation of a high resistance region depletion layer. However, in an IGFET it is also possible to operate the device with the gate biased in the forward direction. This is feasible because the insulating layer prevents the flow of forward current which would occur if the device possessed a real junction. The effect of this forward biasing is to reduce the width of the depletion layer, thus reducing the resistance of the channel and allowing a larger current to flow. Under these conditions the IGFET is operating in an enhancement mode. Both *n*-channel and *p*-channel IGFETs can be constructed to produce either depletion or enhancement types.

The enhancement IGFET is made in such a way that the gate can apply a field which can penetrate the whole of the channel. The channel is lightly doped in the opposite polarity to the source and the drain. With $V_{GS}=0$, the source-to-drain current takes place through the lightly *p*-doped channel and is very small since it is that through a reverse biased diode. In the *n*-channel device, making the gate positive with respect to the source attracts free electrons to the region close to the gate. This causes part of the lightly doped *p*-type region to become effectively an *n*-type material, and current flows along the channel. The lead from the base substrate is normally connected to the source.

Handling Precautions

A gate voltage exceeding the rated value is liable to puncture the thin silicon dioxide layer, and care must be taken to avoid electrostatic potentials occurring which could thus ruin the device. In handling a MOST, the soldering iron should always be earthed, and if possible one of the other device leads touched with the fingers before touching the gate lead with fingers or tools which are not earthed. The gate lead should not be left in a position where it can be influenced by possible high voltage transients, induced or otherwise.

The Use of a Field Effect Transistor as a Chopper

When a wide frequency range is not necessary, it is convenient in low level d.c. amplifiers to employ a chopper technique. The basic principle of the chopper amplifier is to convert the input d.c. signal into a square wave, which is then amplified with an a.c. (R–C coupled) amplifier. Phase-sensitive rectification is employed to convert the amplified a.c. signal back into a d.c. output. In this way the problem of slow drifts associated with a conventional d.c. amplifier is overcome.

Referring to *Figure 6.61*, the switch *S* shorts out the input to the amplifier once per switching cycle, giving rise to a square wave input to the a.c. amplifier. Series resistor *R* prevents short-circuiting of the signal source. The output of the a.c. amplifier approximates to a sine wave. It is rectified and smoothed to yield the required d.c. output. Clearly, the frequency response of the complete system is limited by the frequency of switching and the time constant of the smoothing circuit.

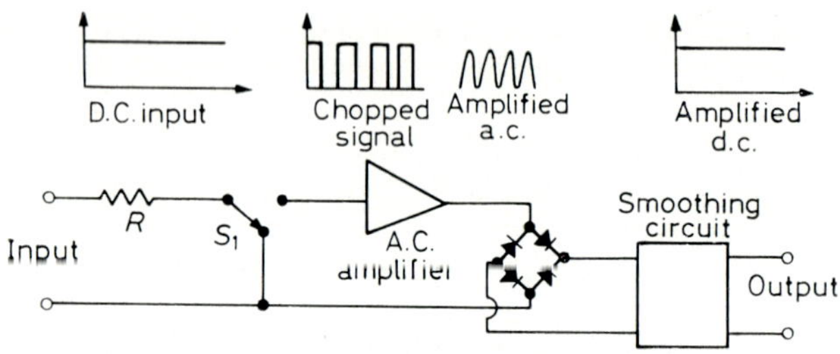

Figure 6.61. Block diagram of a chopper-type d.c. amplifier

In order that the output shall be positive when the input is positive and negative when the input is negative, it is necessary to use a phase-sensitive rectifier. A simple rectifier will give a positive output even though the phase of signal applied to it becomes reversed. The function of the phase-sensitive rectifier is first to rectify, and secondly to cause the output current to flow in one direction through the load when the input voltage is in phase with a reference a.c. voltage. It must cause the output current to reverse when the input and reference voltages are 180 degrees out of phase. The reference voltage is derived from the chopper drive signal voltage.

A phase-sensitive rectifier circuit is shown in *Figure 6.62*. When the reference voltage makes point A positive with respect to point B, all four diodes conduct and the reference voltage divides equally between paths ACB and ADB. With the input polarity shown, the input voltage adds to the reference voltage in arms CB and AD and subtracts from it in arms CA and BD. Assuming all the four diodes to be identical, no output voltage will be produced when the reference voltage alone is applied. The direction of the bridge imbalance depends upon the polarity of the input voltage. The amplitude of the reference voltage must be sufficiently large to prevent the input signal from reducing any of the branch currents in the bridge to zero, since the arms would then stop conducting. The fact that the rectification is in synchronism with the chopper drive signal provides a valuable means of discriminating against random background signals such as noise.

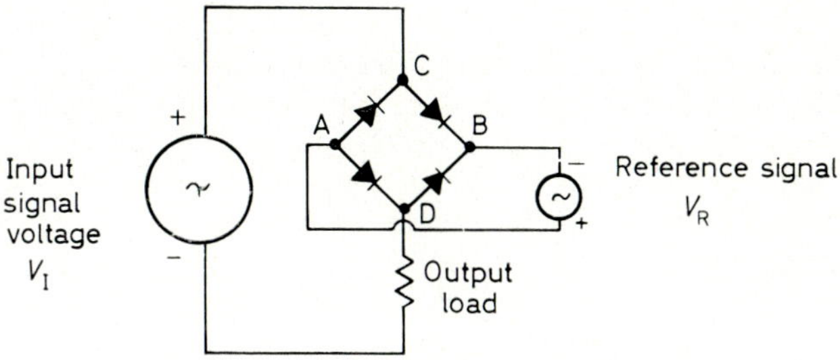

Figure 6.62. Phase-sensitive rectifier circuit

In older models of chopper-type d.c. amplifiers the chopper might have been a high speed relay, or preferably a specially designed low noise mechanical chopper using gold-plated contacts. Such choppers are still used in the d.c. amplifier systems of potentiometric recorders having full scale sensitivities of 1 mV. In principle it is feasible to utilize a bipolar transistor as a chopper. In the case of a conventional bipolar transistor, when it is switched hard ON there will still exist a voltage between the collector and the emitter due to the base current, and this means that in the ON position the output voltage can never fall below this value. In fact this Offset Voltage forms a pedestal upon which is superimposed the output signal. Additionally, carrier storage and capacitance effects result in the production of switching transients as shown in *Figure 6.63.* The switching-on

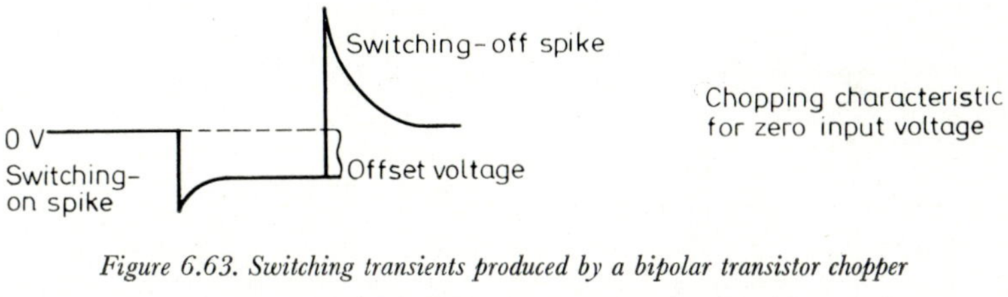

Figure 6.63. Switching transients produced by a bipolar transistor chopper

spike is normally smaller than the switching-off spike since it is damped by the resistance of the signal source in series with the conducting transistor. The time required for the switching-off spike to disappear limits the upper switching frequency of the transistor. Special chopper transistors are available in which the offset voltage is less than 5 mV, but this may be too high for low level signals (Bhola and Murphy, 1967).

FETs are now widely used as choppers (Verill, 1966). A typical FET might have an ON resistance of 8,000 Ω and an OFF resistance of more than 100 M Ω. The ON resistance is not as low as that found with a bipolar transistor, but unlike the transistor, the FET has no offset voltage. Hence it is possible to avoid circuits designed to compensate for the offset voltage and to work with simple arrangements down to microvolt levels. No pedestal appears with the FET since the channel appears as a high resistance when the FET is OFF and a very small resistance when it is ON. There is no non-ohmic leakage

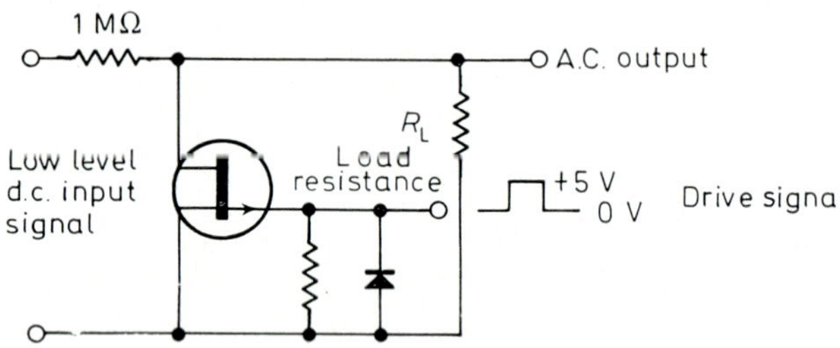

Figure 6.64. Basic arrangement for an FET chopper

current. The drain–source capacitance limits the upper value of the chopping frequency. *Figure 6.64* gives the basic arrangement for an FET low level chopper. It can operate with signals of 10 μV.

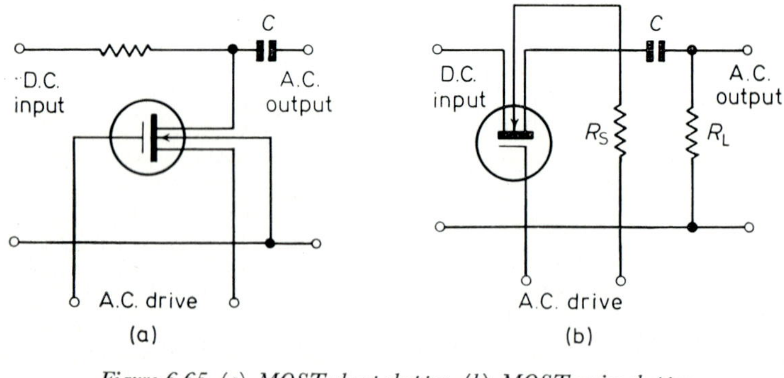

Figure 6.65. (a) MOST shunt chopper. (b) MOST series chopper

The chopping arrangement described so far is a 'shunt' in which the chopper in the ON position acts almost as a short-circuit across the input to the amplifier. The requirement for the ON resistance to be small compared with the load resistor R_L is alleviated if R_L is the high input impedance of a further MOST amplifier stage. *Figure 6.65a* illustrates an MOST shunt chopper. It is a popular configuration since no return path is required for the d.c. input signal, and it can thus be capacitively coupled to the input of the following a.c. amplifier without the need for a choke or input transformer. *Figure 6.65b* gives the alternative type of MOST series chopper. The value of the d.c. return resistor R_S must be large compared with R_L in order to reduce resistive losses. R_L must be large compared with the ON resistance of the MOST, but small compared with its OFF resistance.

Phillips and Dunlop (1969) state that at high switching rates with a MOST chopper, capacitive coupling of the driving waveform from the gate to the signal path produces large transient spikes on the output waveform. When one MOST is used as a series chopper, the switching spikes can be cancelled to a large extent by having a second MOST connected in shunt across the load resistor. The gate of the second MOST is driven in anti-phase to that of the first MOST, so that the combination forms a series shunt chopper and mutual cancellation of the opposite polarity capacitive spikes reduces the spikes on the final output waveform. Phillips and Dunlop (1969) describe a suitable circuit for driving the pair of MOSTs.

THE UNI-JUNCTION TRANSISTOR

The uni-junction transistor forms a very useful switching device and is widely used, for example to fire a silicon-controlled rectifier. As shown in *Figure 6.66*, the uni-junction transistor has three

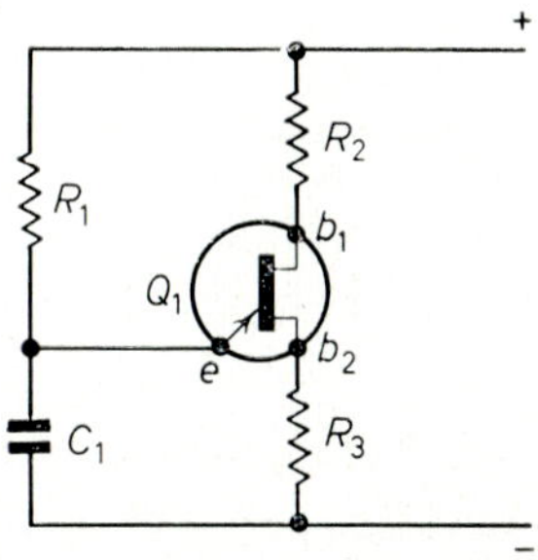

Figure 6.66. Basic uni-junction transistor oscillator circuit

electrodes. Bases 1 and 2 are simple ohmic connections to the silicon material, whilst the emitter is a p–n junction. The resistance between bases 1 and 2 is called the interbase resistance and has values in the range 4·7–9·1 kΩ at 25° C. The voltage existing between the two bases V_{BB} is known as the interbase voltage. When a current flows through the interbase circuit, the potential attained by the emitter will be a function of its relative distance between the two bases. If the emitter *p–n* junction voltage is a fraction η of the interbase voltage, then voltages less than ηV_{BB} will keep the junction reverse biased, whilst voltages greater than ηV_{BB} will bias it in the forward direction. As the emitter junction becomes forward biased, holes are released and move into the region between the emitter and base 1. This effectively reduces the resistance between these two points, so that the emitter current increases as the emitter voltage falls, producing a negative resistance effect. The emitter current is now limited only by the emitter–base 1 resistance.

The basic uni-junction circuit is the oscillator circuit of *Figure 6.66*. In this simple relaxation circuit, capacitor C_1 charges through R_1 until the emitter junction becomes forward biased, when the uni-junction turns on and discharges C_1 through R_3. When the emitter voltage reaches a value of some 2 V, the emitter ceases to conduct, the uni-junction turns off and the cycle recommences. The frequency of oscillation is determined by the values of R_1 and C_1 and is almost independent of the value of the supply voltage. This follows since the emitter turn-on voltage is a fixed fraction η (the intrinsic stand-off ratio) of the interbase voltage. Thus as the supply voltage (and hence V_{BB}) alters, so the emitter turn-on voltage alters in proportion. The value of η lies between 0·51 and 0·82. The period of oscillation $T = R_1C_1 \log_e (1/(1-\eta))$.

The use of a uni-junction transistor to trigger a silicon-controlled rectifier is illustrated by the thermostat circuit of *Figure 6.67*. The thermistor element is used to sense the temperature of, for example, a water bath. The bath heater is controlled by half-wave current pulses derived from the a.c. power supply via a silicon-controlled rectifier whose gate signals are generated by the uni-junction oscillator. The relaxation frequency of the oscillator is stabilized by feeding both the interbase circuit and the timing circuit from a stabilized voltage source consisting of R_3 and the Zener diode Z_1. The thermistor *Th* is connected in parallel with the timing capacitor C_1. The component values are chosen so that when the temperature drops to a preset level, the uni-junction fires and the silicon-controlled rectifier conducts. The SCR acts as a half-wave rectifier extinguishing on the next half-cycle of the a.c. supply. C_1 provides sufficient energy to fire the SCR when the uni-junction turns on, and also introduces a delay in the control function of the thermistor. With this type of circuit it is possible to obtain a temperature control of ±0·01° C over the range 15–35° C using a thermistor having a negative temperature coefficient of −6 per cent per degree Centigrade.

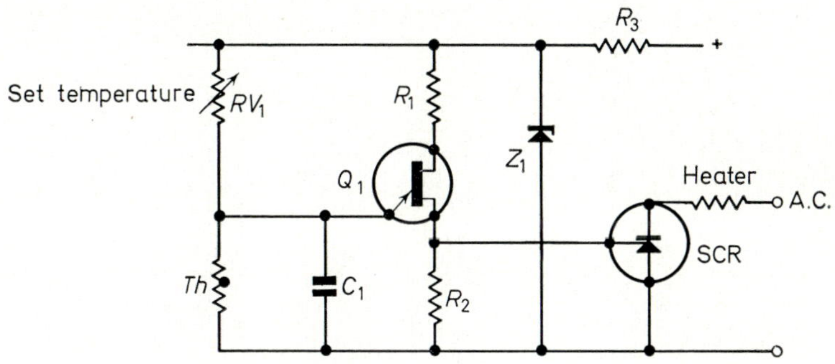

Figure 6.67. The use of a uni-junction transistor and an SCR in a thermostat circuit

A simple integrator, using a uni-junction transistor, for use with a recorder is described by Atkins (1967).

THE PHOTON COUPLER

This interesting device consists of a light-emitting diode and a photo-diode in one package. The light emitted by one diode is, in part, received by the other so that the device acts as an optical coupler. The use of photon coupling can reduce the number of conventional R–C couplings in an amplifier. This is useful, since the long time constants of the R–C couplings required for the passage of low frequency signal components can be 'blocked' for extended periods of time by voltage transients, often caused by switching gain ranges. Optical coupling also provides a high degree of isolation between amplifier stages, and this is desirable in protecting patients from contact with parts of the circuit containing high voltages. Van der Weide and Van Bemmel (1968) describe a photon-coupled amplifier for use with physiological signals.

An equivalent circuit due to Bracale and Marsico (1970) for the photon coupler is shown in *Figure 6.68*. R_{se} is the resistance in series with the light-emitting diode and r_e is the incremental a.c. resistance of that diode at $T°A$ with a d.c. bias current I_1. r_s is the incremental resistance of the photo-diode and R_L the load resistor. η is the current transfer ratio$=I_2/I_1$ (d.c. conditions)$=i_2/i_1$ (a.c. conditions). Under a.c. conditions, $v_1=(R_{se}+r_e)i_1$ and $v_o=R_L\ \eta i_2$. In practice η is approximately 4×10^{-4}, $R_{se}=1\ \Omega$ and r_e is approximately 2·2 Ω at 20 mA. If R_D is the d.c. resistance of the emitting diode, its drive circuit should have an internal resistance much greater than R_D in order to supply a constant current and thus hold the light

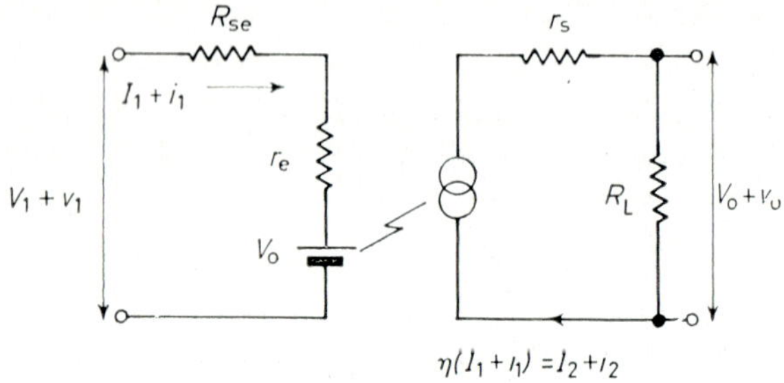

Figure 6.68. Equivalent circuit for a photon coupler
(Reproduced from Bracale and Marsico, 1970, by courtesy of the Editor of *Medical and Biological Engineering*)

intensity constant. The photo-diode acts as a current generator with a high internal resistance due to the low value of η and should be fed into a high input resistance current amplifier in order to produce

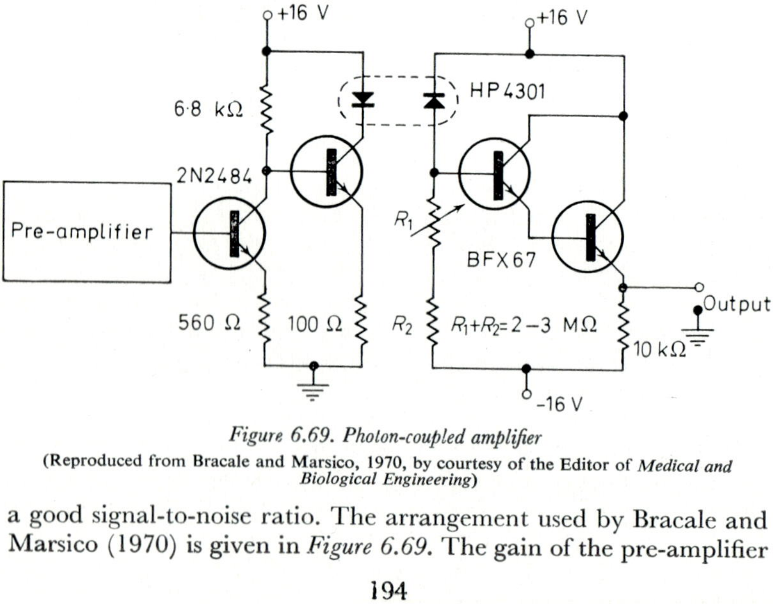

Figure 6.69. Photon-coupled amplifier
(Reproduced from Bracale and Marsico, 1970, by courtesy of the Editor of *Medical and Biological Engineering*)

a good signal-to-noise ratio. The arrangement used by Bracale and Marsico (1970) is given in *Figure 6.69*. The gain of the pre-amplifier was 100 and that of the photon-coupled amplifier was 60. The low frequency cut-off could be set at 0·1 or 10 Hz and the high frequency cut-off at 300, 3,000 or 6,000 Hz, or d.c. coupling could be chosen.

THE PROGRESS OF TRANSISTORIZATION

Now that an indication has been given of the operating principles of transistors, it is of interest to review briefly the rapid progress made in the development of the different types of transistor. The transistor was invented in 1948 (Bardeen and Bratain, 1948). This was the point-contact type which became superseded by the junction type. The method of fabricating junction transistors by alloying was described in 1952 by Law *et al.* The alloy junction transistor is made by melting a sphere of a suitable impurity metal in contact with each side of a semiconductor dice approximately 0·05 in (1·3 mm) by 0·01 in (0·25 mm) thick, by heating in a furnace. On cooling, the recrystallized regions form the *p–n* junctions as the impurity metal is of the opposite type to the original semiconductor material. For a *p–n–p* transistor, the dice contains an impurity giving *n*-type conduction, and the spheres are indium which is a *p*-type deposit. *Figure 6.70* shows the construction of a *p–n–p* alloy junction transistor.

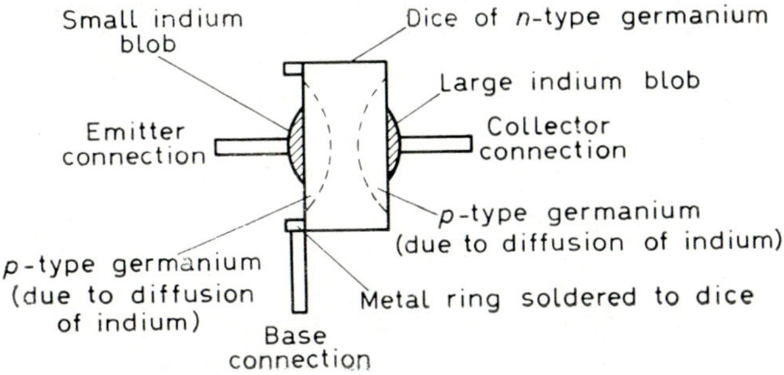

Figure 6.70. The construction of a p–n–p alloy junction transistor

A similar technique is used to prepare *n–p–n* alloy junction transistors. A dice of *p*-type material is used, and pellets of a pentavalent material such as arsenic are alloyed to it.

From 1952 to 1955, the other basic method of junction transistor manufacture was the grown-junction process. The method of forming junctions by the solid-state diffusion of impurities into the crystal

(Hall and Dunlop, 1950) became standard for producing high performance transistors. The high input impedance field effect transistor was proposed by Shockley in 1952. Silicon was not yet in use for transistors, but only for alloy junction diodes (Pearson and Foy, 1952).

The use of transistors in high frequency circuits was advanced by the concept of the graded base or 'drift' transistor (Kremer, 1954). In the Drift transistor, a graduation of the impurity content in the base region produces an enhancing field to decrease the transit time of current carriers across the base. The Surface Barrier transistor (Bradley, 1953) introduced the concept of micro-alloying and of the controlled chemical shaping of the germanium dice.

By 1955, attention was concentrated on the development of diffusion transistor techniques in both germanium and silicon. The greater temperature tolerance of silicon meant that both high frequency and high power devices could be fabricated in this material. Thus there was a 100 kHz 50 W power transistor and a 50 MHz 250 mW high frequency transistor. The high frequency transistors were of the *mesa* type of construction where the diffused collector area is defined by etching a platform from the silicon dice.

In 1960, epitaxially grown silicon and germanium transistors became available. This technique enabled the high resistivity layers suitable for collector regions to be deposited on to low resistivity substrates which served as ohmic connections for the collector, and allowed the collector series resistance of diffused transistors to be drastically reduced. This resulted in epitaxial diffused mesa transistors.

Then followed the appearance of the diffused planar technique. This utilizes the selective diffusion of impurities into silicon using silicon oxide on the surface of the slice as a masking agent. Certain impurities will diffuse only into those regions which have been exposed by removal of the oxide. In this case the area of the device is defined by diffusion, rather than by etching as in the mesa construction. Good diagrams of planar construction are given by Kendall (1963). The diffused planar technique gives a much greater consistency to the device characteristics, and makes it feasible to fabricate a pair of transistors on the same piece of silicon. This is a great advantage in minimizing drifts in d.c. amplifiers. A typical example of a general purpose silicon *n–p–n* silicon planar transistor is the plastic encapsulated Ferranti type ZTX 108. This has maximum collector–base and collector–emitter voltages of 20 V and a maximum emitter–base voltage of 5 V. The maximum peak collector current is 100 mA with a maximum dissipation of 300 mW at 25° C.

The collector–base reverse current is 0·2 μA max with 20 V between the collector and base and zero emitter current. The maximum emitter–base current is 0·2 μA when the emitter–base voltage is −4 V and the collector current is zero. The d.c. current gain h_{fe} is 40 minimum 130 maximum at a collector current of 10 μA, and 110–435 at 2 mA. The gain–bandwidth product is typically 115 MHz. Both the planar silicon field effect transistor and the insulated gate field effect transistor are readily available for high input impedance and chopper applications, sample and hold circuits and very high frequency amplifiers.

Although discrete transistors still have a significant role to play in circuitry, for many instrument applications they are being replaced by integrated circuits where transistors, diodes, resistors and some capacitors are interconnected on one chip of silicon. Similarly, integrated logic circuit modules are widely used in the computer industry and have resulted in the production of compact laboratory computers.

REFERENCES

Adler, E. and Selikson, B. (1962). 'A review of the tunnel diode.' *Electron. Engng* **34,** 8, 32.

Amos, S. W. (1971). 'Negative feedback in transistor amplifiers.' *Wireless Wld* **76,** 37.

Atkins, A. R. (1967). 'A simple recorder integrator using a unijunction transistor.' *Electron. Engng* **39,** 440.

Bardeen, D. C. and Bratain, W. A. (1948). 'The transistor, a semi-conductor triode.' *Phys. Rev.* **74,** 230.

Barton, K. (1913). 'The field effect transistor used as a low-level chopper.' *Electron. Engng* **37,** 80.

Belsey, D. C. and Gabriel, W. P. (1963). 'A direct indicating infra-red radiation meter.' *J. scient. Instrum.* **40,** 526.

Bhola, S. K. and Murphy, R. H. (1967). 'Design of low-level chopper amplifiers.' *Electron. Engng* **39,** 318.

Bolic, S. M. (1960). 'Noise in the metal-oxide semiconductor transistor.' *Electron. Engng* **38,** 40.

Bracale, M. and Marsico, M. (1970). 'A photon-coupled amplifier for measuring and recording physiological signals.' *Med. biol. Engng* **8,** 103.

Bradley, W. E. (1953). 'The surface barrier transistor.' *Proc. Inst. Radio Engrs* **46,** 949.

Butler, F. (1963). 'Controlled rectifiers in stabilized power supplies.' *Wireless Wld* **69,** 480.

Chang, K. K. N. (1964). *Parametric and Tunnel Diodes*. Englewood Cliffs, N. J.: Prentice-Hall.

Chow, W. F. (1964). *Principles of Tunnel Diode Circuits*. New York: Wiley.

Cullis, R. (1965). 'Silicon field effect transistors.' *Electron. Engng* **37,** 606.

Duddridge, G. (1964). 'Silicon avalanche rectifiers.' *Electron. Engng* **36,** 247.

Finlay, D. J. (1966). 'The analysis and performance of transistor choppers.' *Electron. Engng* **38,** 572.

Fogel, L. G. (1963). *Biotechnology: Concepts and Applications*, p. 117. Englewood Cliffs, N.J.: Prentice-Hall.

Gibson, J. M., Gibson, M. M. and Hirsch, H. R. (1970). 'Distortion of neural data by "notch filters".' *Med. biol. Engng* **8,** 95.

Gosling, W. (1967). 'Amplifiers combining bipolar and field effect transistors.' *Electron. Engng* **39,** 478.

Gregory, N. L. and Lewin, J. E. (1962). 'A semi-conductor current amplifier.' *Electron. Engng* **34,** 155.

Grigson, C. W. B. (1964). 'Some precision direct coupled transistor amplifiers and their approximate design.' *Electron. Engng* **36,** 454.

Gutzwiller, F. W. (Ed.) (1961). *SCR Manual*. 2nd edn. New York: General Electric Co.

Hall, R. W. and Dunlop, C. W. (1950). '*p–n* junctions prepared by impurity diffusion.' *Phys. Rev.* **76,** 467.

Hastings, A. E. (1946). 'Analysis of a resistance–capacitance parallel-T network and application.' *Proc. Inst. Radio Engrs* **34,** 126P.

Hilbourne, R. A. and Miles, J. F. (1965). 'The metal-oxide-semiconductor transistor.' *Electron. Engng* **37,** 156.

Jones, E. L. (1963). *A Direct Coupled Amplifier Using Silicon Planar Transistors*. Application Note MK173X. Footscray: I.T.T. Ltd.

Kendall, J. T. (1963). 'The future of transistors.' *J. Inst. elect. Engrs* **9,** 508.

Kremer, H. (1954). 'The drift transistor.' *Arch. elekt. Ubertr.* **8,** 223.

Law, R. R., Mueller, C. W., Pankowe, J. I. and Armstrong, L. D. (1952). 'Developmental germanium *p–n–p* junction transistor.' *Proc. Inst. Radio Engrs* **40,** 1352.

Lowry, H. R., Giorgis, J., Gottlieb, E. and Weischedel, R. C. (1961). *General Electrode Tunnel Diode Manual*. New York: General Electric Co.

Mason, D. T. and Braunwald, E. (1963). 'A simplified plethysmographic system for the measurement of systemic arterial pressure and peripheral blood flow.' *Am. Heart J.* **64,** 796.

Miles, J. F. and Tumber, A. J. (1964). 'Simple voltage-reference circuit.' *Mullard tech. Commun.* **7,** 290.

Murari, B. (1967). 'ECG and EEG pre-amplifiers.' *Wld med. Electron.* **5,** 264.

Oberg, P. A., Persson, A. and Sjostrand, U. (1967). 'A high input impedance low-level d.c. amplifier utilizing a solid-state operational amplifier.' *J. scient. Instrum.* **44,** 870.

Pearson, G. L. and Foy, P. W. (1952). 'Silicon *p–n* junction diodes prepared by the alloying process.' *Phys. Rev.* **87,** 190.

Phillips, V. J. and Dunlop, J. (1969). 'A series shunt MOST chopper with complementary drive circuit.' *Electron. Engng* **41,** 29.

Richards, J. C. S. (1965). 'A d.c. differential amplifier using field effect transistors.' *Electron. Engng* **37,** 598.

Rigg, B. (1962). 'The characteristics and applications of Zener diodes.' *Electron. Engng* **34,** 736.

Shockley, W. (1952). 'A uni-polar field effect transistor.' *Proc. Inst. Radio Engrs* **40,** 1365.

Straub, G. F. (1958). 'A voltage variable capacitor.' *Electron. Inds, Philad.* **1,** 69.

Towers, T. D. (1968). 'How modern diffused silicon transistors and f.e.t.s are used to amplify d.c. low level currents and voltages.' *Wireless Wld* **74,** 269.

Van der Weide, H. and Van Bemmel, J. (1968). 'A photon coupled amplifier for the transmission of physiological signals.' *Med. biol. Engng* **6,** 447.

Verill, R. (1966). 'A very high input impedance chopper d.c. amplifier.' *Electron. Engng* **38,** 802.

Vierhout, R. R. and Vendrik, A. J. H. (1964). 'An electronic scanner for transistor pairs used in balanced pre-amplifiers.' *Electron. Engng* **36,** 630.

Wallmark, J. J. and Johnson, H. (1966). *Field Effect Transistors.* Englewood Cliffs, N.J.: Prentice-Hall.

Watson, J. (1966). *Semiconductor Circuit Design.* London: Hilger & Watts.

Webb, R. E. (1966). 'Field effect transistor for biological amplifiers.' *Electron. Engng* **37,** 803.

Yarker, C. A. (1962). 'A simplified assessment of transistor amplifier performance.' *Electron. Engng* **34,** 554.

Chapter 7

Operational Amplifiers

Operational amplifiers were originally developed for use in circuits designed to perform various mathematical functions such as addition, subtraction, differentiation and integration upon analogue signals. Analogue signals are continuous with time and are often proportional to some definite quantity such as a force or a velocity. Analogue computers continuously process the input analogue signals fed into them in order to perform the required computations and produce an analogue output signal which is proportional to the final result. This is in contrast to digital computers, which operate upon a set of discrete numerical values. An analogue-to-digital converter is used to sample an analogue input signal at a regular rate in order to produce a series of digital values which can be fed into digital instrumentation such as a digital computer.

Early operational amplifiers used discrete components in valve circuits. They were expensive and often were of the chopper amplifier type. The introduction of integrated circuit techniques has brought the price of operational amplifiers down to the region of £1 sterling for standard types. This has led to their almost universal use in low frequency circuitry and extended their application far beyond computing. In effect, they represent stable packages of gain, and it is far simpler and cheaper in most cases to use these modules rather than to design from scratch using discrete components.

Before proceeding with the applications of operational amplifiers, it is worth while to give something of the development of integrated circuits.

MONOLITHIC INTEGRATED CIRCUITS

The great strides made in recent years in the practical application of diffusion techniques to transistor construction have led to the development of monolithic integrated circuits. It is now possible to lay down a complete amplifier on a single chip of silicon. As an example, a complete high fidelity pre-amplifier and power amplifier can be produced on a chip of silicon 1·25 mm (0·05 in) square and 0·25 mm (0·01 in) thick. The chip contains 13 transistors (including two power types), two diodes, one Zener diode and 18 resistors, formed simultaneously in the silicon by a series of diffusions. The chip is encapsulated in a solid plastic package which holds a metal heat sink and the connecting pins. The maximum amplifier output is 5 W r.m.s. The main amplifier is d.c. coupled throughout, and complete freedom from thermal runaway is claimed due to the close thermal coupling between the output transistors and the bias diodes. Three transistors are used in the pre-amplifier and ten in the main amplifier.

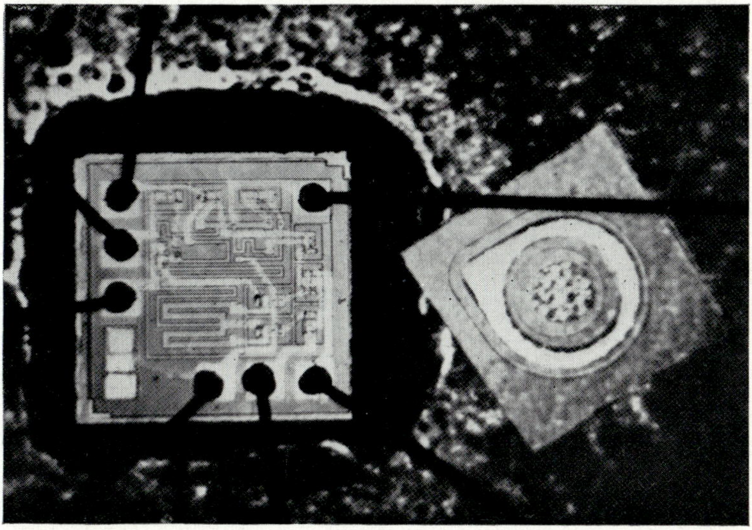

Figure 7.1. Comparison of the size of a first generation monolithic integrated circuit operational amplifier with that of a silicon planar transistor

(By courtesy of SGS-Fairchild Ltd.)

Essentially, integrated circuit operational amplifiers are high gain (typically 100,000 up to 8 kHz) differential input amplifiers having a low value of output impedance and the ability to have up to 100 per cent negative feedback applied over a stated frequency range without spurious oscillation occurring. It is usual to add the resistors forming the feedback network external to the integrated circuit, and this also applies in the more inexpensive amplifiers to the stabilizing capacitors. *Figure 7.1* compares a type BFY56 epitaxial silicon transistor with a type A702 completed integrated circuit operational amplifier.

As well as linear amplifiers, a wide range of logic circuits is available in integrated circuit form. Their availability has resulted in a dramatic reduction in the physical size of counting equipment used in departments of nuclear medicine, and also in the size of digital computers. These are now readily available in a 483 mm (19 in) rack format suitable for building into patient monitoring equipment.

THIN AND THICK FILM INTEGRATED CIRCUITS

The range of resistor values that can be laid down in a monolithic construction integrated circuit is limited to the lower values. A greater range is possible by means of the 'thin film' technique. In this case a ceramic substrate is used and the resistors are laid down on it by the controlled evaporation of a material such as Nichrome. An extension of this idea is the 'thick film' technique. This also allows for the deposition of conducting and insulating films to form capacitors. At present, an arbitrary subdivision exists which distinguishes thick film circuits (film thickness greater than 1,000 nm) from thin film circuits (film thickness less than 1,000 nm).

Thick film circuits are generally produced by a stencil screen printing process, line widths of 0·25 mm (0·01 in) or less being readily achievable. A number of processes have been employed in the production of thin film circuits, including deposition through masks made of metal, resin or an adherent inorganic substance. These are additive processes. Subtractive processes provide for deposition over the complete area followed by the removal of unwanted material by chemical or mechanical means, electron beam machining or spark erosion. Trimming is required in order to produce resistors to better than a 5 per cent tolerance.

In thick film circuits (Loasby, 1971), the materials used to provide the resistive, conductive and dielectric elements are delineated directly by the screen process. A choice of different resistivities is available, but the temperature stability of a thick film circuit is not so good as that of a thin film circuit. After firing, these materials effectively become an integral part of the substrate. This can consist of alumina, high temperature glass or mica. Resistor compositions consist of suspensions of noble metals or their oxides together with a glass frit in media suitable for screen printing. A new development is the use of ruthenium oxide. By a suitable choice of the glaze, film resistances of 100–300 Ω per square can be achieved for fired films 12,500 nm thick. Resistance tolerances of ±20 per cent are easily possible, whilst better than ±10 per cent can be attained under closely controlled conditions. A peak firing temperature of 580–650°C is recommended.

Materials for conductors have a similar composition to those used for resistors but have a higher metal content. Materials for dielectrics consist of pastes of high permittivity glass powder. The carefully controlled application of these materials to suitable substrates, followed by the appropriate firing in a continuous furnace to a closely controlled temperature profile, enables passive circuits to be produced. Active components (transistors) can be preformed into sub-assemblies to which the passive circuit substrate is attached. The availability of 'flip-chip' semiconductors without leads enables the direct attachment of active devices on to suitable contact regions in the passive circuit.

A flip-chip consists of a piece of silicon containing a transistor, a diode, a resistor or a combination of these. It is inverted and then bonded on to the circuit, sometimes a printed circuit board, without any encapsulation or wire bonds. The chips are usually provided with solder-dipped bonding pads and are fixed to a well fluxed circuit board merely by the controlled application of heat. In some cases, ultrasonic bonding is used in conjunction with aluminium contacts.

Capacitors for use with integrated circuits can take the form of additional discrete components, can be laid down (printed) by a thick film process, or can have a flake construction. Where substrate and package size permit, almost all types of small discrete capacitor can be used, providing that they can withstand the short-term stoving operation which is part of the encapsulation process. The most useful and popular components of this type are miniature tantalum capacitors. Flake capacitors are thin ceramic wafers which have two faces metallized. A suitable conductor pattern is laid down on the circuit substrate, to which one face of the capacitor is bonded. The top face of the capacitor must be connected via a wire link to the appropriate part of the circuit. Capacity values range from 20 to 4,700 pF, with a working voltage of 200 V as standard. Various types of dielectric are available from high stability to high permittivity ceramics.

Printed capacitors can be classified into two quite different types.

In the first, a predetermined area of conductor material is printed on both sides of the substrate, thus forming a capacitor whose capacitance is determined by the permittivity and area of the substrate. The second type is the printed glaze dielectric capacitor. A conducting electrode is first printed on to the substrate, followed by a layer of printed dielectric glaze and finally by the second electrode. A tolerance of 1–2 per cent is possible in the capacity range 20–50,000 pF.

Thin film circuits are used in the latest types of implanted cardiac pacemakers. In order to attain the required time constants, external capacitors are used with the thin film circuit. The whole of the circuitry can now be hermetically sealed in a metal case, which provides protection against the ingress of body fluids through the conventional epoxy resin encapsulation and also against damage which might result from a leakage of the mercury batteries used to power the pacemaker.

TERMINOLOGY

In order to clarify the position in regard to device construction, it is useful to consider the terms which are encountered in the literature.

Semiconductor Device Terminology

Base width—The separation between the emitter and collector regions of a transistor, typically 0·5–1·5 μm for a planar transistor.

Bipolar transistor—A conventional transistor containing *p–n–p* or *n–p–n* junctions as opposed to a field effect transistor.

Charge storage—The effect which enables a *p–n* junction to act as a capacitance, the depletion layer acting as a dielectric.

Depletion layer—The cross-over (junction region) where *p*-type material merges into *n*-type material. The junction does not contain many free holes or electrons due to the cancelling effect, and thus it has a high resistivity.

Dopant—A substance which, when added to a semiconductor such as silicon, will produce *n*-type or *p*-type material. Common *n*-type dopants are arsenic, antimony and phosphorus, while boron is a common *p*-type dopant.

Epitaxial growth—The deposition of a material, typically silicon, on to a substrate. Although the grown layer may differ in type or material from the substrate, it will follow the same crystal orientation.

Etching—Selective etching preferentially removes one material from a sandwich structure without affecting any other material.

Junction—The region between *p*-type and *n*-type material, which is deficient in holes and electrons and has rectifying properties.

Planar process—The planar process for fabricating semiconductor devices is based upon the use of a single surface for referencing each successive operation. It depends upon the repeated use of silicon dioxide from the surface to control the location of diffusions.

Integrated Circuit Terminology

Bonding (wire bonding)—The connection of very fine gold or aluminium wires to the ohmic contact areas of circuits and thence to the lead-out terminals of the package. Soldering can be used in thin film circuits, but thermal compression or ultrasonic welding is more common.

Dice bonding—The attachment of the dice or chip to the substrate or circuit board. Dice bonding is performed prior to wire bonding.

Bonding pads—Small area (typically of gold for thin film circuits and of aluminium for semiconductor integrated circuits) to which are bonded the fine lead-out wires.

Cermet—A combination of ceramic and metallic powders used in the manufacture of thin and thick film resistors.

Discrete components—Conventional circuit components having lead wires as opposed to integrated components.

Dual-in-line package—A popular form of package for integrated circuits. It has two rows of outlet leads separated by 7·5 mm (0·3 in). The leads in each row are in line and separated by 2·5 mm (0·1 in). This is compatible with 2·5 mm (0·1 in) matrix perforated circuit boards.

Fan-in—The number of inputs a logic gate can handle.

Fan-out—The number of stages a logic gate can drive.

Flat-pack—A very compact form of package for integrated circuits. One example is $\frac{1}{4}$ in (6·25 mm) square by $\frac{1}{16}$ in (1·56 mm) thick. The lead-out wires are located in the plane of the package and are designed for welding into a circuit.

Flip-chip—A piece of silicon containing a transistor, a diode, a resistor or a combination of these, designed to be inverted and bonded into a circuit.

Hybrid integrated circuit—A complex circuit fabricated from semiconductor integrated circuits together with thin film circuits. The integrated circuits may be in the form of flip-chips. Strictly speaking, film circuits are integrated, but the term is tending to be used specifically for semiconductor integrated circuits of the monolithic type.

Large-scale integration—The process of fabricating complex circuits by interconnecting adjacent circuits on a wafer of silicon to form larger circuits on a single substrate.

Monolithic integrated circuit—An integrated circuit in which all the components have been fabricated from a single piece of material.

MTBF (*mean time between failures*)—A term particularly used when referring to the reliability of integrated circuits.

Multi-chip circuits—As opposed to monolithic circuits, these are fabricated from several silicon chips each containing circuit elements. These chips may be flip-chips or may be interconnected by wire bonding.

Ohmic contact—A contact which does not have rectifying properties and obeys Ohm's law.

Probing—The testing of integrated circuits prior to wire bonding. Contact is made with the contact areas of the circuit via several small accurately positioned probes.

SCIC—Abbreviation for Semiconductor Integrated Circuit.

SIC—Abbreviation for Silicon Integrated Circuit—a circuit formed entirely on a silicon chip.

Thick film circuit—A circuit made by depositing paint by a silk screen process on to an insulating substrate and then burning off the organic material to leave a mineral component.

Thin film circuit—A circuit in which all the components have been made by depositing thin films of various kinds on to an insulating substrate.

INTEGRATED CIRCUIT OPERATIONAL AMPLIFIERS

Until the appearance of monolithic operational amplifiers in quantity production in the late 1960s, operational amplifiers had to be made from discrete components on the lines of the circuit shown in *Figure 7.2*. This uses positive and negative supply lines with a long-tailed pair balanced input stage followed by a second long-tailed pair which acts as a level shifter to return the single-ended output to a d.c. level of zero (Towers, 1971).

Figure 7.3 gives the circuit of the well-known Fairchild μA 709 amplifier introduced in 1965. This is more complex than the circuit of *Figure 7.2* because monolithic fabrication techniques had difficulty in producing directly the high value resistors and high gain transistors used in the discrete component amplifier. In *Figure 7.3* the input transistors Q_1 and Q_2 form a balanced long-tailed pair with a fixed 40 μA tail current provided by Q_{11}. This is biased as a constant

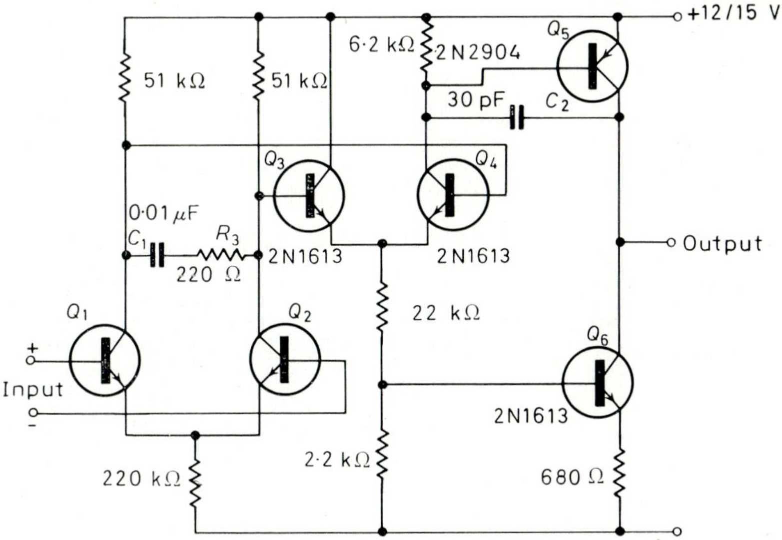

Figure 7.2. Discrete component operational amplifier
(Reproduced after Towers, 1971, by courtesy of the Editor of *Wireless World*)

current source by R_{11} and Q_{11}, which is connected as a diode and forward biased by the current through R_8 and R_{10}. A balanced output is taken from the collector resistors R_1 and R_2. Q_7, R_5, Q_3, R_3 and Q_{15} provide a balanced stabilization against both temperature and supply voltage changes. A single-ended output is taken from across R_2 and amplified by the Darlington pair Q_4 and Q_6. An output is taken from across R_6 and used to drive Q_8, which is an emitter follower. Q_8 controls, via the common base stage Q_9, the pre-output common emitter driver Q_{12}. The collector of Q_{12} is connected directly to the bases of the complementary symmetry class B output transistors Q_{13} and Q_{14}. A final output is taken from the common emitters of

Q_{13} and Q_{14}. The output d.c. level has been brought back to zero via Q_4, Q_6, Q_8, Q_9, Q_{12}, Q_{13} and Q_{14}.

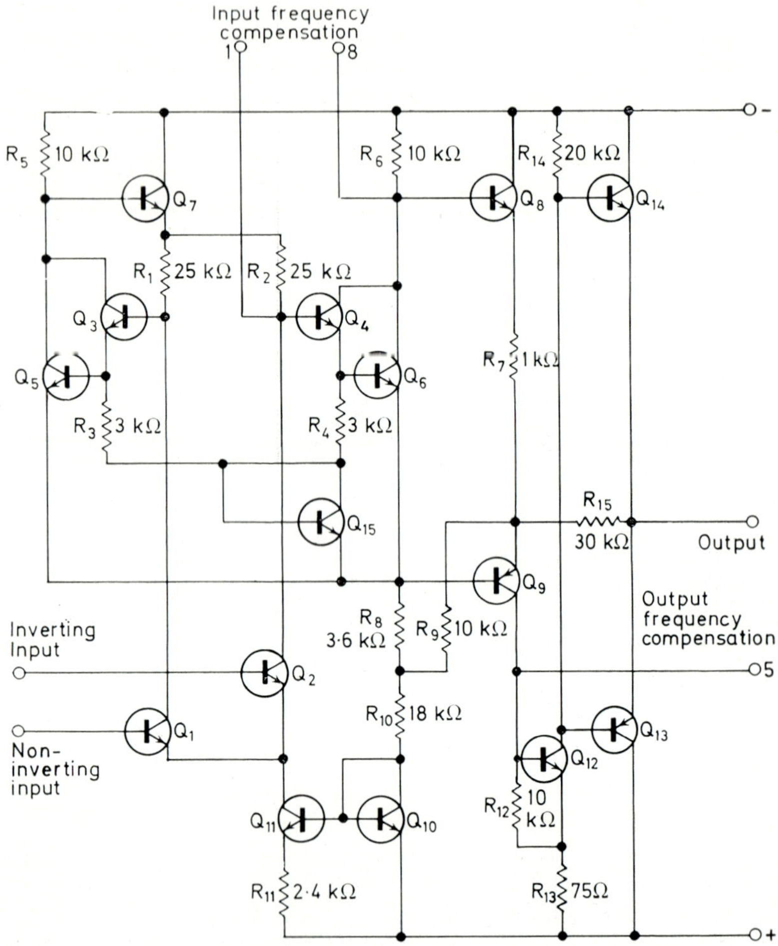

Figure 7.3. First generation monolithic amplifier—the μA 709

(By courtesy of SGS-Fairchild Ltd.)

In the discrete component amplifier of *Figure 7.2*, capacitors C_1 and C_2 act to limit the upper frequency response in order to prevent high frequency instability. In the amplifier of *Figure 7.3*, terminals 1, 8 and 5 are provided so that external capacitors may be connected.

Ideally, an operational amplifier should possess an infinite gain, zero input voltage and current offset, infinite input impedance, zero output impedance and zero response time (infinite bandwidth). In practice, at ±15 V supply and 25° C, the μA 709 has typically an open loop d.c. voltage gain of 50,000, an offset voltage (10 kΩ source resistance) of 2 mV, input offset current of 100 nA, a differential input resistance of 250 kΩ, an output resistance of 150 Ω, and output voltage available swing of ±12 V with a 10 kΩ load and a common mode rejection ratio of 90 db. This type of amplifier has been very widely used and a lot of thought went into its design. A non-Darlington differential input pair of transistors is preferred to a Darlington input since it has a lower sensitivity to temperature changes and a lower offset. The input stage has to be operated at low values of collector current but without the need for high value resistors, since these do not accord with integrated circuit manufacturing techniques. A constant current source is provided for Q_1 and Q_2 by the combination of Q_{11} and Q_{10}, which is connected as a diode. The method is based upon imposing the emitter–base voltage of the diode-connected transistor across the emitter–base junction of the second transistor Q_{11} (*Figure 7.4*). If the two transistors

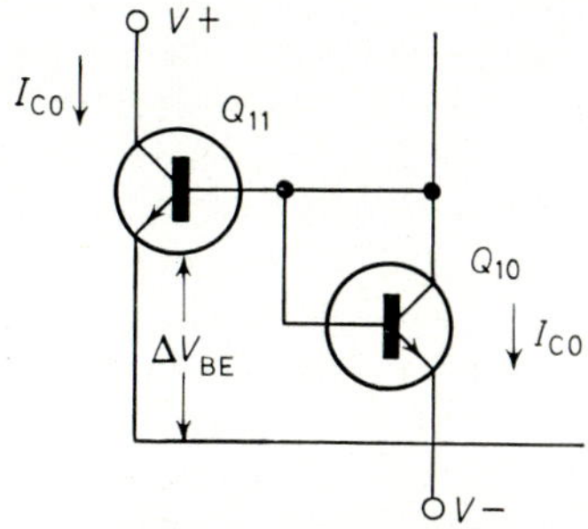

Figure 7.4. A current source for generating a very small current using moderate value resistors
(By courtesy of SGS-Fairchild Ltd.)

are identical, the two collector currents will be equal and the current drawn from the current source is determined by the supply voltage and resistor R_1.

In discussing this design, SGS-Fairchild Ltd. (1967) point out that if Q_{10} is operated with a collector current of 1 mA, then Q_{11} can be run at a stable collector current of 10 μA by arranging an emitter–base voltage difference of 120 mV between the two transistors at room temperature. This is obtained by placing a 12 kΩ resistor in the emitter lead of Q_{11}. A number of other interesting techniques are employed in the complete amplifier, and readers are referred to SGS-Fairchild Ltd. (1967).

Towers (1971) records that in practice this type of amplifier was found to possess certain disadvantages. The input resistance of 50 kΩ was rather low, the amplifier was liable to damage if the output was short-circuited, the quiescent current consumption of 2·5 mA was too large, and at least two external compensation capacitors were required to stop oscillation under open loop conditions. The next improvement in this first generation type of amplifier was to provide a diffused internal frequency compensation capacitor. This was followed by second generation circuits which had an order of magnitude improvement in bias and offset currents. Both bipolar and field effect transistors are used in a complete amplifier, together with components such as lateral *p–n–p* transistors and 'pinch' resistors which have developed as a result of integrated circuit technology. Pinch resistors make available resistance values of up to 100 kΩ by means of a technique which reduces or 'pinches' the cross-sectional area of a conventional diffused resistor by means of an emitter diffusion on top of it. Towers (1971) states that whereas the first generation amplifiers had input bias and offset currents of 1,500 nA and 500 nA maximum, the corresponding values for the second generation had been reduced to 250 nA and 20 nA respectively. By 1970, a third generation of amplifier technology had succeeded in reducing the values by yet another order of magnitude to 2 nA and 0·2 nA maximum respectively.

The achievement of these small current values arises from the use of 'super-gain' or 'punch-through' transistors at the input of the amplifier. The current gain of an *n–p–n* transistor in a monolithic circuit depends partly upon the length of time allowed for the diffusion of the emitter during the fabrication process. If the diffusion is carried on for an unusually long time, current gains of 4,000 can be obtained but at the expense of a low collector breakdown voltage, perhaps 4 V. A pair of super-gain transistors are used as the input transistors and each is operated in a cascode arrangement with a conventional transistor which protects it from voltage breakdown. The super-gain transistors are operated with an almost zero collector–base voltage. Their use makes possible input impedances of the order of 30 MΩ compared with 50 kΩ for the first generation, a voltage gain of 94 db minimum compared with 84 db, a common mode rejection ratio of 80 db minimum compared with 65 db, and a reduction in supply current from 2·5 to 0·15 mA.

Figure 7.5 gives an example of a circuit for use with super-gain integrated circuits which is due to Widlar (1969). Basically, a high gain 'primary' transistor is operated in a common emitter configuration driving a common base 'secondary' transistor which has a high breakdown voltage. This cascode arrangement provides the output

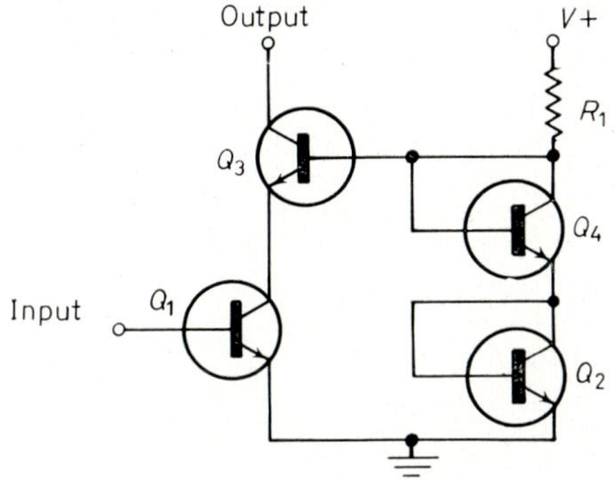

Figure 7.5. Protective circuit for use with super-gain transistors

(Reproduced after Widlar, 1969, by courtesy of the National Semiconductor Corporation, Santa Clara, California)

voltage capability of the secondary transistor but has retained the high current gain of the primary transistor. Although additional transistors are required, this presents no problems in the manufacture of the integrated circuit. In *Figure 7.5* the secondary transistors are depicted with a wider base than the primary transistors.

APPLICATIONS OF OPERATIONAL AMPLIFIERS

For many purposes, one side of the amplifier's input and output is common to earth (*Figure 7.6a*). In this case, the earth line is usually omitted from the diagram as shown in *Figure 7.6b*.

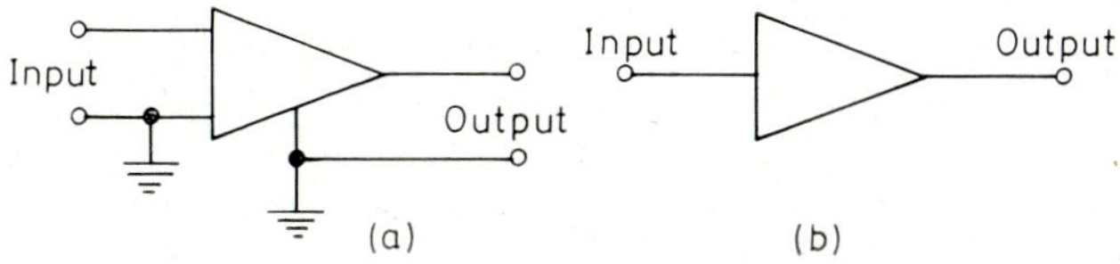

Figure 7.6

Suppose that the maximum output voltage of the amplifier is deliberately limited to 10 V and that the gain is 50,000. Because of this, the input terminal of the amplifier cannot differ from earth by more than (10/50,000) = 0·2 mV. For the majority of applications this is sufficiently small to be neglected and the input terminal can be considered to be at earth potential. It is said to constitute a 'virtual earth' since it is not physically connected to earth. The input terminal of the amplifier is the base connection of one of the pair of input transistors forming the input differential stage. In the following discussion it will be referred to as the amplifier input in order to distinguish it from the stage input, which is the input to the complete operational amplifier stage. The use of various external components with operational amplifiers will now be described.

Unity Gain Inverter

In *Figure 7.7*, two resistors R_i and R_{fb} are connected respectively to the amplifier input and from the amplifier output to its input.

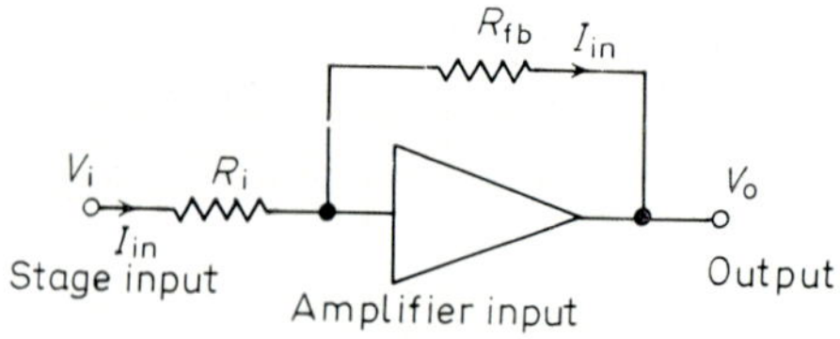

Figure 7.7. The use of an operational amplifier as a unity gain inverter

R_{fb} is a feedback resistor. Let the value of each resistor be 1 MΩ and a d.c. voltage of +5 V be applied to the input of the stage. Since the potential at the amplifier input is effectively zero, a current of $5/10^6$ A, i.e. 5 μA, will flow from left to right through the input resistor R_i. Since the operational amplifier is designed to draw a negligible input current, it is clear that a current of 5 μA must also flow through R_{fb}. The value of R_{fb} is also 5 MΩ, so that the potential of the amplifier output must be −5 V with respect to the amplifier input, that is, −5 V with respect to earth. If this were not so, the amplifier input would change its potential slightly, causing the amplifier to amplify, until the condition was satisfied. In the simple situation described, the output voltage is the inverse of the input voltage to the stage, that is, the stage is acting as a unity gain inverter.

It is often necessary to introduce a stage of sign reversal when several operational amplifiers have to be connected in series as in an analogue computer.

Summer

A useful extension to the simple inverter stage is obtained by providing a number of inputs to the stage as shown in *Figure 7.8*. Let +5 V be applied to the first input and +3 V to the second. The total input current is now 8 μA, so that the potential of the output

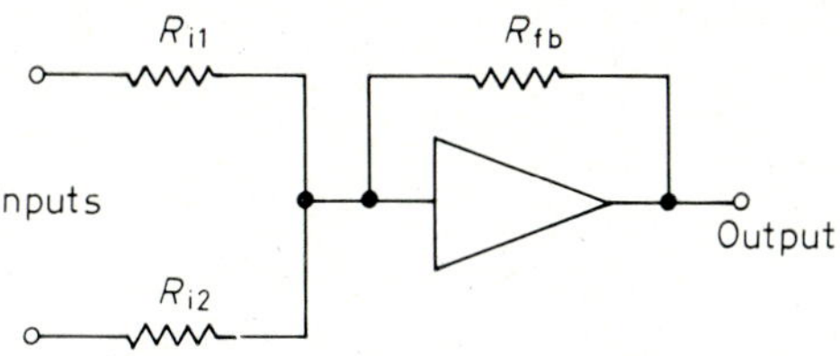

Figure 7.8. The use of an operational amplifier as an equal gain summer

terminal becomes −8 V. The output voltage is now the inverse of the sum of the input voltages. If the second input had been −3 V instead of +3 V, the current in that input resistor would have been reversed, causing the output voltage to become −2 V. Thus the output from such a 'summer' is equal to the inverse of the algebraic sum of the inputs. In general, $V_{out} = -(V_1 + V_2 + \ldots V_n)$.

The various input signals can be added in different proportions by suitably adjusting the values of the input resistors (*Figure 7.9*).

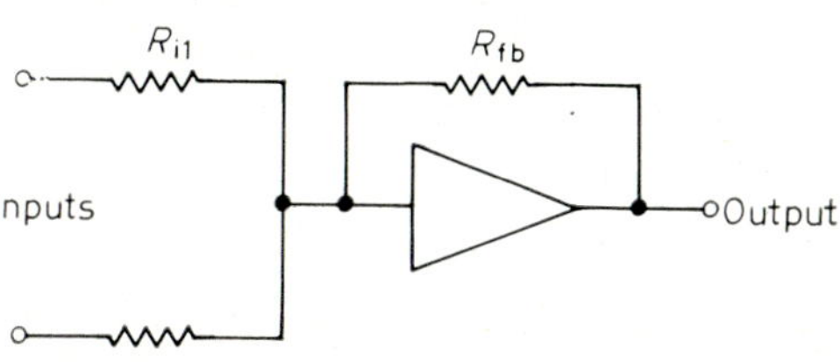

Figure 7.9. Summing circuit with different gains

Suppose that $V_1 = V_2$, then the current flowing in the second input resistor must be ten times that flowing in the first. Hence $V_{out} = (V_1 + 10V_2)$. When a number of input resistors are used, the point at which they are joined and connected to the input terminal of the amplifier is known as the Summing Junction.

Referring to *Figure 7.9*, the amplifier is used to provide an inverted output, so that $V_{out} = -I_{in}R_{fb} = -V_{in}(R_{fb}/R_I)$, so that the effective closed loop gain of the amplifier is $V_{out}/V_{in} = -R_{fb}/R_{in}$. Neglecting effects due to stray capacity, the input impedance $Z_{in} = V_{in}/I_{in} = V_{in}/(V_{in}/R_{in}) = R_{in}$. The output impedance must be approximately zero, since if V_{out} were not determined solely by the feedback components, a voltage which was not zero would appear at the virtual earth point at the amplifier input, and this is not permissible with the basic assumptions that have been made for the circuit operation.

Voltage Follower

When the output of the operational amplifier is connected directly back to the input (the inverting input of the amplifier) the circuit functions as a voltage follower. Since the input current to the amplifier is almost zero, the gain of the circuit is almost unity, hence the output voltage follows changes in the input voltage. Because of the very small input current, the input impedance is high, whilst since the two amplifier input terminals are almost at the same potential, the output impedance is very small. *Figure 7.10*

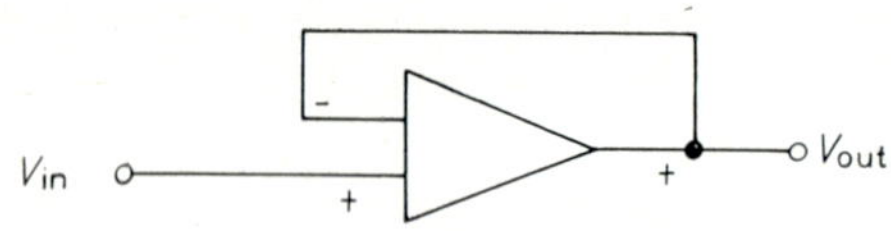

Figure 7.10. The use of an operational amplifier as a voltage follower

shows the arrangement. It is widely used as an impedance converter when a high input and a low output impedance are required, perhaps for driving a long cable to some distant equipment.

Non-inverting Amplifier

In this case the input signal is applied to the non-inverting input

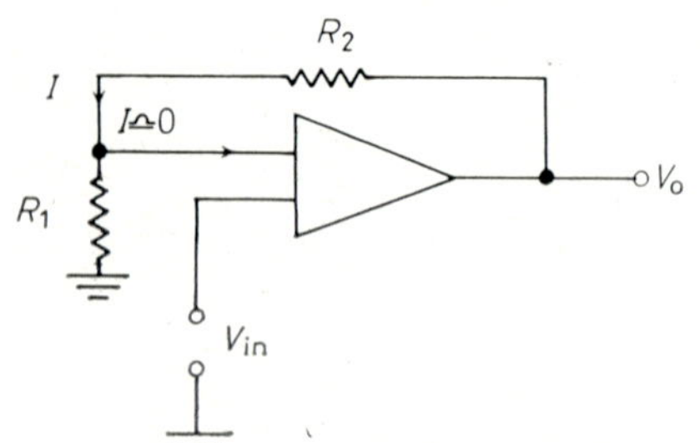

Figure 7.11. The use of an operational amplifier as a non-inverting amplifier

of the amplifier. Since it is a differential amplifier, it will set itself up so that the voltage difference between the inverting and non-inverting inputs is almost zero. Under these conditions, $V_{R_1}=V_{in}$ and $I_{R_1}=V_{in}/R_1$. $V_{R_2}=I_{R_1}R_2=V_{in}(R_2/R_1)$. $V_{out}=V_{R_1}+V_{R_2}=V_{in}(1+(R_2/R_1)$ (*Figure 7.11*).

Integrator

Referring to *Figure 7.12*, it is seen that the feedback resistor which has been used previously has now been replaced by a capacitor. Assume that the circuit is fed with only one, positive, input signal.

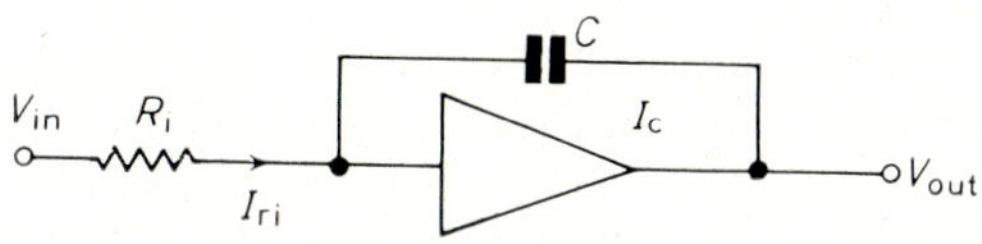

Figure 7.12. Operational amplifier integrator circuit

For a given value of the input resistor, a certain constant input current will flow, and this must also flow in the feedback path since the amplifier draws a negligible input current. Since the feedback capacitor is now charged by a constant current, its charge will increase at a uniform rate, and so will the potential difference developed across it. As the summing junction side of the capacitor is held at the virtual earth potential, it follows that the output voltage will increase negatively at a constant rate. Let Q be the charge contained in the capacitor C, then the voltage appearing across it will be $V=Q/C$ and the charging current will be $I=\mathrm{d}Q/\mathrm{d}t$. Differentiating with respect to time, $\mathrm{d}V/\mathrm{d}t=(1/C).(\mathrm{d}Q/\mathrm{d}t)=I/C=V_{in}/R_1C$. Integrating,

$$V=\int_0^t \mathrm{d}V/\mathrm{d}t=\int_0^t V_1/R_1C=K\int_0^t V_1.$$

Thus the output voltage is proportional to the integral with respect to time of the input voltage. The constant of proportionality is $K=1/R_1C$, where the product of the input resistor (MΩ) and the feedback capacitor (μF) is equal to the time constant of the integrator in seconds. Typically, an integrator stage in an analogue computer might be provided with switched capacitors in order to give time constants of 1, 0·1 and 0·01 seconds. If a time constant of one second is chosen and an input of +1 V applied to the integrator, the output will become increasingly negative at a rate of one volt per second.

Unless otherwise stopped, the fall in the output voltage will cease when the maximum amplifier excursion is reached.

Setting the Initial Conditions for an Integrator

In a practical integrator, it is often necessary to make provision for starting integration with the integrating capacitor already containing a certain amount of charge. In effect this corresponds to a constant of integration. After the integration has been performed, it is necessary to reset the integrator, and this is done by switching it into the 'Reset' mode. The circuit is now effectively connected as a unity gain summing amplifier, the capacitor being connected across the feedback resistor. An initial condition voltage applied to the input of the integrator gives rise to a similar voltage of opposite polarity at the output terminal. As a result, the capacitor is charged to this voltage before the integration commences. A 'Set initial condition' potentiometer allows the appropriate initial condition voltage to be obtained. By disconnecting the input resistor from the summing junction, the integrator is placed in a 'Hold' mode. The effect now is that the charge held in the integrating capacitor is stored. Thus the output voltage is held at the value which obtained at the instant of switching the mode from 'Integrate' to 'Hold'. The low input current requirements of good operational amplifiers make it feasible to store analogue signal voltages in this way.

Differentiation

Figure 7.13 illustrates an operational amplifier arranged to generate an output voltage which is proportional to the differential with respect to time of the input voltage. A capacitor is connected between

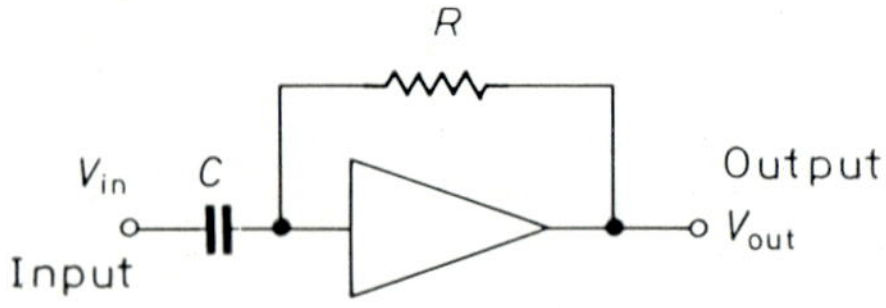

Figure 7.13. Operational amplifier differentiator circuit

the input to the differentiator and the amplifier input, whilst a feedback resistor is connected between the inverting input of the amplifier and the output.

Suppose that the input voltage V_{in} is suddenly increased by an amount dV_{in}. This will produce a flow of charge dQ/dt into the capacitor C during the time interval dt. Then $dV/dt = 1/C.(dQ/dt) = I/C$ where I is the current flowing. This also flows in the feedback resistor. The corresponding output voltage change is $-V_{out} = I.R = RC(dV/dt)$. The product RC is the differentiating time constant. Since the output from a differentiator is proportional to the time rate of change of the input voltage, the arrangement will obviously favour the more rapidly changing components of the input signal. Thus any transient noise spikes present will give rise to marked artefact components at the output. For this reason, differentiating circuits need to be used with care and are usually followed by a filter to limit the effective bandwidth.

Angelakos (1964) describes the use of semiconductor pressure micro-transducers for the measurement of intraventricular pressures. The output signal from the transducer is differentiated once to give an output proportional to the blood velocity and then a second time to yield an output proportional to the blood acceleration. A differentiator is also used to give the rate of change of left ventricular pressure as a step in the calculation of the Isometric Time Tension Index for monitoring changes occurring in the myocardial contractility (Ty Smith, 1969). Differentiators are also employed as part of circuits for identifying the occurrence of the R-waves in an electrocardiogram.

The Use of an Operational Amplifier as a Perfect Rectifier

Sandman (1969) describes the use of an operational amplifier to form a 'perfect rectifier' as in *Figure 7.14*. When the input goes negative, the output voltage becomes positive and diode D_2 conducts.

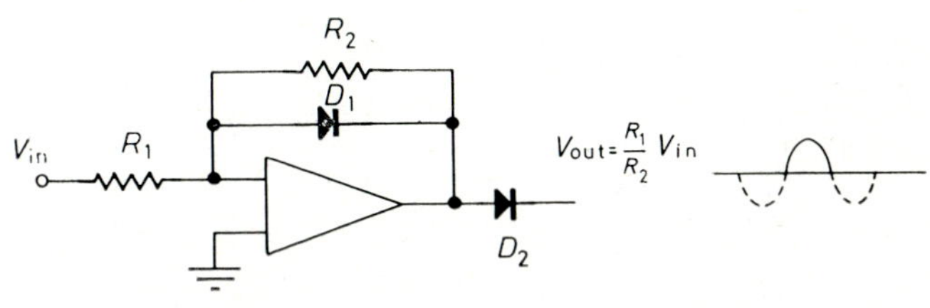

Figure 7.14. The use of an operational amplifier as a 'perfect' rectifier

(Reproduced after Sandman, 1969, by courtesy of the Editor of *World Medical Instrumentation*)

The voltage drop (approximately 0·5 V) developed across it is absorbed by the effect of the amplifier gain. D_1 is non-conducting under these conditions. However, when the input goes positive, D_2 cuts off and the output falls to zero. The fact that D_1 now conducts is an essential feature, since if it did not, the inverting input of the amplifier would swing violently away from zero and the output would go positive via R_2.

The Use of an Operational Amplifier as a Perfect Switch

The circuit of *Figure 7.15* (Sandman, 1969) acts as a closed switch for negative inputs and an open switch for positive inputs when transistor Q_1 is OFF. It is possible to switch the circuit OFF for all inputs by arranging to drive Q_1 hard ON. When this occurs, the 200 mV across Q_1 means that the 0·5 V required to make D_2 conduct is not available. Provided the inverting input to the amplifier

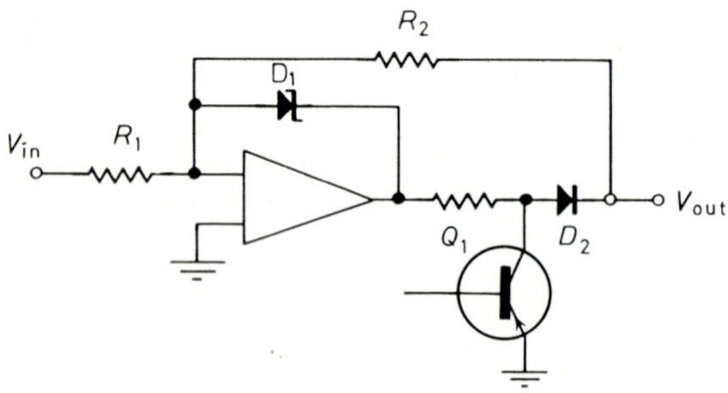

Figure 7.15. The use of an operational amplifier as a 'perfect' switch

(Reproduced after Sandman, 1969, by courtesy of the Editor of *World Medical Instrumentation*)

is maintained at a virtual earth, no output will appear. The Zener diode D_1 conducts when Q_1 is ON and maintains the virtual earth condition by preventing the amplifier output from being overloaded.

THE FREQUENCY COMPENSATION OF OPERATIONAL AMPLIFIERS

The Possibility of Oscillation

In general, the gain of an amplifier in which a fraction β of the output signal is fed back to the input as negative feedback is given by open loop gain/(1 + closed loop gain). The gain with negative feedback is reduced when the closed loop gain is positive. However, the gain with negative feedback becomes infinite if the loop gain

Aβ becomes equal to −1. When this occurs, the phase shift through the amplifier will be 180 degrees. The amplifier now supplies its own input even if the external input is zero. The system is thus self-sustaining and will oscillate continuously at the frequency for which the gain becomes −1. In spite of the original negative feedback connection, the effect now is to change the negative feedback into positive feedback. In order for a negative feedback operational amplifier to be conditionally stable at all frequencies within a stated range, it is necessary that the gain with negative feedback should not approach −1 too closely. The magnitude of the modulus of the loop gain when the phase shift is 180 degrees provides a 'gain margin' criterion, i.e. gain margin (g.m.)=20 $\log_{10}$ $(1/|A\beta|)$/db. The gain margin provides an indication of the amount by which the loop can be permitted to increase before oscillations occurred. The phase margin provides another criterion of stability. It has the value of 180 degrees minus the phase shift of the open loop amplifier when the open loop gain is unity.

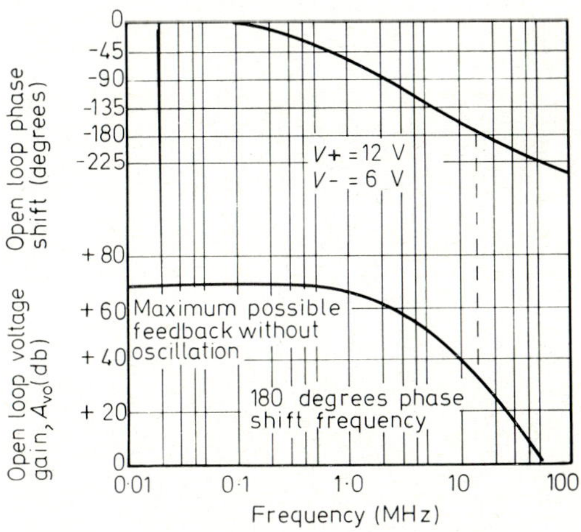

Figure 7.16. Typical open loop gain and phase shift characteristics for the μA 702A operational amplifier

(By courtesy of SGS-Fairchild Ltd.)

It is usual to plot the frequency response characteristic of an amplifier on a decibel–log frequency diagram. If the slope of the diagram is 6 db per octave, the loop phase shift cannot exceed 90 degrees, so that instability cannot occur. By limiting the slope of the diagram it can be ensured that an excessive amount of phase shift cannot occur. For example, the slope might be limited to 10 db per octave, corresponding to a maximum phase shift of 150 degrees. A fall of 12 db per octave corresponds to a phase shift of 180 degrees. One possibility is to include a phase advance circuit in series with the loop in order to reduce the slope of the db–log frequency plot over a particular frequency range. The critical point for stability occurs where the db–log frequency plot passes through zero, i.e. where the loop gain passes through unity. If the phase shift is here less than 180 degrees, there is a phase margin and the system is stable.

The open loop gain and phase responses of the Fairchild μA 702A operational amplifier are given in *Figure 7.16*. It is seen that

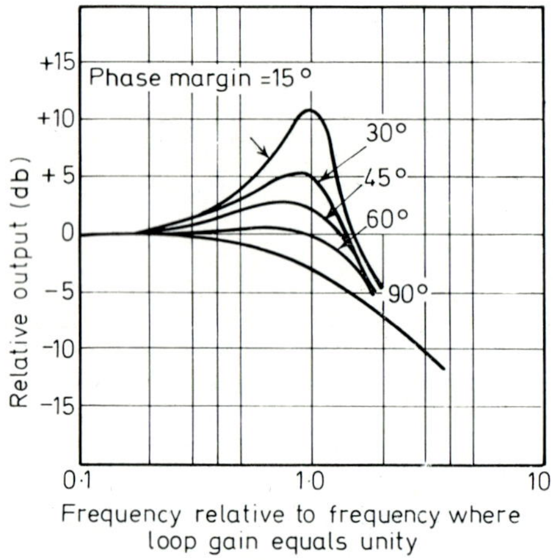

Figure 7.17. Peaking in the closed loop response of the μA 702A amplifier for various phase margins

(By courtesy of SGS-Fairchild Ltd.)

the gain falls off at the 0·8 MHz first breakpoint with a slope of approximately 6 db per octave. There is a second breakpoint at approximately 4 MHz, followed by a third at 40 MHz. The 180 degrees phase shift frequency is approximately 14 MHz, corresponding to a gain of approximately 34 db. Thus not more than 34 db of negative feedback can be applied at this frequency without oscillation starting. As has been previously mentioned, in practice this much feedback could not be applied since the 180 degrees phase criterion becomes exceeded by small deviations in the amplifier or external circuitry. Phase margins of less than 90 degrees will give rise to peaking in the closed loop response at that frequency for which the loop gain becomes unity (*Figure 7.17*). This arises because $(1+A\beta)$ becomes less than unity due to phase shift in $A\beta$. A satisfactory phase margin would be 45 degrees, giving less than 3 db peaking. This means that only 20 db of feedback can be applied to the basic μA 702A amplifier.

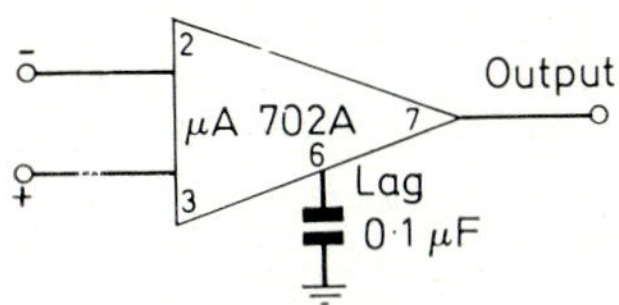

Figure 7.18. The use of a simple capacitor lag frequency compensation

(By courtesy of SGS-Fairchild Ltd.)

The amplifier frequency and phase response are limited by internal capacitances, so that the only practical way to increase the amount of feedback which can be used is deliberately to limit the amount of phase shift which can occur by adding additional components to the amplifier. The simplest technique is to shunt some signal point in the circuit to earth by means of a single relatively large capacitor.

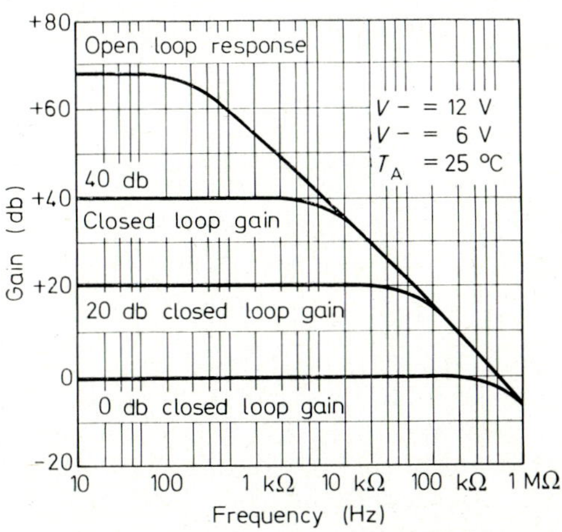

Figure 7.19. Frequency response of the μA 702A amplifier with a simple lag compensation

(By courtesy of SGS-Fairchild Ltd.)

If the reduction in gain due to this capacitor starts at a sufficiently low frequency, the loop gain can fall to unity at a frequency below that at which other circuit components produce additional phase shift. The maximum phase shift produced by a single R–C network is 90 degrees, so that the circuit cannot become unstable.

The connection of a 0·1 μF capacitor between the base of one of the output transistors of the μA 702A and earth is shown in *Figure 7.18*. This is known as a simple Lag Compensation. The capacitor attenuates the high frequency signal components and produces the required roll-off in response. *Figure 7.19* shows the effect for various closed loop gains. Maximum negative feedback over wide bandwidth can be obtained by using the natural roll-off with frequency of the amplifier to provide part of the compensation. The series R–C compensation network (*Figure 7.20*) produces a roll-off

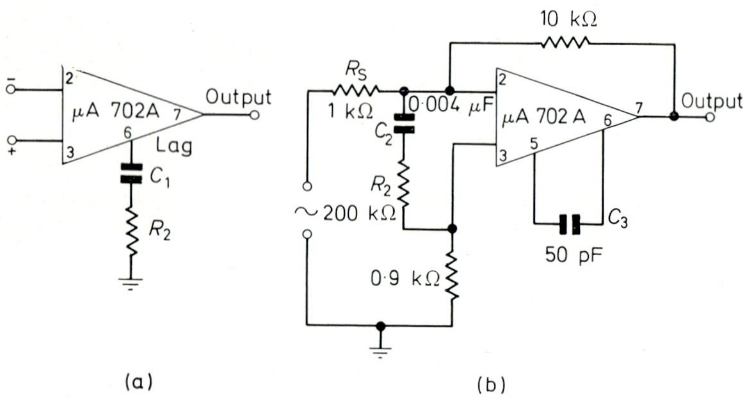

Figure 7.20. Compensation for maximum bandwidth using a lag network

(By courtesy of SGS-Fairchild Ltd.)

which starts at a lower frequency and breaks into the natural roll-off of the amplifier. The amplifier's internal roll-off then provides the additional attenuation required to ensure that at unity there is an adequate phase margin. This is illustrated in *Figure 7.21*.

A significant disadvantage of placing frequency compensation components near the output of an amplifier lies in the fact that now the maximum high frequency output swing is reduced. The latest types of monolithic integrated circuit operational amplifiers incorporate the frequency compensation components in the circuit, the capacitors being sited in the centre of the chip.

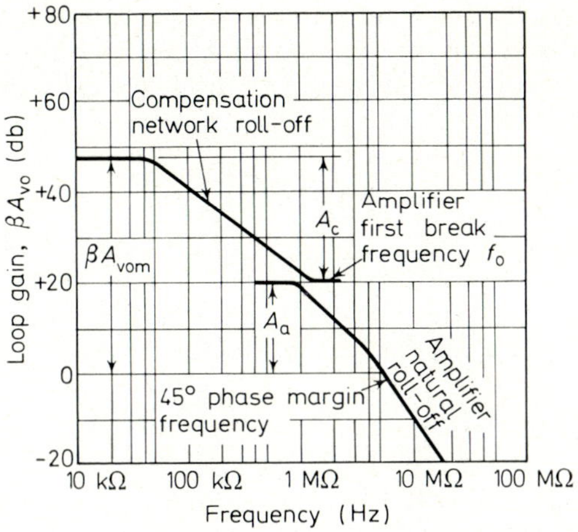

Figure 7.21. The lag network roll-off breaking out into the amplifier's natural roll-off

(By courtesy of SGS-Fairchild Ltd.)

THE USE OF AN OPERATIONAL AMPLIFIER WITH A D.C. BRIDGE CIRCUIT

It is convenient to use operational amplifiers to amplify the out-of-balance voltage generated by d.c. bridge circuits, typically from an unbonded strain gauge type of blood pressure transducer, for

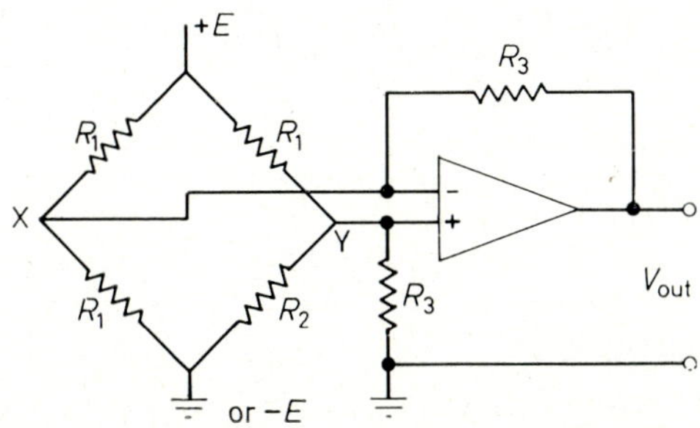

Figure 7.22. The use of an operational amplifier with a bridge circuit having an earthed or floating supply

example the well-known P23 series. Clayton (1969) describes various circuits suitable for use with the bridge energizing voltage earthed or floating (*Figure 7.22*). The action of the operational amplifier is to maintain the corners X and Y of the bridge network at the same potential by supplying the current required to balance the bridge. Assuming that negative supply for the bridge is earthed, then summing the currents at point X gives

$$\frac{E-V_x}{R_1}-\frac{V_x}{R_1}+\frac{V_{out}-V_x}{R_3}=0.$$

For point Y,

$$\frac{E-V_y}{R_1}-\frac{V_y}{R_2}=0.$$

At balance, $V_x=V_y$, and if $R_2=R_1\,(1+\beta)$,
then

$$V_{out}=E\beta\frac{R_3}{R_1}\beta\;\frac{1}{(1+\beta)\,[1+(R_1/R_3)]+1}$$

THE USE OF AN OPERATIONAL AMPLIFIER AS A PHASE-INVERTING A.C. AMPLIFIER

Referring to *Figure 7.23*, the capacitor C blocks any d.c. level from reaching the input. The gain of the amplifier is equal to R_{fb}/R_I with the gain 3 db down at a frequency equal to $1/(2CR_i)$. The upper

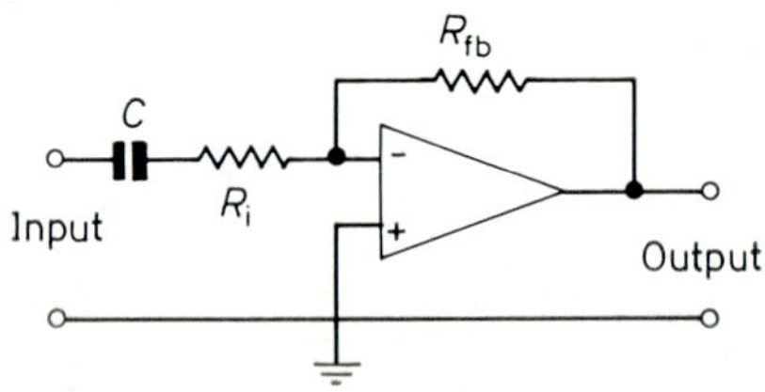

Figure 7.23. Phase-inverting a.c. operational amplifier circuit

frequency bandwidth for the amplifier will be dependent upon the loop gain and the extent to which the open loop frequency response has been compensated.

THE USE OF AN OPERATIONAL AMPLIFIER AS A NON-INVERTING A.C. AMPLIFIER

The input resistance of the circuit (*Figure 7.24*) is R_i and this provides a path for d.c. bias. The gain is $(1+R_{fb}/R_2)$, and the lower 3 db point of the frequency response is set by the shorter of the time constants R_2C_2 and R_iC_i. It is possible to raise the effective value of the input impedance by bootstrapping R_i as shown in *Figure 7.25*. Positive feedback is applied to the end of R_i via R_{FB}, C_2 and R_2.

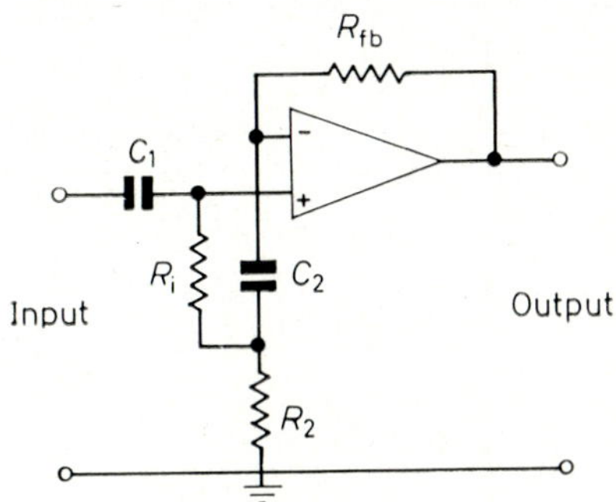

Figure 7.24. Non-inverting a.c. operational amplifier circuit

The low potential end of R_i is thus driven with a potential which is in phase with, and almost the same amplitude as, the output signal. The gain is $(1+R_{FB}/R_2)$ and the effective input impedance is raised by a factor equal to the ratio of the open loop gain to the closed loop gain.

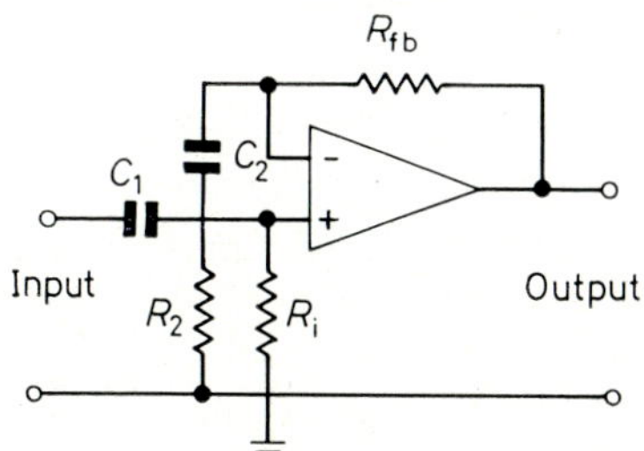

Figure 7.25. Bootstrapped high input impedance a.c. operational amplifier circuit

A FREQUENCY SELECTIVE OPERATIONAL AMPLIFIER CIRCUIT

The circuit shown in *Figure 7.26* is an inverting amplifier with a frequency selective twin-T network placed in the feedback path. At the tuned frequency, the impedance of the network is at a

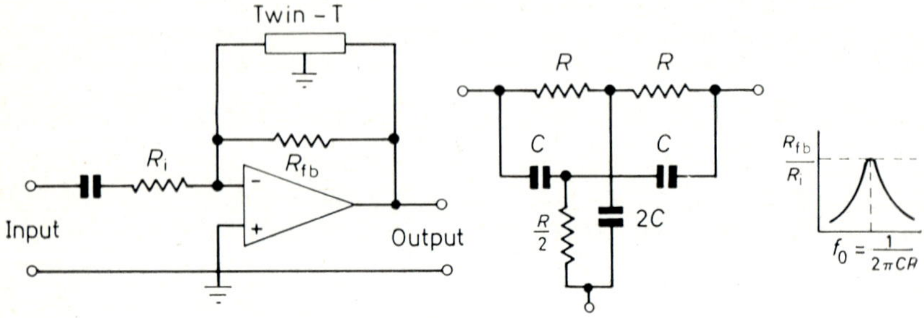

Figure 7.26. Frequency selective operational amplifier circuit

maximum, so that the negative feedback is at a minimum and the gain peaks as shown.

TERMS USED IN OPERATIONAL AMPLIFIER PRACTICE

Input offset voltage—The voltage which must be applied between the two input terminals to obtain a zero output voltage.

Input offset current—The difference between the current flowing into the two input terminals when the output voltage is zero.

Input bias current—The average of the two input currents.

Input voltage range—The range of voltage which can be applied to either input terminal for the amplifier to work normally.

Input common mode rejection ratio—The ratio of the input voltage range to the maximum change in the input offset voltage over this range.

Large-signal voltage gain—The ratio of the maximum output voltage swing across a load to the change in input voltage required to drive the output voltage from zero to that value.

Latch-up—The saturation of an input transistor via the feedback network due to a large output voltage swing. The inverting input now acts as a non-inverting input, positive feedback results and the amplifier latches up in this condition.

Output voltage swing—The peak output voltage swing, referred to earth, which can be obtained without clipping.

Output resistance—The resistance measured looking back into the output with the output voltage zero.

Power consumption—The d.c. power supply consumption required to operate the amplifier when the output voltage is zero and no load current.

Slew rate—The output response for a full output swing; it is the maximum slope of the rate of change of the output voltage and is usually quoted under the condition of unity gain, in volts per microsecond.

Supply voltage rejection ratio—The ratio of the change in input offset voltage to the change in supply voltage producing it.

Transient response—The closed loop step function response of the amplifier under small-signal conditions.

REFERENCES

Angelakos, E. T. (1964). 'Semiconductor pressure micro-transducers for measuring velocity and acceleration of intraventricular pressures.' *Am. J. med. Electron.* **3,** 226.

Clayton, G. B. (1969). 'Operational amplifiers—application.' *Wireless Wld* **76,** 270.

Loasby, R. G. (1971). 'The development of thick film technology.' *Physics Bull.* **22,** 76.

Sandman, A. (1969). 'Practical operational amplifiers.' *Wld med. Instrum.* **7,** 20.

SGS-Fairchild Ltd. (1967). *The Application of Linear Microcircuits,* 2nd edn. London: SGS-Fairchild Ltd.

Towers, T. D. (1971). 'Elements of linear microcircuits. 4. Three generations of operational amplifiers.' *Wireless Wld* **76,** 23.

Ty Smith, N. (1969). 'Cardiac function evaluation.' In *Techniques in Clinical Physiology,* p. 125. Ed. by J. W. Bellville and C. S. Weaver. London: Collier-Macmillan.

Widlar, R. J. (1969). *Super Gain Transistors for Integrated Circuits.* Data Sheet TF11. Santa Clara, California: National Semiconductor Corporation.

Chapter 8

Oscillators

PRINCIPLES OF OSCILLATORS

The basic operating principle of a feedback oscillator for generating a sinusoidal output signal is shown in *Figure 8.1*. Suppose that an alternating voltage of magnitude v volts r.m.s. is applied to the input of a linear amplifier having a voltage gain A_v. The output of the

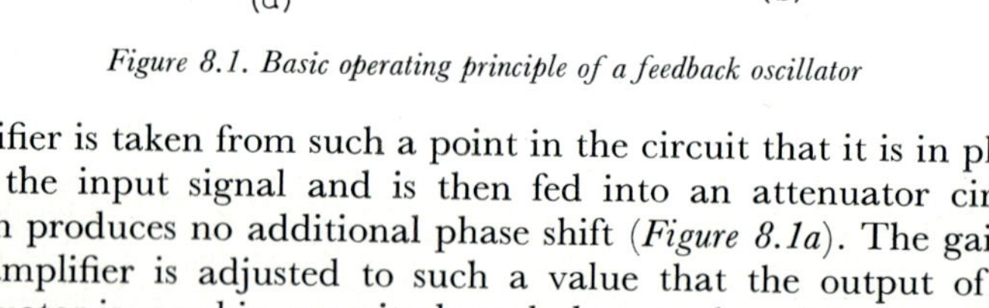

Figure 8.1. Basic operating principle of a feedback oscillator

amplifier is taken from such a point in the circuit that it is in phase with the input signal and is then fed into an attenuator circuit which produces no additional phase shift (*Figure 8.1a*). The gain of the amplifier is adjusted to such a value that the output of the attenuator is equal in magnitude and phase to the original amplifier input voltage. On connecting the output from the attenuator to the input of the amplifier as shown in *Figure 8.1b* the amplifier will supply its own input, maintaining the circuit in a continuous closed loop operation and supplying the original input v at the original frequency. This is a case of positive feedback.

In general, if a fraction of the amplifier output is fed back to the input, the circuit will oscillate at a frequency for which the feedback signal is equal in magnitude and phase to the input signal. With this simplest type of arrangement, there may well be more than one possible frequency for which oscillation occurs. Since an oscillator is normally required to generate an oscillation at only one particular frequency, it must therefore incorporate a frequency determining circuit, whether in the amplifier itself or more usually in the feedback network.

For an amplifier voltage gain of Av and an input r.m.s. voltage of v, the output voltage will be $A_v v$. If the feedback network attenuates the output voltage by a factor β, then the voltage fed back in-phase to the input is $\beta A_v v$. For continuous oscillation, $\beta A_v = v$, that is, $A\beta = 1$, i.e. the loop gain must be unity, and the voltage feedback must be in phase with the input signal. Should $A\beta$ be made much greater than unity, considerable overloading will occur before the gain falls to the value where $A\beta = 1$, and the output waveform will be distorted. To ensure the production of a pure sine wave output, the feedback factor must be adjusted so that the circuit is only just oscillating. The output from the oscillator is then usually amplified to the desired level by means of a linear amplifier. The use of an oscillator to supply power is detrimental to its frequency stability and this also leads to the concept of a master oscillator–power amplifier combination.

The frequency determining element can be either (*a*) an inductive–capacitive (L–C) circuit, (*b*) a resistive–capacitive (R–C) network, or (*c*) a crystal. Application of the necessary positive feedback can occur either externally via a transformer or through a suitable internal feedback path in the circuit. The biasing of the amplifier maintaining oscillation can be arranged (*a*) so that the amplifier conducts over each complete cycle (Class A operation); (*b*) by increasing the bias to near the cut-off point, so that the amplifier conducts for approximately only one half of each cycle (Class B operation); or (*c*) by applying a large bias so that the amplifier conducts only on the positive or negative going peaks of the waveform, depending on the polarity of the transistors (Class C operation). The pulses of energy supplied by the amplifier under Class B or C operation once per cycle are sufficient to 'kick' the tuned circuit of an L–C oscillator and maintain it in a resonant condition. The oscillatory 'tank' current flowing backwards and forwards in the tuned circuit provides a reservoir of power from which a sinusoidal output signal can be drawn.

In practice, if the loop gain $A\beta$ is less than unity, any slight transient at the input will give rise to a damped oscillation at the output. When the loop gain exceeds unity, the amplitude of the oscillation will build up until it is limited by non-linearity of the maintaining amplifier. This limiting is essential for stable operation.

It is usual to arrange that $|A\beta| \simeq 1{\cdot}05$ in order that variations in circuit parameters shall not cause $|A\beta|$ to fall below unity.

L–C CIRCUIT OSCILLATORS

Common Emitter L–C Oscillator

The tuned collector circuit (*Figure 8.2*) determines that the frequency of oscillation will be approximately 10 kHz. The secondary winding of the transformer provides positive feedback from the collector to the base. The bypassed emitter resistor provides d.c.

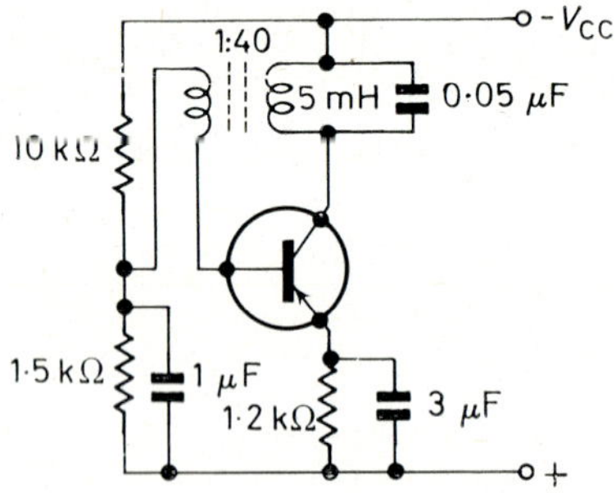

Figure 8.2. Transistor common emitter L–C oscillator

bias, and stabilization is provided by the base potentiometer network. The frequency of oscillation is approximately that of the resonant frequency of L and C, i.e. $f_0 = 1/(2\pi\sqrt{LC})$ Hz when L is in henrys and C is in farads. There is a 180 degrees phase difference between the collector and base signals, so that the direction of the transformer secondary must be arranged to provide the additional 180 degrees phase change to achieve oscillation. As an alternative, the secondary winding can be placed in the emitter lead of the transistor, but then the transformer must be connected so as to produce 0 degrees rather than 180 degrees phase change.

The Hartley Oscillator

In the Hartley oscillator (*Figure 8.3*) the tuned circuit is connected between the collector and the base, a series capacitor being employed to prevent the passage of d.c. The emitter is connected via the low impedance of the power supply to a tapping on the inductance in order to introduce a 180 degrees phase shift into the feedback.

Again the frequency of oscillation is approximately

$$f_o = 1/(2\pi\sqrt{LC})\ \text{Hz.}$$

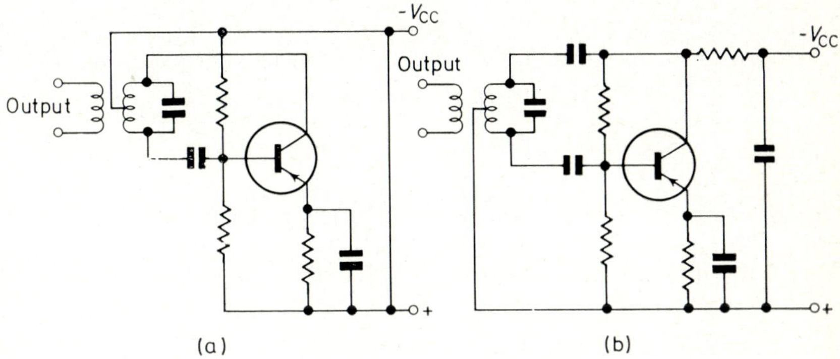

Figure 8.3. Transistor Hartley oscillator. (a) Series fed. (b) Shunt fed

The Colpitts Oscillator

Referring to *Figure 8.4*, the emitter is connected to a tapping on the capacitance of the tuned circuit. The voltage appearing across C_2 supplied the signal input to the base. The frequency of oscillation

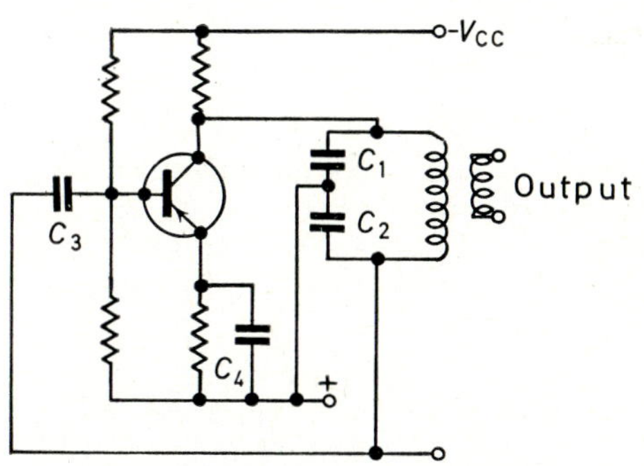

Figure 8.4. Transistor Colpitts oscillator

is approximately equal to $f_o = 1/(2\pi\sqrt{LC})$ Hz where C is now the capacity of C_1 and C_2 in series. There is a tendency to prefer the Colpitts circuit at higher frequencies.

BIAS ARRANGEMENTS

The shock of switching ON is normally enough to start the tuned circuit oscillating, and oscillations then build up in amplitude. Class A bias conditions in the maintaining amplifier give rise to the minimum distortion, whilst Class C bias gives the maximum efficiency. A simple R–C bias circuit is shown in *Figure 8.5.* The capacitor *C* charges on each negative signal pulse applied to the base–emitter diode and discharges slightly on each positive cycle as the diode is non-conducting. In this way, over a number of

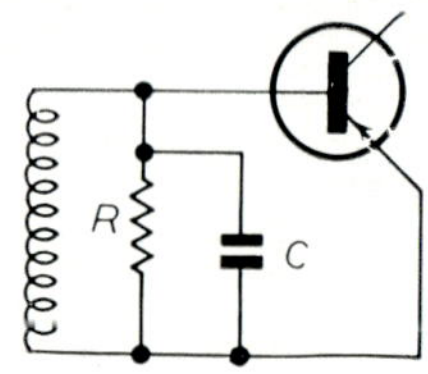

Figure 8.5. Simple R–C bias circuit

oscillatory cycles, the bias voltage developed across *R* builds up to a steady level. If the positive bias level built up is sufficiently large, it is overcome only on the peaks of the negative cycles of the oscillation signal, causing Class C operation with pulses of emitter current flowing. By making the time constant *CR* long compared with the periodic time of oscillation, the capacitor can retain its charge between successive charging half-cycles and a steady positive bias voltage is produced.

SQUEGGING

When the time constant in the base–emitter circuit is excessive, regular or irregular interruptions of the oscillation may arise. This phenomenon is most likely to occur when the amount of positive feedback is greater than is required just to maintain oscillation. In this case on switching ON, oscillations build up rapidly and

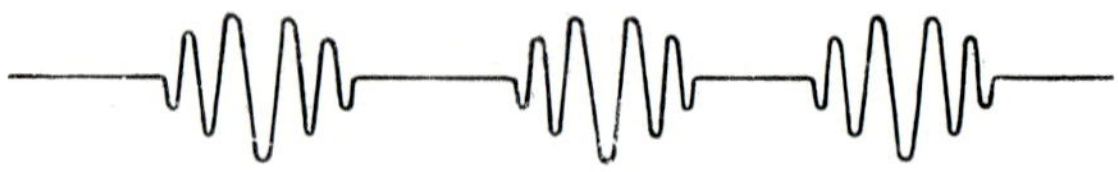

Figure 8.6. A squegging waveform

eventually sufficient bias is built up to cut the transistor off. Normally the time constant in the base–emitter circuit would be small enough for the bias to decrease during the next half-cycle, allowing oscillation to recommence. When the time constant is long, the transistor will stay cut off for a considerable time until the capacitor has been able to discharge sufficiently for conduction to restart. As a result, continuous oscillation becomes markedly interrupted as shown in *Figure 8.6*. This is a typical waveform observed when squegging occurs.

CRYSTAL OSCILLATORS

When a precise frequency is required, a crystal-controlled oscillator is employed. Typical applications occur in the generation of the carrier frequency in some types of medical radio telemetry transmitter and of the timing waveforms used in digital computers.

In a crystal oscillator, the frequency determining element is a thin wafer of single crystal quartz which has been cut in a special direction with respect to the crystal axes. It is connected to the circuit by means of metal electrodes placed on the flat surfaces of the crystal. The application of an alternating electric field across the crystal causes it to vibrate. This is known as the Piezo-electric Effect. The crystal behaves as a resonant circuit, its electrical equivalent circuit being given in *Figure 8.7*. The series circuit L,

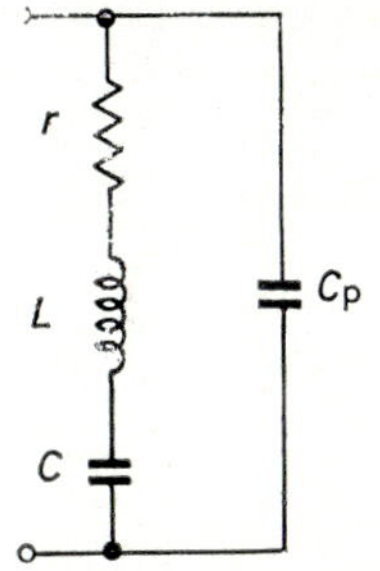

Figure 8.7. Equivalent electrical circuit for a crystal

C and R resonates at the mechanical (natural) resonant frequency of the crystal. For a 104·8 kHz crystal, $L=115$ H, $C=0{\cdot}02$ pF, $Cp=2{\cdot}5$ pF and $r=5{,}000\Omega$. The magnification factor $Q=2\pi fL/r=15{,}000$. For timing purposes, a 1 MHz crystal oscillator might be used and sub-multiples of it generated in the form of pulse trains by using synchronized frequency dividing circuits.

Crystal oscillators are very stable, and the crystal can be cut in such a way that the frequency it generates is little affected by changes occurring in the ambient temperature. This arrangement is encountered in the simpler types of digital frequency meter, but for the most precise frequency stability the crystal is mounted in a small thermostatically controlled oven.

A simple Pierce-type crystal oscillator is shown in *Figure 8.8*. When the oscillator is required to supply a power output, the crystal oscillator is run at a low power level and an emitter follower 'buffer'

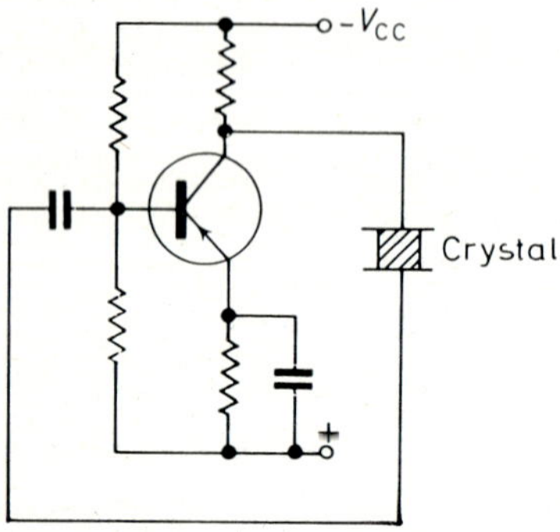

Figure 8.8. Pierce transistor crystal oscillator

stage interposed between it and the following power amplifier. This arrangement prevents variations in the loading of the output stage from 'pulling' the crystal frequency away from its normal value.

When output power is drawn off from an oscillator circuit, care must be taken to ensure that the amplifier provides enough power not only for the external requirements but also to cover the losses occurring in the feedback path and supply the required input to the amplifier for oscillation to occur. This fact is illustrated in *Figure 8.9*,

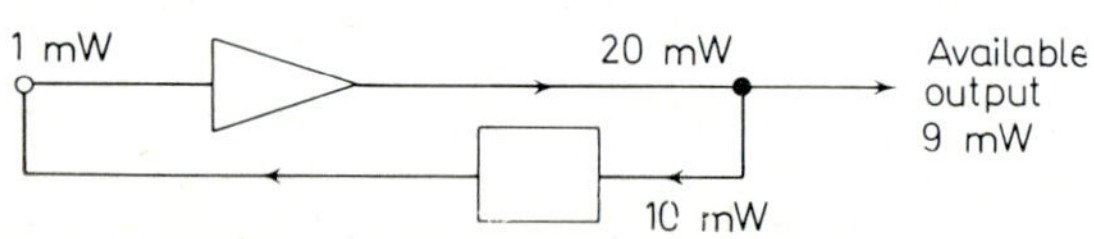

Figure 8.9. The abstraction of output power from an oscillator

where the amplifier has a power gain of 20. For a total output power of 20 mW, an input of 1 mW must be supplied. If the loss in the feedback network is 10 mW, the power available for external use is 20–10–1=9 mW.

FEEDING ARRANGEMENTS FOR THE POWER SUPPLY

The power supply can be placed either in series or in parallel with the maintaining amplifier and feedback network as shown in

Figure 8.10. *Figure 8.3* also shows a series fed and a parallel fed Hartley oscillator. In the parallel (shunt) fed case, the supply voltage is kept away from the tuned circuit components.

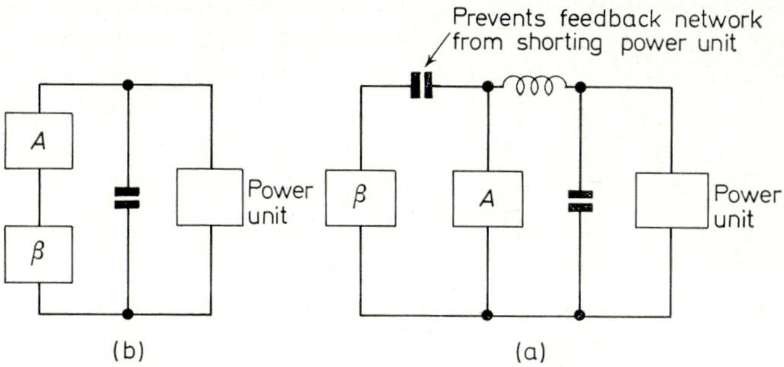

Figure 8.10. (a) Series fed and (b) shunt fed Hartley oscillator

RESISTANCE–CAPACITY OSCILLATORS

Essentially, an R–C oscillator consists of an amplifier which has a flat frequency response over a wide range of frequency and a negative feedback path consisting of an R–C network only. It is arranged that the phase shift introduced by the R–C network will be either 0 degrees or 180 degrees (depending upon the configuration of the maintaining amplifier) at the desired oscillation frequency and that the amplifier gain will exceed the network loss. Under these conditions the circuit will oscillate at the chosen frequency. The fact that the feedback path contains only resistors and capacitors and no inductors confers a number of advantages. Using a linear amplifier, minimal distortion of the sinewave signal results, since there is no question of saturating cores and thus introducing non-linearity. A good frequency stability can be obtained since the running frequency is determined only by resistors and capacitors which can be obtained with low temperature coefficients. Laboratory oscillators of the R–C type are commonly available with frequencies variable in the range from 1 Hz to 1 MHz.

The Wien Bridge Oscillator

The feedback network used in a Wien bridge oscillator is shown in *Figure 8.11*. If a sinusoidal signal is applied to the input, the input and output voltages will be in phase at a frequency given by $f=1/(2\pi RC)$ Hz. At this frequency the attenuation introduced by the network is such that the output signal is one-third of the input. Hence in order to maintain oscillation with this network, the maintaining amplifier must have a gain of at least three. A two-stage amplifier is used in order that the input and output of the network may be connected to two points where the signal is in phase.

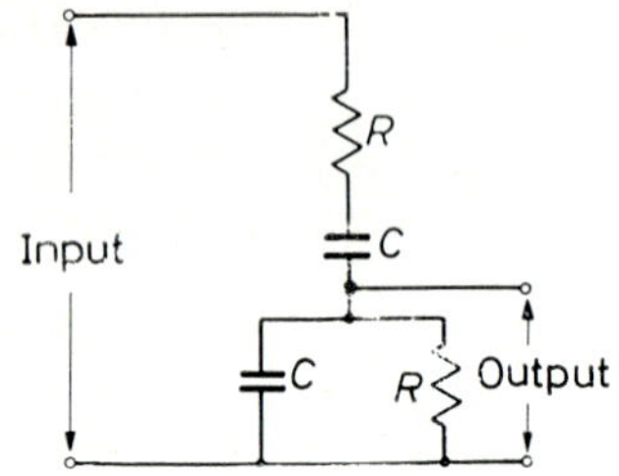

Figure 8.11. Feedback network for a Wien bridge oscillator

Figure 8.12 outlines a simple two-transistor Wien bridge oscillator. Coarse frequency ranges are provided by simultaneously switching the capacitors C in steps, whilst a fine adjustment is provided by means of the ganged rheostat R. The gain control RV_1 allows the output waveform to be adjusted for amplitude and distortion.

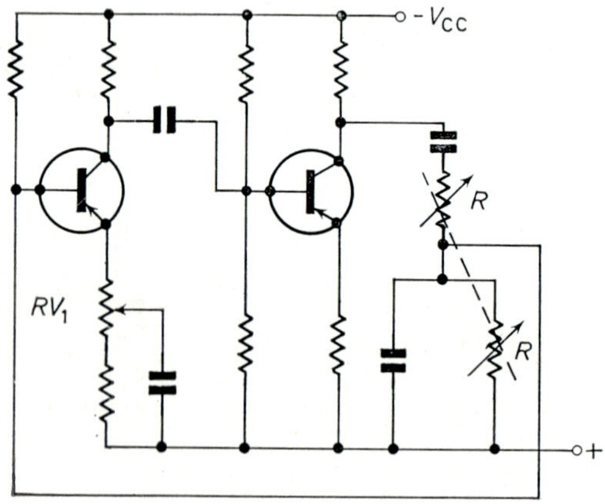

Figure 8.12. Outline circuit of a transistor Wien bridge oscillator

In many oscillators a thermistor is also included in the negative feedback path. It acts to maintain the output amplitude almost constant over the frequency range. If the output increases, the thermistor warms up and its resistance decreases. This produces more negative feedback and reduces the output amplitude to approximately its original level. The limits are set by the frequency range over which no phase shift occurs through the amplifier. A frequency range of 1·5 Hz to 150 kHz might be covered in five ranges.

In addition to the pure sine wave output, it is convenient also to provide a square wave output. This is arranged by over-driving an amplifier stage and clipping the resultant grossly distorted sine wave with Zener diodes in order to provide a flat-topped square wave. Watson (1966) points out that for the best results a Wien bridge network should be fed from a low impedance voltage source and should work into a very high input impedance.

The Single-stage R–C Oscillator

If a single-stage maintaining amplifier is used, the R–C feedback network must introduce an additional 180 degrees phase shift between its input and output terminals. This can be accomplished by means of three C–R combinations (*Figure 8.13*). The attenuation

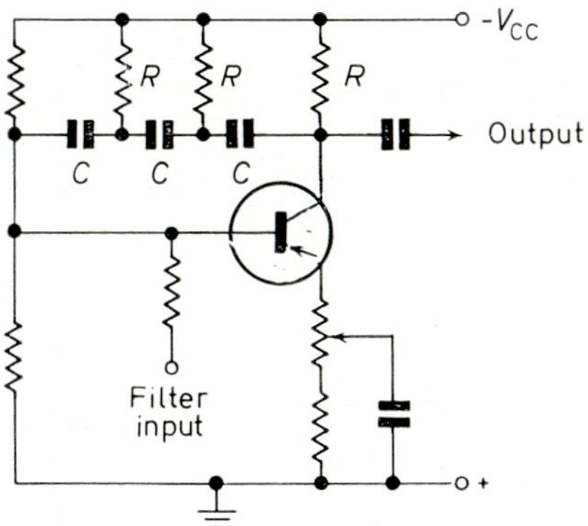

Figure 8.13. Transistor single-stage R–C oscillator

introduced by the network is 29 at the frequency where its input and output are 180 degrees out of phase. For oscillation to occur, the gain of the amplifier must be at least equal to 29. The frequency at which the network produces a 180 degrees phase shift is $f = 1/(2\pi CR\sqrt{6})$ Hz. This type of oscillator is best suited to the generation of a single fixed frequency for use as a timing wave or for the energization of a bridge or transducer. A high gain transistor

($h_{fe}=60$) is required, and the calculated frequency of oscillation is modified by the presence of the input and output impedances of the amplifier. In one case, the circuit actually oscillated at 800 Hz rather than a calculated 650 Hz. The gain of the maintaining amplifier is adjusted in *Figure 8.13* by altering the amount of the emitter resistance which is bypassed and thus the amount of negative feedback. The gain is adjusted so that the circuit just oscillates and distortion is low.

If the gain of the amplifier is reduced to the point where the circuit does just not oscillate, it can function as a tuned amplifier. In the circuit of *Figure 8.13*, the input signal to the filter is input via a high resistance to the base of the transistor. Banks of these filters have been used in electroencephalogram frequency analysers covering the range 1–30 Hz in 1 Hz steps.

THE USE OF AN OPERATIONAL AMPLIFIER IN AN OSCILLATOR CIRCUIT

A conventional operational amplifier configuration is shown

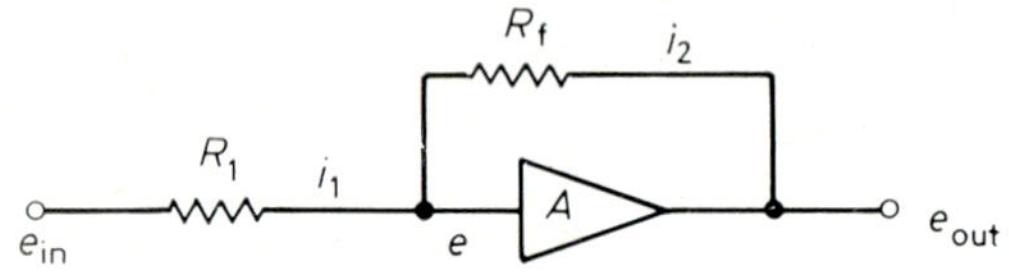

Figure 8.14. Conventional operational amplifier circuit

in *Figure 8.14*. Assuming that the amplifier does not draw any input current, the following relationships obtain.

$$I_1+I_2=0.$$

$$\frac{e_{in}-e}{R_1}+\frac{e_{out}-e}{-R_f}=0$$

and $e_{out}=A_v.e$ where A is the gain of the amplifier. Eliminating e,

$$A_v=e_{out}/e_{in}=-R_f\Big/\left(R_1-\frac{R_1+R_f}{A_v}\right)$$

where A_v is the voltage gain of the circuit.

In a conventional operational amplifier stage, negative feedback is employed and A_v is assumed to be large and negative. However, in order to produce oscillation A_v must be positive and is assumed still to be large.

The equation

$$A_v = -R_f \Bigg/ \left(R_1 - \frac{R_1+R_f}{A_v}\right)$$

can be written as

$$e_{out}\left(R_1 - \frac{(R_1+R_f)}{A_v}\right) = -R_f e_{in}.$$

This equation is also satisfied when $e_{in}=0$, i.e. when there is no externally connected input, provided that $R_1=(R_1+R_f)/A_v$, and e_{out} is not necessarily zero. Since A_v is a positive number, this is a state of positive feedback with the implication that an output is obtained for zero input.

With a direct coupled operational amplifier, this arrangement would simply produce a rapid change in the voltage levels throughout the circuit which would continue until it was stopped by saturation or cut-off occurring in one of the amplifier stages. The output voltage e_{out} would then remain at either the positive or the negative supply line voltage, depending on the direction of the signal which happened to be fed back to the input.

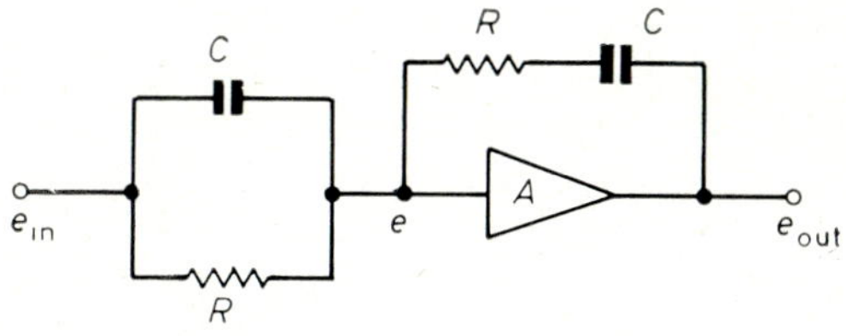

Figure 8.15. Operational amplifier Wien bridge oscillator

If frequency-dependent networks are substituted for R_1 and R_f, it is possible for continuous oscillation to be maintained. Let R_1 be replaced by the combination of C and R in parallel and R_f by C and R in series (*Figure 8.15*). The condition for oscillation to be maintained is that oscillation will occur at a frequency $f=1/2\pi CR$ if A_v is a positive number equal to 3. In practice, with A_v positive and greater than 3, oscillation is still maintained but the waveform is no longer sinusoidal. For example, with $A_v=5$ the circuit goes into a relaxation oscillation mode, producing a square wave output. However, the gain of the circuit can be adjusted accurately and oscillations of a sine wave nature can be produced with a gain of 3·1. This arrangement is seen to be an operational amplifier Wien bridge oscillator. With a Wien bridge oscillator based on a conventional amplifier, a gain of 3·1 would be too low to allow the oscillations to be built. For this reason a thermistor is usually included in the feedback path so that the gain is initially high and as oscillation builds up, the thermistor is warmed and its resistance falls. This is arranged to reduce the gain and maintain a low distortion output waveform. With an operational amplifier this is not necessary.

An interesting account of a precision operational amplifier oscillator based on the use of an a.c. bridge in the feedback path is that of Brach (1966). The frequency range was from 1 Hz to 10 kHz with a frequency change of 3 Hz per 1,000 from 15 to 40° C.

RADIO TELEMETRY SYSTEMS

Small modulated radio frequency oscillators are being increasingly used as transmitters in radio telemetry systems designed to send physiological signals via a radio link from experimental animals, exercising subjects or patients in bed. The freedom from connecting wires provided by the wireless system makes for much more natural circumstances in the data collection. For example, industrial workers can be monitored during a normal factory shift, or patients can be ambulant in a ward. In the United Kingdom, the bands 102·2 to 102·35 MHz and 102·36–102·39 MHz are set aside for medical telemetry purposes. The maximum deviations allowed are ±50 kHz and ±3 kHz respectively. The carrier frequency accuracy and stability must be better than one part in 10^5. The permissible output power is expressed in terms of the allowable field strength, e.g. 10 V/m at 200 m.

Particularly in EEG studies, up to 16 channels of information may have to be transmitted. Each input signal is caused to modulate the frequency of its own audio frequency sub-carrier. The modulated sub-carriers are then applied as a modulation to the main carrier of the transmitter. Frequency modulation is generally preferred to simple amplitude modulation because of its freedom from artefacts produced by extraneous noise signals. An eight-channel EEG radio telemetry system is described by Kamp (1963).

Ko *et al.* (1971) describe an integrated circuit micropower radio telemetry transmitter using active dry electrodes for ECG monitoring. The transmitter power consumption is only 180 μW and the range is 1.5–6m (5–20 ft) without an external aerial at 143 MHz. The supply voltage is 2·6 V and pulse width modulation is employed. Two signal inputs can be used, each with a bandwidth of 0·1 to 100 Hz. The input impedance is 1–2 MΩ. Silicon oxide electrodes are used, each carrying its own integrated circuit FET and source follower. The Si-SiO_2 insulated electrode is mounted on a ceramic base forming the lid of the flatpack containing the electrode circuitry.

A good general review of biomedical telemetry systems, especially implanted types, is that of Mackay (1968). Bellet and Muller (1965) discuss the use of a radio link for the monitoring of the ECG during exercise.

Endoradiosondes or 'radio-pills' are in regular use to measure intestinal pressures and temperatures and have also been used to monitor bladder pressures in women. The transmission frequency is usually in the region of 400 kHz. The pH-sensitive Heidelberg capsule (Noller, 1962) uses a transistor Hartley oscillator at 1·9 MHz powered from a 1·5 V collector supply battery. A base bias battery is formed by an outer antimony electrode separated by a dialysing membrane from the inner silver chloride electrode of the collector battery. The base bias battery is pH-sensitive and varies the oscillator frequency. The resulting frequency change is virtually linear from pH 2 to pH 7. Another account of pH-sensitive endoradiosondes is that of Watson and Paton (1965).

The use of endoradiosondes for the detection of bleeding in the gut has been described by Kimoto *et al.* (1964), and the application of implanted pressure sensor–transmitters for the measurement of intracranial pressures is discussed by Atkinson, Shurtleff and Foltz (1967). Endoradiosondes need not be of an active nature, i.e. actually containing a radio transmitter. They can contain merely a passive tuned circuit which is interrogated periodically by an external pulsed transmitter. The resulting damped oscillation set up in the tuned circuit depends on the environment, such as intestinal pressure, to which the pill is exposed and can be detected outside the body (Nagumo, 1965).

Franklin *et al.* (1966) have devised a telemetry system for recording blood flow velocity changes in unrestrained animals, whilst Robinson (1964) has designed a telemetry system for following changes occurring in body temperature.

Figure 8.16, from Roy *et al.* (1971), gives the circuit diagram of an implanted transmitter used to telemeter the ECG and body temperature of the white-footed mouse. The weight of the transmitter and mercury battery is only 2 g. The output stage of the transmitter is a blocking oscillator whose pulse repetition rate is determined by the combination of the capacitor in the base circuit and the thermistor resistance. This is temperature-dependent, so measurement of the repetition rate enables the body temperature to be monitored. In fact, the oscillator frequency of about 400 kHz is modulated by two signals. The modulation, which is affected by body temperature, is arranged to be in the range 0–0·5 Hz, whilst

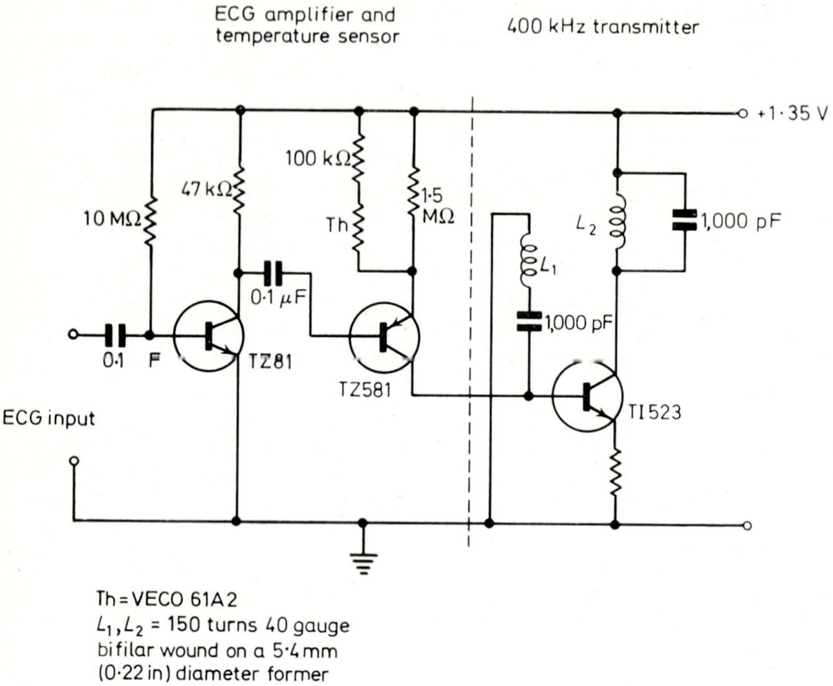

Figure 8.16. An ECG–temperature transmitter

(Reproduced from Roy *et al.*, 1971, by courtesy of the Editor of *Medical and Biological Engineering*)

that due to the ECG is in the range 1–10 Hz. The main interest was in heart rate.

SURGICAL AND THERAPEUTIC DIATHERMY UNITS

Surgical diathermy units are widely used in the operating room both for cutting tissue and for the coagulation of bleeding points. *Figure 8.17* shows a typical modern diathermy unit. It contains two separate radio frequency oscillator systems. For cutting purposes a valve oscillator is used having a maximum power output of 300 W

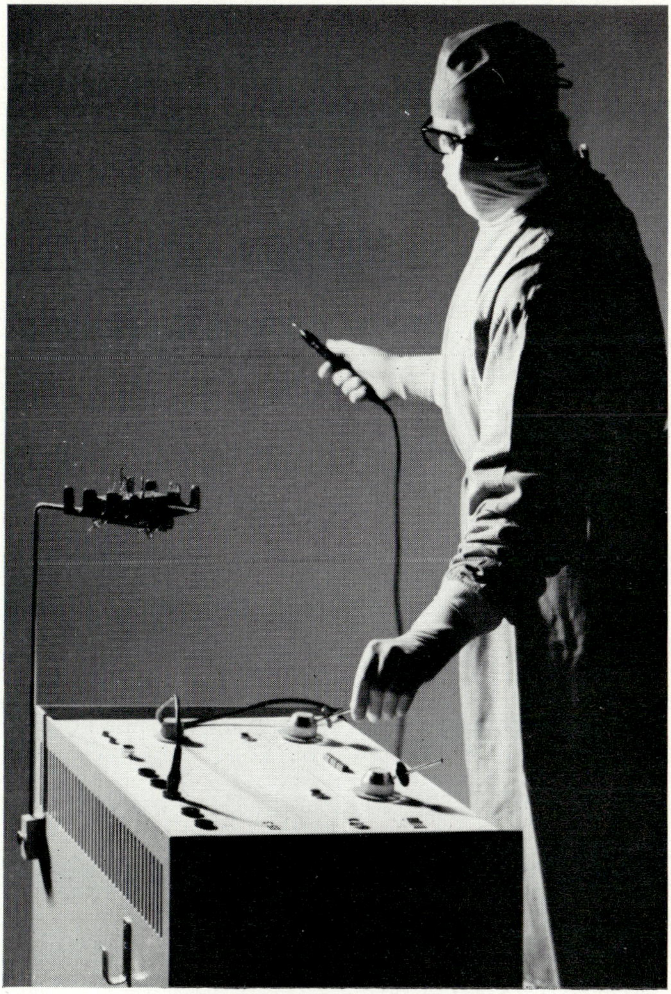

Figure 8.17. Philips ES3 surgical diathermy unit
(By courtesy of Philips Medical Systems Ltd.)

into a patient load of a nominal 150 Ω. The frequency is in the region of 1·75 MHz. Full wave solid state rectifiers are used in the power supply, so that the waveform is a sine wave with 100 Hz modulation. A coupling coil is used to draw power out from the oscillator tank circuit and ten tappings are provided for power adjustment.

When coagulation is needed, the output is taken from a 300 W spark gap oscillator. An outline circuit of a spark gap oscillator is given in *Figure 8.18*. The a.c. mains supply voltage is stepped up to 1,500 V by the mains transformer and then applied across several spark gaps arranged in series. Twice per mains cycle (on the positive and the negative peak) the voltage appearing across the gaps is sufficiently high to ionize the air and break down the gap, causing

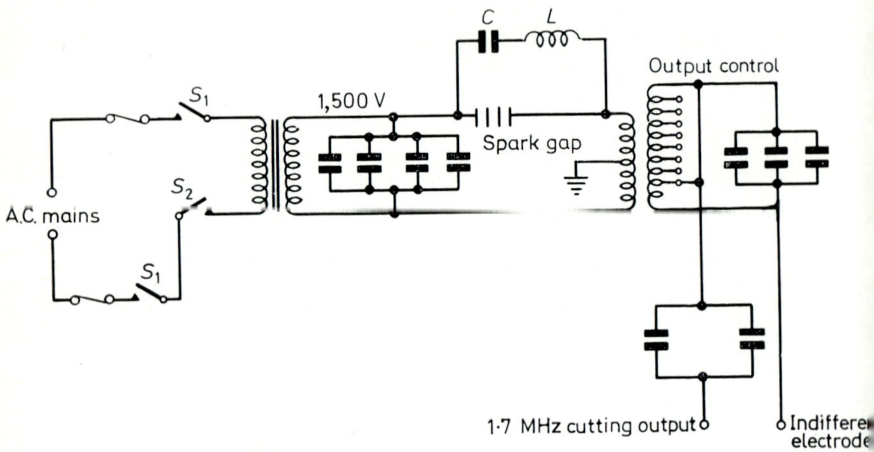

Figure 8.18. Outline circuit of a spark-gap type diathermy unit

sparking. As a result, capacitor C discharges in a regular fashion, the combination of L and C being chosen to oscillate at about 1·7 MHz. The output from the oscillator then consists of bursts of damped radio frequency oscillations at intervals of 10 ms (the periodic time of the 50 Hz mains being 20 ms). Tappings on the output coil allow the power to be adjusted.

In the diathermy unit of *Figure 8.17*, provision is made for mixing the outputs from the valve and spark gap oscillators. This facility is recommended for the control of haemorrhage from the edges of wounds and for the trans-urethral resection of the prostate. At the start of the resection, the outputs are mixed in such a ratio that excessive bleeding is avoided and the view through the urethroscope is not obstructed. Towards the end of the resection the coagulating current is considerably reduced, resulting in a clean wound bed. Any remaining bleeding sites are then coagulated individually. The output impedances of the oscillators are low enough to provide the heavy currents required for swift cutting and coagulation in a fluid-filled bladder.

The operation of surgical diathermy presents a number of problems in regard to the protection of the patient from radio frequency burns or electrocution and the minimizing of interference with patient monitoring equipment from the 100 Hz (50 Hz units with half wave rectification) modulation.

Therapeutic diathermy units are widely used in departments of physical medicine for the treatment of affected joints and other areas, lumbago and abscesses (Zeiter, 1950). They usually operate at 27 MHz with a maximum output power of about 300 W. Although the higher frequency is easier to filter out, the units radiate more effectively than do surgical diathermies, and radiated interference may be picked up at a distance. Microwave diathermy units are employed when a preferential heating of superficial tissue layers of good conductivity is required, with only a slight heating of fatty tissues (Herrick *et al.*, 1950). A good detailed account of therapeutic diathermies is that of Nightingale (1959).

REFERENCES

Atkinson, J. R., Shurtleff, D. B. and Foltz, E. L. (1967). 'Radio telemetry for the measurement of intracranial pressure.' *J. Neurosurg.* **27,** 428.

Bellet, S. and Muller, O. F. (1965). 'The electrocardiogram during exercise: its value in the diagnosis of angina pectoris.' *Circulation* **32,** 477.

Brach, E. J. (1966). 'A precision oscillator based on an operational amplifier.' *Electron. Engng* **38,** 724.

Franklin, D. E., Watson, N. W., Pearson, K. E. and Van Citters, R. L. (1966). 'Technique of radio-telemetry of blood flow velocity from unrestrained animals.' *Am. J. med. Electron.* **4,** 108.

Herrick, J. F., Martin, G. M., Krusen, F. H. and Wakim, K. G. (1950). 'Physical medicine: diathermy, microwave.' In *Medical Physics*, Vol. 2, p. 710. Ed. by O. Glasser. Chicago: Year Book Publishers.

Kamp, A. (1963). 'Eight channel E.E.G. telemetering.' *Electroenceph. clin. Neurophysiol.* **15,** 164.

Kimoto, S., Watanuki, T., Hori, M., Suma, K., Nagumo, J., Ouchi, A., Takahashi, T., Kumano, M. and Watanabe, J. (1964). 'Endoradiosonde for bleeding detection.' *Med. Electron. biol. Engng* **2,** 81.

Ko, W. H., Yon, T., Greenstein, E., Hynecek, J. and Conrad, D. (1971). 'A micropower telemetry system with active electrodes.' *Solid-State Circuits Conference Digest*, p. 102. New York Institute of Electrical and Electronics Engineers.

Mackay, R. S. (1968). *Bio-medical Telemetry.* New York: Wiley.

Nagumo, J. (1965). 'Echo capsules for medical use.' *Jap. Electron. Engng* **12,** 2.

Nightingale, A. (1959). *Physics and Electronics in Physical Medicine.* London: Bell.

Noller, H. G. (1962). 'Results of examinations of stomach functions with the endoradio capsule. The Heidelberg capsule—a new appliance for assisting stomach diagnosis.' *Fortschr. Med.* **80,** 351.

Robinson, S. G. (1964). 'A temperature telemetering system with constant accuracy.' *Med. Electron. biol. Engng* **2,** 81.

Roy, O. Z., Gaertner, R. A., Hart, J. S. and Charbonneau, J. R. (1971). 'Techniques used in the study of the white-footed mouse under semi-natural conditions.' *Med. biol. Engng* **9,** 1.

Watson, J. (1966). *Semiconductor Circuit Design.* London: Hilger & Watts.

Watson, W. C. and Paton, E. (1965). 'Studies in intestinal pH by radio-telemetering.' *Gut* **6,** 606.

Zeiter, W. (1950). 'Physical medicine: diathermy.' In *Medical Physics,* Vol. 2, p. 710. Ed. by O. Glasser. Chicago: Year Book Publishers.

Chapter 9

A.C. Interference and Patient Safety

The limit to the amount that wanted signals can be amplified is set by the presence of unwanted random background signals—electrical 'noise'. The wanted signal can also be spoiled by the appearance of unwanted signals from the preparation (an unwanted electrocardiogram or electromyogram, for example), or by unwanted pick-up signals (interference). Interference can normally be reduced to acceptable proportions by the taking of suitable precautions and arrives by three main routes—electrostatic induction, electromagnetic induction and conduction. Interference at the frequency of the mains supply shows up as a 'hum' or 'ripple' on the recording.

ELECTROSTATIC PICK-UP WITH A SINGLE-SIDED AMPLIFIER

The laws of electrostatic induction show that if a charged body is brought up close to an uncharged body, a charge is induced on the previously uncharged body (this could be the input resistor of an amplifier). Marked electrostatic effects can arise when someone wearing nylon outer clothing walks past an unshielded high input impedance amplifier, and cables carrying an alternating mains voltage can induce an alternating input voltage into an amplifier through the coupling action of stray capacities. Electrostatic pick-up is voltage dependent and can arise from cables which are not carrying a current. For this reason, cables not in use should be disconnected at the supply end.

Consider the case of a patient lying on an examination couch (*Figure 9.1*). A capacity C_2 exists between the patient and earth. There will also be a coupling capacity C_1 between the patient and any unshielded mains cables in the room. Suppose that an attempt is made to use a single-sided amplifier to record the patient's electrocardiogram. The resistors R_1 and R_2 represent the electrode–skin contact resistances. This is an a.c. resistance, typically measured in the band 1–20 Hz where capacitive effects are negligible. There is a capacity C_3 between the amplifier and the mains and C_4 between the amplifier and earth. If $C_1=C_2$, the patient acquires an alternating potential of 115 V r.m.s., but because of the high impedance

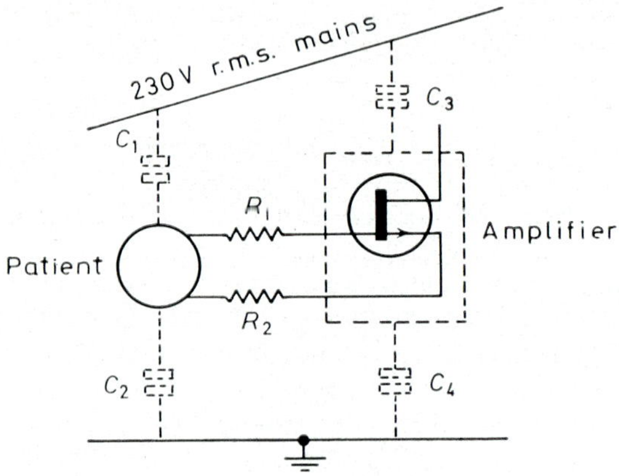

Figure 9.1. The effect of capacitive pick-up with a single-sided amplifier

of the capacitances only a minute current flows. The four capacitances C_1, C_2, C_3 and C_4 form an a.c. bridge circuit which will, in general, not be balanced. The out-of-balance a.c. voltage from the bridge is applied across the resistors R_1 and R_2 and hence to the input of the amplifier. The interference is only made worse by earthing the case of the amplifier, since this shorts out C_4. A significant interference occurs even though C_1 may have a value of only a few pico-farads. The mains frequency interference could have been eliminated by using a battery-powered amplifier and placing it and the patient inside a wire mesh cage.

It is obviously not always feasible to work in a screened enclosure, and hence balanced (differential) rather than unbalanced amplifiers are commonly used for this type of application. When very low level signals have to be recorded, the use of a screened enclosure can eliminate radiated interference from 27 MHz therapeutic diathermy apparatus or that from a local television station. The design of screened enclosures is discussed by Leadbitter (1963), and *Figure 9.2* shows a typical screened room in use for electrophysiological experiments.

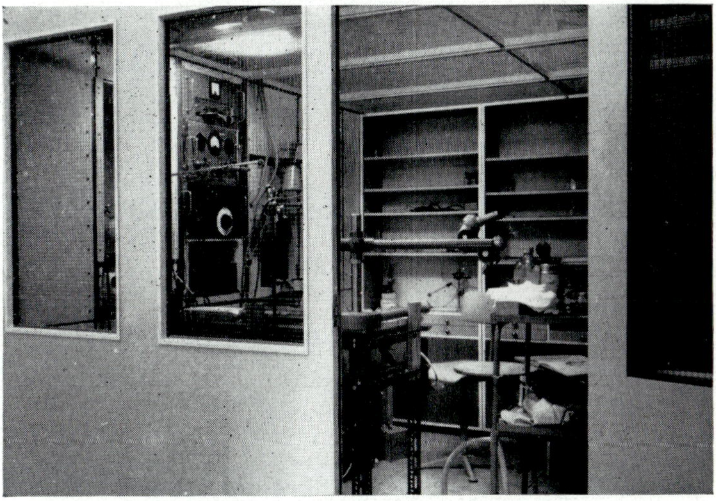

Figure 9.2. Screened room in use for electrophysiological experiments
(By courtesy of the University of Nijmegen)

THE USE OF A BALANCED AMPLIFIER

The use of a common emitter resistor in a long-tailed pair stage of a balanced amplifier allows the amplifier to discriminate against an unwanted signal which is in-phase at the two active input terminals. In discussing the emitter follower, it was shown that the signal voltage developed across the emitter resistor acts to produce negative feedback. The emitter moves in the same direction as the base, and it is the emitter–base voltage which controls the base current and thus the emitter current. If this feedback is not required, the emitter resistor is bypassed with a large capacitor whose reactance is small at the signal frequencies concerned. This is not practical at low frequencies of a few hertz. However, in the balanced amplifier stage, the voltage drop developed across the common emitter resistor remains constant when there are two equal anti-phase inputs and there is now no negative feedback. For two in-phase inputs, there is a change in the total emitter current and negative feedback occurs. The gain of the stage is thus markedly lower for the unwanted in-phase signals than it is for the wanted anti-phase signals. This is achieved by making the common emitter resistor large, comparable in size with the collector load resistors. The use of a 'long' tail to the stage requires that it be connected to a correspondingly large supply voltage. In a number of designs, such as that of Murari (1967), the emitters are fed from a transistor constant current source. This provides an ample reserve of current to cope with any marked imbalance of the stage d.c. conditions which may arise with maximal common mode or differential input signals.

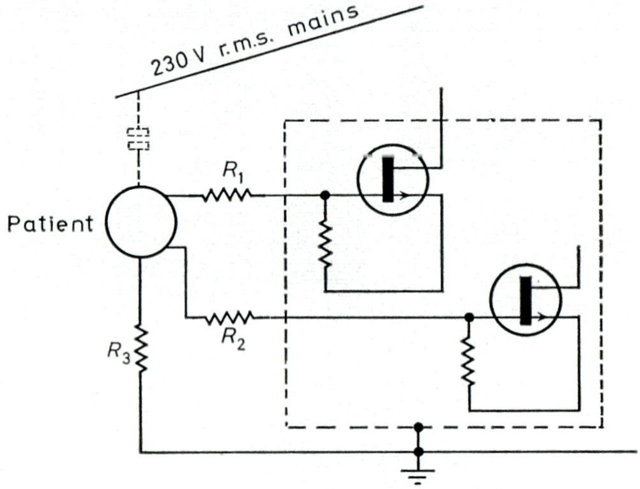

Figure 9.3. The use of a balanced amplifier

The use of a balanced amplifier is illustrated in *Figure 9.3*. The case of the amplifier is earthed and the patient is connected to earth via an additional electrode which has a skin contact resistance of R_3 ohms. The skin contact resistances of the active electrodes are respectively R_1 and R_2. The patient is now effectively connected between the mains power wiring and earth by a potentiometer network consisting of the impedance Z_1 of C_1 and the resistance R_3. Hence the patient develops an alternating voltage with respect to earth equal to the mains voltage multiplied by a factor $R_3/(Z_1+R_3)$. This voltage divided by the discrimination factor of the amplifier represents the unwanted in-phase signal which is amplified. The discrimination factor is defined as the ratio of the amplifier gain for differential (anti-phase) signals to the gain for common mode (in-phase) signals. For a well designed amplifier alone it may have a value of 1,000 (60 db) or more. It should be remembered that it is the discrimination factor of the recording system as a whole which is important. This will also depend on the values of the electrode skin contact resistances R_1 and R_2.

In *Figure 9.4*, V_h represents the voltage signal generated by the heart. V_e represents the unwanted common mode electrostatic signal picked up from the mains wiring. R_I is the total input resistance of the electrocardiograph amplifier, whilst R_1 and R_2 are the skin contact resistances of the electrodes. The signal frequencies are assumed to be sufficiently low to allow the effects of shunt capacities to be ignored and resistances to be used instead of impedances. The resistances represent the resistances of blood and other tissues, and these are taken as negligibly small compared with the other resistances.

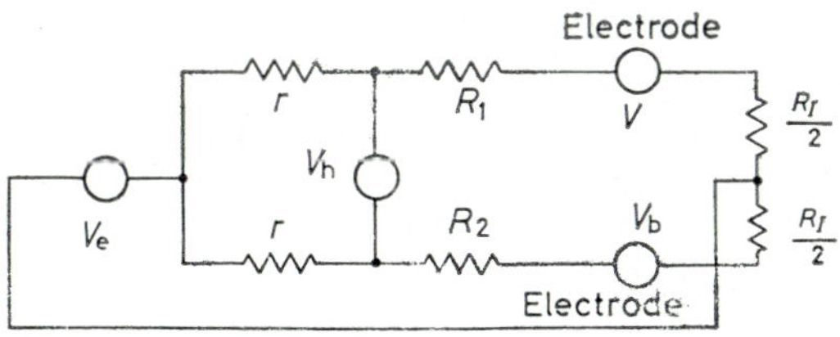

Figure 9.4. Equivalent circuit for ECG recording

If the amplifier were perfectly balanced, the equal common mode voltages V and V_b at the electrodes would give rise to a zero amplitude output signal. However, the voltages V and V_b depend in practice upon the values of R_1 and R_2. It can be shown that the electrostatic interference signal V_e will give rise to the same value of output signal as would a wanted signal from the patient having an amplitude $V_e(R_2-R_1)$ $(R_I/2)$. Hence the discrimination factor between the wanted and unwanted signals is given by $(R_I/2)/(R_2-R_1)$. For the case where the total input resistance R_I equals 2 MΩ and the electrode skin contact resistances are 5 kΩ and 3 kΩ respectively, the discrimination factor is 500. The expression shows that in order to obtain high discrimination factors, the amplifier input resistance should be high and the electrode skin contact resistances should be low and as nearly equal as possible. With a good technique of abrading the outer horny layer of the skin and the application of electrode jelly or cream, skin contact resistances of the order of a few thousand ohms can be obtained. *Figure 9.5* shows the effect of an imbalance in electrode skin contact resistance on the discrimination factor of an electrocardiograph.

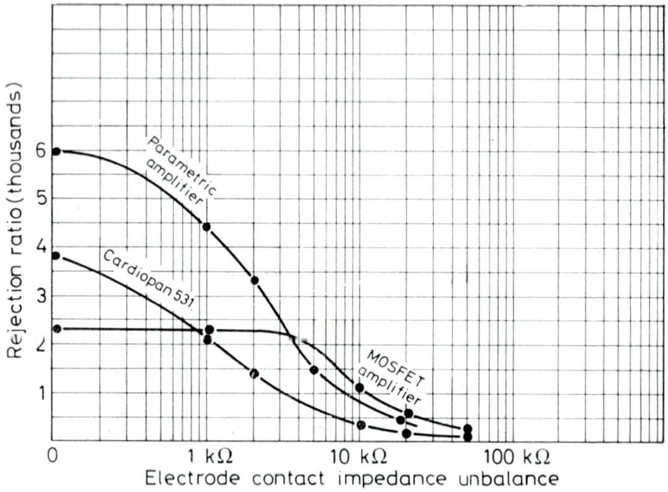

Figure 9.5. The effect of an imbalance in electrode skin contact resistance on the discrimination of a Philips type 531 electrocardiograph

(Reproduced from Hill and Khandpur, 1969, by courtesy of the Editor of *World Medical Instrumentation*)

In EEG recording, it is good practice to use a simple ohmmeter type of resistance tester to check the scalp contact resistances of the electrode montage before the commencement of recording. In cases of extreme interference, it may be desirable to employ an additional series resistor in order to balance up markedly unequal electrode skin contact resistances. Gentille (1956) draws attention to the fact that a high value of skin contact resistance can distort an electrocardiogram, and the subject is also discussed by Hill and Khandpur (1969). In some older types of electrocardiograph, provision has been made for cancelling any residual mains frequency signal by the injection later in the amplifier of an equal amplitude anti-phase signal.

THE USE OF A BALANCED INPUT TRANSFORMER

A balanced (symmetrical) transformer having a centre-tapped primary winding will discriminate against common mode input signals. Each half of the primary is carefully balanced with respect to the earthed centre-tap. If two equal amplitude in-phase signals are applied to the ends of the primary winding, they will cancel and there will be zero output from the secondary winding. On the other hand, if two equal amplitude differential signals are applied to the primary, there will be an output from the secondary.

The use of a simple transformer arrangement has been applied to EMG recording where the signal frequencies are reasonably high (Battye, 1962).

Mundl (1970) describes an EEG amplifier which uses an input transformer. He points out that such an amplifier has a very high rejection ratio for common mode input signals, a fast recovery from overvoltages since direct coupling can now be employed between stages, and a limited response at low frequencies. These properties are particularly useful when recording an EEG whilst simultaneously applying electrical stimulation, and when recording an EEG in the presence of movement artefacts. The response of Mundl's amplifier was 2 db down at 3 Hz and 50 Hz.

When a response down to d.c. is required, recourse may be made to a 'chopper' technique. In the well-known Offner Dynograph, a 400 Hz low noise mechanical chopper is employed. The upper limit of frequency which can be handled with this chopper is about 100 Hz. Dobbie (1967b) reports an interesting case of electrical interference encountered with an Offner Type T Dynograph EEG recorder. This arose from a beating between the chopper frequencies and signals picked up from the hospital's inductive loop staff location system.

EARTH LOOPS

In the construction of high gain amplifiers it is usual to connect all the points in the circuit which have to be earthed to an insulated

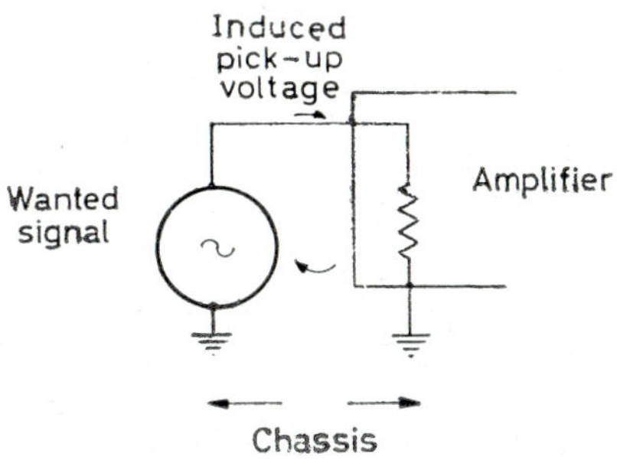

Figure 9.6. The formation of an 'earth loop'

busbar. This earth 'bus' is connected to a good earth at only one point. As a result, earth currents cannot flow through the chassis. Multiple earthing in a circuit can give rise to the formation of an unwanted 'earth loop' as illustrated in *Figure 9.6*. The loop circuit has induced in it an unwanted interference signal.

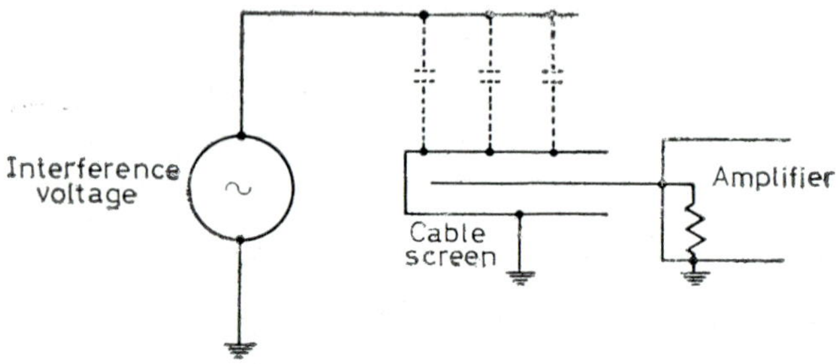

Figure 9.7. The action of a screened cable

Electrostatic coupling exists between the source of the interfering voltage and the mesh of the cable screen. The action of the screen is to ensure that there can be no electrostatic field inside it (*Figure 9.7*). Thus a correctly screened cable is protected from the induction of electrostatic pick-up voltages. Pick-up occurs at the unscreened electrodes connected to screened cables if the impedance between them is sufficiently high. Screened cables are used on the input leads and mains cables of high gain recording systems.

THE IMPEDANCE OF THE SIGNAL AMPLIFIER TO EARTH

It must be emphasized that not only must the input impedance of the signal amplifier be high, but also the impedance to earth of the recording leads.

The common mode electrostatic interference signal is applied in *Figure 9.8*, effectively across two voltage-dividing networks $R_1+(R_I/2)$ and $R_2+(R_I/2)$. R_1 and R_2 are the electrode skin contact resistances and R_I is the amplifier input resistance. If R_I is much greater than R_1 or R_2, the common mode signals applied to each input terminal are almost equal and rejection occurs. Suppose, however, that the impedances to earth, Z_1 and Z_2 (*Figure 9.8b*), of the electrodes are significant compared with R_1 and R_2. Then if R_1 and R_2 are not equal, different magnitudes of interference signal

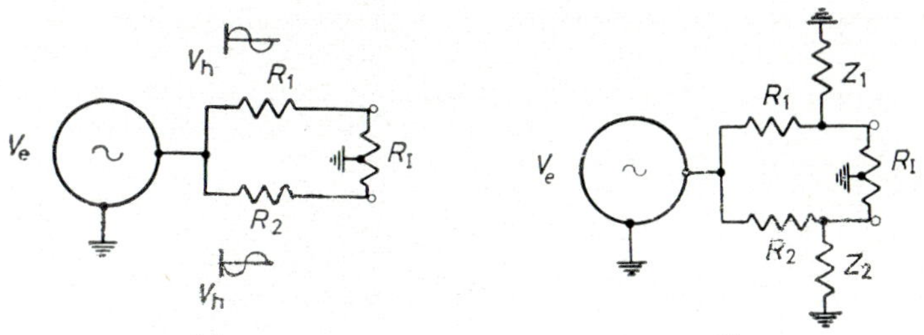

Figure 9.8. Balanced amplifiers. (a) Active elements completely isolated from earth. (b) Active elements having a significant impedance to earth

will be applied to the amplifier input terminals, and an output will result for the interference signal.

ELECTROMAGNETICALLY INDUCED INTERFERENCE

An alternating current flowing in a cable has associated with it an alternating magnetic field which can induce unwanted interference voltages in neighbouring conductors. Dobbie (1967a) reports two cases of hospitals experiencing 50 Hz interference. In each case it was found to be due to a leakage current flowing from the neutral wire of the mains to earth as a result of misconnections joining the neutral to earth. In one case the neutral wire was at a potential of 2 V relative to earth and carried a current of 2 A. The unwanted connection of the neutral to earth was traced to the control unit of a sterilizer. This resulted in a current to earth flowing through a water pipe under the floor of a laboratory, giving rise to the interference. Currents flowing to earth via unplanned routes can give rise to a loop of current similar to that provided in an induction loop staff location system. Thus a considerable space can be filled with a fairly uniform 50 Hz magnetic field. The heavier the current flowing, the greater the interference.

Electromagnetic interference can occur particularly from mains power transformers. The best solution is to move the apparatus concerned as far away from the transformer as possible. It may also be possible to alter the orientation of the transformer core in order to reduce the interference to a minimum. In extreme cases it may be necessary to locate a ‘neutral point’ in the field and to site the apparatus there. Screening from induced magnetic pick-up is usually harder than screening from electrostatic pick-up. One can generally provide a satisfactory screening for the electrostatic case by placing the circuit concerned inside a wire mesh or a light metal enclosure and incorporating filters in any leads entering the enclosure. Shielding from electromagnetic interference is usually performed by placing the circuit concerned within a box made of a 'soft' magnetic material such as mumetal.

CONDUCTED INTERFERENCE

As well as supplying power, mains cables commonly conduct interference to the equipment they are supplying in the form of radio frequency currents and voltage transients. When a mains supply has to be fed into a screened enclosure, it is essential to take it in via a good radio frequency filter. Voltage transients can be a source of much trouble, such as the breakdown of transistors in power supplies. Protective diodes may be employed together with adequately rated components. Fluorescent lamps should be excluded from areas where low level recordings have to be made since they can generate radio frequency signals. Sparking at thermostat contacts and electric motor brushes is another source of high frequency interference. A series resistor–capacitor combination placed across the contacts or the armature supply will usually remove the interference.

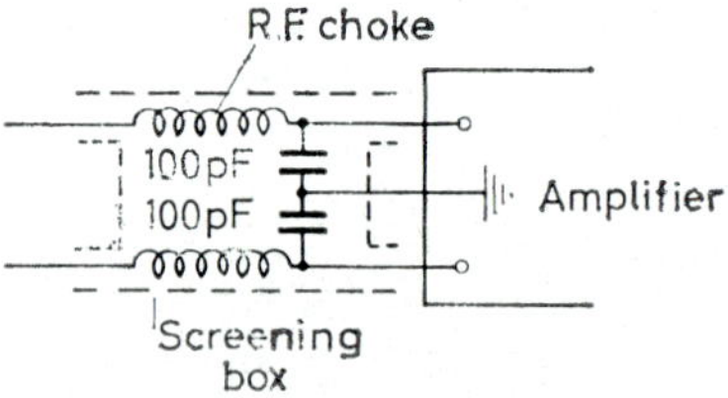

Figure 9.9. Balanced interference suppressor arrangement

The mains transformer of each equipment should be fitted with an electrostatic screen between the primary and the secondaries to stop radio frequency interference getting across to the secondary windings. A balanced suppressor choke and capacitor arrangement, as shown in *Figure 9.9*, should be fitted to the mains cable.

THE USE OF A BALANCED MAINS TRANSFORMER

The use of a carefully balanced mains transformer placed outside the recording room offers several advantages. With a 1:1 transformer, the output consists of two equal voltages exactly out of phase (*Figure 9.10*). This results in a cancellation of the electrostatic and electromagnetic fields from the wires connected to the secondary.

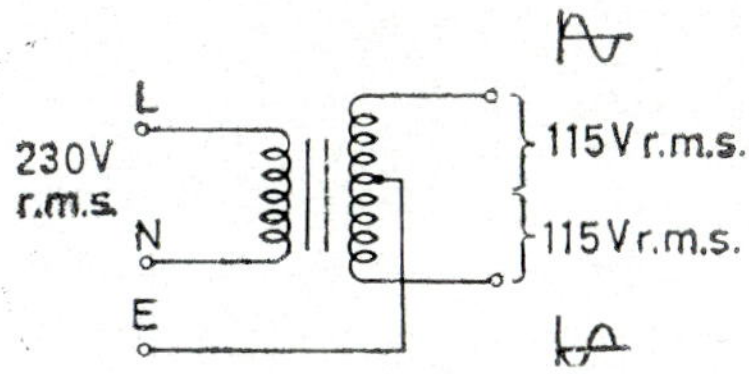

Figure 9.10. The action of a balanced mains transformer

A typical balanced transformer might have each half of its secondary winding matched to within ±1 per cent for both amplitude and phase over the range 0–80 per cent of its full 3 kW rating. With a 1:1 ratio, the peak voltage existing between either end of the secondary and earth is only half of that between the corresponding end of the primary and earth, so that the risk of an electric shock is reduced. Since the secondary centre tap is earthed, this arrangement does not constitute an 'isolating transformer' and give an earth-free mains supply.

INTERFERENCE FROM DIATHERMY UNITS

When a surgical (1·75 MHz) or a therapeutic (27 MHz) diathermy unit is activated, considerable interference may be experienced by neighbouring physiological recording systems. The usual trouble arises from the radio frequency signal being modulated at 50 or 100 Hz (60 or 120 Hz in the U.S.A. and Canada). The modulation arises from the inefficient smoothing provided in the h.t. supply. The modulation is detected (demodulated) by the first non-linear impedance (valve or transistor) in the recording amplifier and is fed to the pens. The pen galvanometers will respond to the modulation frequency. Many diathermy sets make use of a half-wave rectified, unsmoothed power supply so that the output waveform of the set will be 100 per cent modulated at the mains frequency.

In 1969, the Department of Health and Social Security in the United Kingdom issued a specification limiting the modulation factor of short wave therapeutic diathermy units to 30 per cent. In practice, some sets now have a modulation of less than 10 per cent. Even if good power supply smoothing is provided and the diathermy output is almost a pure sine wave, this can overload one or more of the recording amplifier stages, giving rise to non-linearity and rectification and thus producing a d.c. signal which could overload the pens.

Radiated interference tends to be more severe in the case of the 27 MHz diathermies because they are in use for longer periods for therapeutic purposes. Fortunately, at 1·75 MHz the leads connected to a surgical diathermy represent an inefficient aerial, but interference may be conducted away via the mains cable. The most severe interference problems arise when recordings are being taken from a surgical patient with diathermy in use. The direct connection of the diathermy to the patient provides a level of interference which it is almost impossible to remove completely. The use of input filters on the recording channels can allow *R*-waves to be recognized although *P*-waves will be obliterated. In order to save spoiling the record at least, one solution is to fit the diathermy unit with an additional relay. When the foot pedal of the unit is depressed, the relay is activated and transfers the output of the recording amplifier from the galvanometers to resistive dummy loads, thus muting the tracings. An alternative arrangement is that of Mapleson (1961). His device consists of a transistor radio receiver which picks up the radiated diathermy signal and energizes a relay to switch in the resistive loads.

A study carried out by the Electrical Engineering Division of the Department of Health and Social Security in the United Kingdom has shown that interference from surgical or therapeutic diathermies can be virtually eliminated by the use of simple R–C filter networks placed in the input leads and at the input of the recording amplifiers (Dobbie, 1965). A series resistor of 10 kΩ is recommended in combination with a shunt capacitor of 470 pF. A set of these components should be fitted to each of the input transistors, as close to the base as possible. In the case of electromyographs it is not feasible to use as large a value of capacity as 470 pF owing to the higher upper frequency of the EMG signals. Dobbie recommends 10 kΩ for the series resistor and 22 pF for the shunt capacitor in this case.

The wavelength of a 2 MHz surgical diathermy unit is 150 metres, so that the leads connected to it, perhaps 1·5 metres long, will represent only a small fraction of a wavelength and will not radiate efficiently. However, even with good mains filters, some interference can be expected when EEG recording has to be made in a room situated close to the operating room, possibly on the floor above or below.

When an EEG recorder has to be operated as close as 3·05 m (10 ft) from a surgical diathermy, Dobbie suggests a double filter arrangement. The EEG machine head box has incorporated into each lead a series 1,000 Ω resistor at each input lead terminal, followed by a capacitor of 330 pF in parallel to earth and a further 1,000 Ω resistor in series with the appropriate lead to the multi-core cable connecting the head box to the console (*Figure 9.11*). Each amplifier input connection is fitted with a series 1,000 Ω resistor and a 330 pF capacitor between base and emitter. In Dobbie's opinion, conditions of interference are seldom likely to be so severe as to warrant the purchase of an expensive screened room.

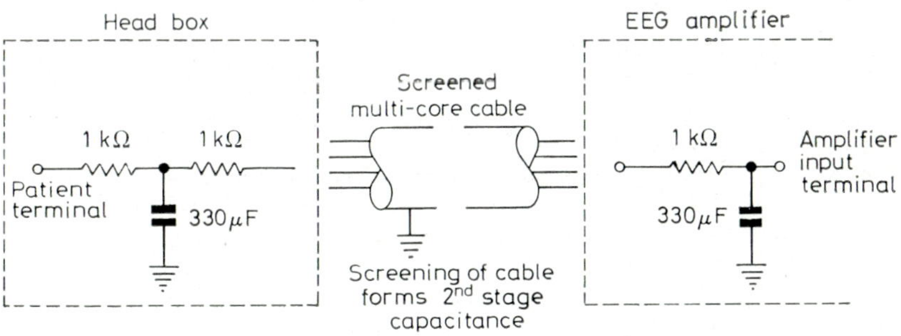

Figure 9.11. The use of radio frequency rejection components fitted to the input of an EEG recorder

(Reproduced from Dobbie, 1965, by courtesy of Pergamon Press)

Dobbie also recommends the use of modified hearing aids for tracking down sources of interference. For the detection of modulated radio frequency fields, a valve hearing aid is used with a 457 mm (18 in) long telescopic aerial connected in place of the microphone via a high pass C–R network to the grid of the first valve, where the modulation is detected and subsequently amplified. For the detection of electrostatic fields, a valve hearing aid is fitted with a probe consisting of a 76 mm (3 in) square metal plate mounted 102 mm (4 in) away from the hearing aid case. The probe is connected via a low pass R–C network (in order to reject radio frequency signals) to the grid of the pentode input valve, which has a 47 M Ω grid resistor. The unit can detect the electrostatic field from a fluorescent lamp at a distance of 3·05 m (10 ft). Low frequency magnetic fields can be detected by the use of a transistorized hearing aid having a pick-up coil wound on to a ferrite rod. With the output for the hearing aid taken to a rectifier moving coil meter, a full-scale deflection is obtained when the probe is held against a wire or pipe carrying a current of as little as 100 mA r.m.s.

PATIENT SAFETY

In the design of equipment which is intended for connection to patients, every precaution must be taken to exclude the possibility of the patient receiving a dangerous shock. The situation is aggravated in operating rooms and intensive care units where an increasing amount of electrical equipment is in use, and additionally surgical patients will be anaesthetized and often paralysed by the use of muscle relaxant drugs. Because of this they will be unable to indicate that they are receiving a shock or to move away spontaneously an extremity which comes into contact with a live object. A paper that bears this out is that of Said and El-Shiribiny (1962). This discusses the case of a patient who received eleven electric shocks resulting from an accidental connection made under general anaesthesia. As a result, repeated ventricular fibrillation occurred. Such incidents usually arise from the connection of a lead carrying a dangerous voltage to the patient who is earthed (grounded), perhaps by the indifferent plate electrode of a diathermy unit.

A special set of high risk circumstances arises when the current can be passed directly into the myocardium. This could occur due to leakage currents flowing through a saline-filled cardiac catheter.

Thresholds of Shock Currents

When an electric current flows through the surface of the body, the resulting threshold of sensation depends upon the current density. A current as low as 50 μA can be sensed with a point contact whilst 1 or 2 mA may be required with a larger electrode (Hopps, 1969). A sensation of pain is apparent with currents of 0·1 to 10 mA, depending on the size of the contact. The ability to move the affected portion of the body away from the conductor is lost when the current reaches 9–20 mA (Dalziel and Massoglia, 1956) and at higher currents there will be muscle cramps, respiratory paralysis and, finally, ventricular fibrillation. Hopps (1969) states that this can occur with currents from about 70 mA to 7 A.

At mains supply frequencies, the impedance existing b
pairs of skin electrodes is likely to lie in the range 1–10 kΩ.
one electrode becomes inserted within the body, the inter-ele
impedance falls markedly and a current as low as 20 μA can induce ventricular fibrillation (Weinberg, 1964). The danger limit for the current has now fallen by a factor of several thousand.

Leakage Currents

Whilst a direct contact with a high voltage conductor is an obvious shock hazard, a more subtle situation arises with the flow of leakage currents from apparatus into the patient. Suppose that a capacitance of 0·02 μF exists between the primary winding of the mains transformer and the core. With a mains voltage of 240 V r.m.s. at 50 Hz, the reactance of the leakage capacitance is approximately 150 kΩ and the leakage current will be 1·7 mA r.m.s. If the core and chassis of the apparatus are earthed, this current will simply flow to earth. If the earth has become disconnected, then it will flow through the patient to earth, assuming that he is earthed, perhaps by touching some earthed object such as a trolley. If the contact is made within the patient, the impedance to earth can be as low as 500 Ω. The 150,000 Ω leakage reactance represents a constant current source, and the current of 1·7 mA could be dangerous if it passed in or near the heart.

For these reasons, a great deal of attention is now being paid to the design of 'isolated front-ends' for monitoring equipment connected to patients. Isolation can be achieved by the use of a photon coupler or of a modulation arrangement and a coupling transformer. The latter arrangement can be employed to introduce the supply voltages for the pre-amplifier, thus avoiding contact with the high voltages in the mains power supply unit. Provision must be made for protective diodes to prevent voltage transients from damaging transistors and causing them to short-circuit.

Internal Current Connections

A number of possibilities arise including external mains-powered cardiac stimulators, blood pressure transducers and dye or contrast medium injection catheters. The radio-opaque contrast medium is likely to have a greater degree of conductivity than saline solution, and there is also the possibility of a catheter containing a metal guide wire. Leakage currents may flow from an improperly earthed power injector, or to the earthed injector from an improperly earthed cardioscope. Cases of this sort have been reported by Bousvaros, Don and Hopps (1962) and by Hopps and Roy (1963).

Earthing

The effective earthing of the case or chassis of monitoring equipment provides a lower impedance path to earth than exists via the patient and thus bypasses leakage currents from within the apparatus. The signal leads connected to the patient should be well isolated from earth and from any dangerous voltages. The patient is normally earthed during surgery by the plate electrode of the diathermy unit.

It is desirable that the various chassis and the patient should be connected to a good earth point and not to the mains earth lead. Normally the single phase a.c. mains supply consists of three leads—line, neutral and earth. In a well-balanced system the neutral should lie within 1 or 2 V of earth. The line alternates between the positive and negative values of the peak voltage (±325 V for a 230 V r.m.s. supply). Hence, mains circuit insulation has to be able to withstand these peak voltages. There exists a possibility of the earth lead of an apparatus being connected in error to the line lead of the mains. To guard against this happening, the mains line and neutral leads are connected via a double pole switch and fuses, as shown in *Figure 9.12*, to the primary winding of the equipment's mains transformer. The earth lead of the mains input cable is connected only to the core, frame and screen of the transformer and to the frame of the mains switch. The switch and the transformer are mounted on an insulated panel (*Figure 9.12*). Even if the line

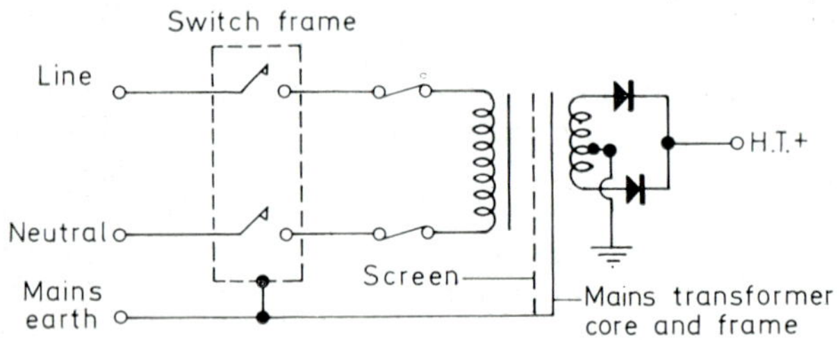

Figure 9.12. Electrical safety precautions at the input to a mains powered medical electronic apparatus

and the mains earth are interchanged, the line voltage is prevented from reaching the patient. If the mains lead becomes disconnected and there is a breakdown in the switch insulation or between the transformer primary and the core, the panel still protects the patient. As a routine precaution, the mains earth lead of each piece of electrical equipment should be regularly tested, preferably by passing a high current, for continuity. It is quite possible for personnel or trolleys in the operating room to invalidate earth leads by cutting or disconnecting them.

The earth lead from the patient is connected to the chassis of the apparatus and to a central earth terminal. The latter should be connected via a copper busbar to a series of copper plates buried in damp ground.

In equipment connected to patients, it is important to segregate the mains circuits from the patient's circuits. *Hospital Technical Memorandum No. 8*, published by the Department of Health and Social Security, sets out the precautions to be taken in this respect. The mains transformer must have an earthed metallic screen interposed between the primary and secondary windings, or else completely separate bobbins must be used for the primary and secondary windings. In the chassis, the mains wiring must be double insulated and consist of stranded wire which is doubly secured at soldering tags by a mechanically sound joint which is subsequently sleeved over the tag or secured by lacing. Electrical strength and insulation tests are specified in addition to the physical separation requirements.

An alternative approach to the risk of the mains line voltage coming into contact with an earthed patient is to use an isolated (earth-free) mains supply in the operating room (Dobbie, 1966). The operating room outlets are fed from an isolating transformer. Any leakage from the mains to earth is continuously monitored by a core-balance transformer unit which will give an indication if there is an imbalance of more than 5 mA between the currents flowing in the power lines from the transformer, resistors limiting this current to a maximum of 12 mA. Dobbie (1966) also describes an alternative relay circuit for detecting an earth leakage situation. The earth-free mains system is recommended in patient monitoring situations where a number of separate equipments may be connected to a patient, for example in intensive care units and during cardiac surgery and neurosurgery.

Burns from Therapeutic Diathermy

When using a 27 MHz therapeutic diathermy unit, care must be taken to avoid the build-up of localized areas of high current density which could give rise to burns. If a patient's hand is placed too near to one of the high frequency cables or to the earthed case of the machine, the high frequency current can take an unwanted path through the small capacitance existing between the hand and the cable or case. A high current density may be attained at the wrist or fingers. Similarly, care must be taken to avoid excessive heating of metallic objects carried in a patient's pocket, or of metallic implants as used in orthopaedics. These situations are discussed by Nightingale (1959) and Scott (1957).

Burns from Surgical Diathermy

The peak-to-peak output voltage from a surgical diathermy unit off-load may be of the order of 1,000 V, maximum power output occurring when the machine is working into a load of about 200–300 Ω. A typical cutting current would be 250 mA, whilst 500 mA would be typical for coagulation using forceps, and contact with a retractor might produce a current of 900 mA.

When surgical diathermy is employed, the patient's body is maintained at a potential as near earth as possible by means of the earthed indifferent electrode. In older installations this is a flexible lead plate about 152 × 127 mm (6 × 5 in) in area, kept in a cloth bag which should be soaked in saline solution or, failing that, in water. The diathermy current flows through this electrode, which must have a low contact impedance with the patient. If it does not, then local heating may produce a burn at the site of the plate electrode. A plate electrode contained in a saline-soaked bag can have a contact impedance as low as 1 Ω at the diathermy frequency, and in a water-soaked bag this may rise to 5 Ω. If the plate is dry, the contact impedance rises to approximately 100 Ω. Alternatively, a polished stainless steel flexible plate electrode may be used. No cloth bag is required, the formation of a film of perspiration between the electrode and the skin ensuring a low value of contact impedance. An aluminium foil electrode has recently been developed, and this is transparent to x-radiation.

If the plate electrode is not placed in position or becomes disconnected, the patient's body may assume a potential as high as 300 V when the live electrode is applied. Accidental burns can arise from contact between the patient's body and metal objects which are earthed or virtually at earth due to an appreciable capacitance to earth at the diathermy frequency. Modern diathermy sets utilize a low voltage d.c. current to monitor the continuity of the plate electrode lead. A stoppage of the current flow causes a light to flash and a buzzer to sound.

ANAESTHETIC EXPLOSIONS AND FIRES

If potentially flammable anaesthetic agents such as cyclopropane, ethylene, trichloroethylene or ether are in use, particular care must be taken to avoid the occurrence of a fire or explosion. The widespread use of non-explosive anaesthetic agents such as halothane and methoxyflurane has reduced this risk to the degree that electrocution represents a greater hazard. Nevertheless it would be very unwise to relax precautions against the build-up of static charges or sparking from current circuits (Macintosh, Mushin and Epstein, 1963).

The build-up of static charges is prevented by adequate humidity in the operating room atmosphere and by the use of conducting rubber for boots, shoes, trolley wheels and anaesthetic tubing. *Figure 9.13* shows a modern operating room. A resistance to earth of the order of 1 MΩ is to be aimed at, since this will leak away static charges without providing a low enough impedance to earth for the patient to be exposed to a current flow shock hazard. With the exception of ethylene, flammable agents are heavier than air and thus would tend to accumulate near the floor of the operating room. For this reason, the air extraction vents should be placed towards the bottom of the walls and the air inlets towards the top. As an additional precaution, any electrical apparatus which is not spark-proof should be mounted at a height of 1·37 m (4 ft 6 in) above floor level in the United Kingdom or 1·52 m (5 ft) in the U.S.A. and Canada.

The most dangerous region in the operating room will be in the vicinity of the anaesthetic machine, tubing, relief valve, reservoir bag and the patient, particularly his head (Bulgin, 1953). This high risk zone extends out horizontally for about 305 mm (1 ft) and downwards to floor level. There is an additional low risk zone extending out for about a further 914 mm (3 ft) horizontally and downwards. Beyond this, the concentrations will generally be below the limit for ignition. If there is any doubt about the sparking risk of a particular piece of equipment, it should be sited more than 1·22 m (4 ft) away from the patient and the anaesthetic machine.

In the United Kingdom, the mains supply outlets in the operating room are specified to be of the mercury switch interlocking type. The plug cannot be removed from the socket whilst the switch is ON. Bruner (1967) and Hill (1971) discuss the problems involved in the use of electrical equipment in the operating room and the risks involved with various volatile anaesthetic agents. Bulgin (1953), Forrest (1953) and Quinton (1953) describe the measures which can be employed to reduce the risk from electrostatic sparks when explosive or flammable agents are in use. Although the danger of an explosion during surgery has been greatly reduced since the introduction of non-explosive anaesthetic agents, the risk of fire has still to be seriously considered in hyperbaric tanks. In a closed environment, the results could be catastrophic within a matter of seconds. Pure oxygen can give rise to deadly flash fires (Denison, Ernsting and Cresswell, 1966), and this hazard is reduced by

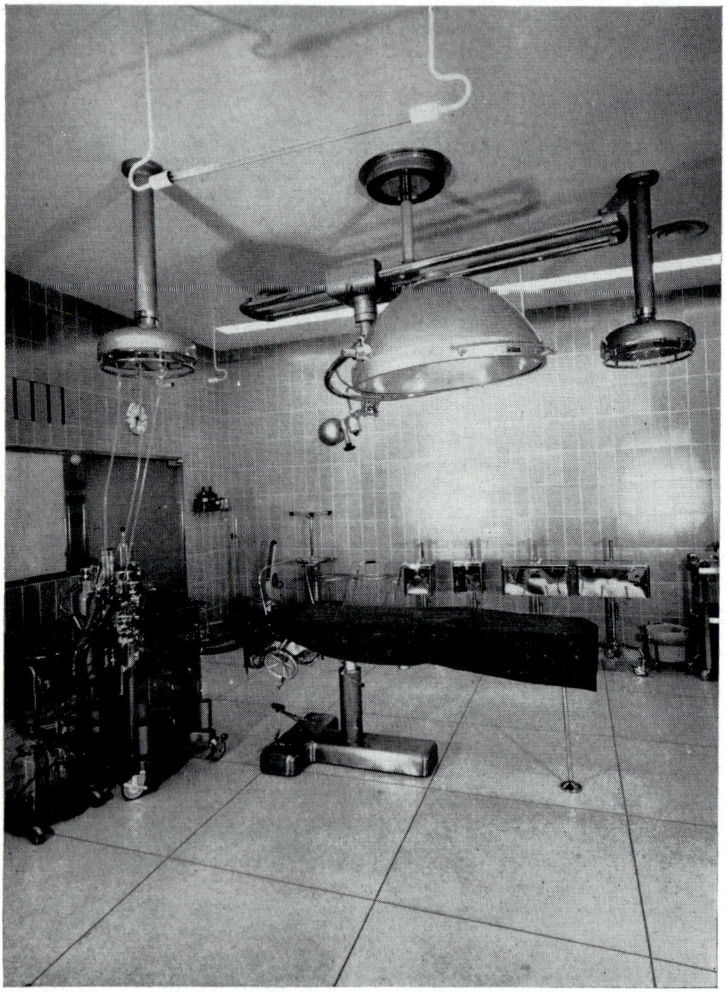

Figure 9.13. Modern operating room showing ceiling pendants which can be raised or lowered by compressed air and supply suction, anaesthetic gases and electrical power

(By courtesy of Drägerwerk, Lübeck)

pressurizing the chamber with air and having only the patient(s) breathe pure oxygen. Brennand (1969) describes special interface circuits which limit the voltage and current applied to equipment

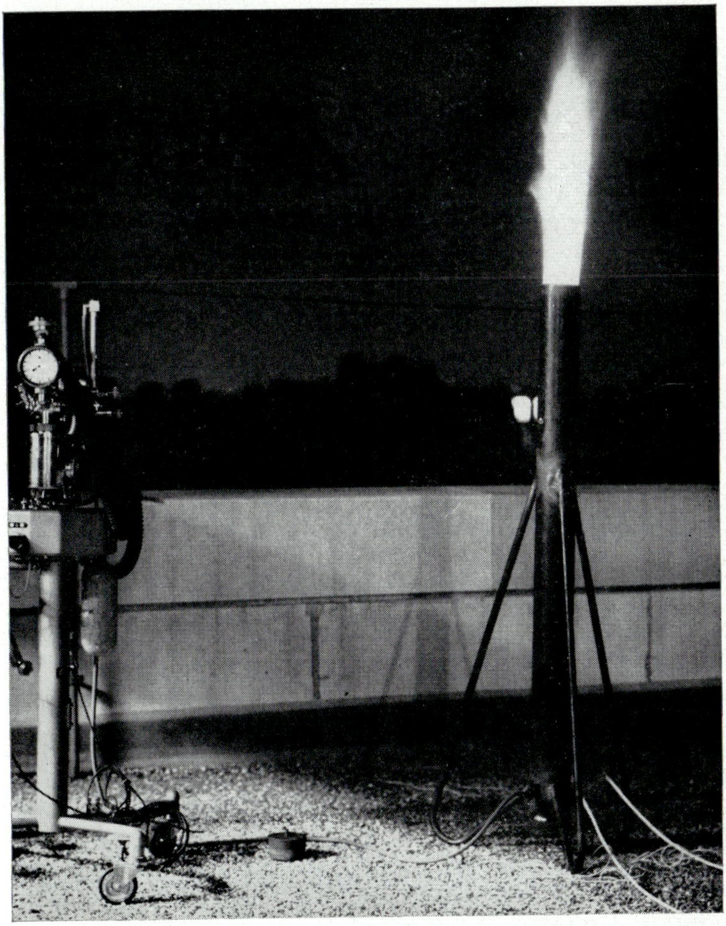

Figure 9.14. Demonstration explosion using an anaesthetic cyclopropane–oxygen mixture

used in the chamber to safe levels at which sparking cannot occur, and Segal (1966) deals with fire precautions necessary with hyperbaric chambers.

Information on explosion hazards in the operating room is given in the following: Hospital Technical Memoranda No. 1, *Anti-static Precautions: Rubber, Plastics and Fabrics* (H.M.S.O., London); Hospital Technical Memoranda No. 2, *Anti-static Precautions: Flooring in Anaesthetizing Areas* (H.M.S.O., London); Ministry of Health Report, 1956, *Report of a Working Party on Anaesthetic Explosions* (H.M.S.O., London); and by Macintosh, Mushin and Epstein (1963).

In the U.S.A. the use of electrical apparatus in conjunction with volatile anaesthetic agents is governed by N.F.P.A. Code No. 56, *A Code for the Use of Flammable Anaesthetics* (*Safe Practice for Hospital Operating Rooms*), June 1959 (National Fire Protection Association, 60 Batterymarch Street, Boston 10, Mass.).

In Germany the relevant regulations are *Normen-Verzeichnis und VDE-Vorschriften der Radiologie und Electromedizin* as laid down by the Verband Deutscher Electrotechniker in August 1950 and published by Beuth-Vertrieb G.m.b.H., Berlin, W.12.

As a final warning, *Figure 9.14* reveals the strength of a demonstration cyclopropane–oxygen explosion.

STERILIZATION OF ELECTRICAL EQUIPMENT

Electrical apparatus which is designed to be completely spark-proof is normally enclosed within a gas-tight enclosure so that it cannot come into contact with the atmosphere. However, electronic apparatus which is not sealed is notoriously dust-catching, and the situation is aggravated when it employs local fan cooling as in the case of visual display units.

Figure 9.15 illustrates a chamber in which complete electronic consoles can be placed to be sprayed with formalin vapour. Bacteriological tests have confirmed that this is an effective method of sterilization. Transistor circuits sprayed with formalin vapour each day for five working days still performed perfectly at the finish and no corrosion was observed after several months. The circuit contained transistors, resistors and capacitors.

Few studies seem to have been made on the possible contamination of electronic equipment used in operating rooms and intensive care areas. In many cases it would seem desirable to wash down the cases and controls with an antiseptic solution, and the effect of this on the efficient functioning of the equipment must be borne in mind.

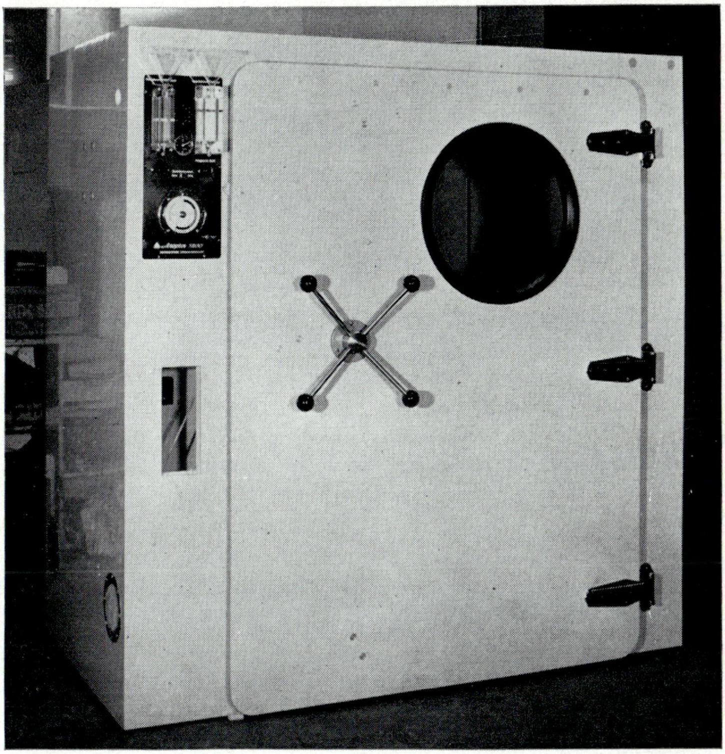

Figure 9.15. Formalin vapour sterilization chamber suitable for treating medical electronic apparatus

(By courtesy of Drägerwerk, Lübeck)

REFERENCES

Battye, C. K. (1962). 'A telemetering electromyograph with a single frequency modulated channel.' *Electron. Engng* **34,** 398.

Bousvaros, G. A., Don, C. and Hopps, J. A. (1962). 'An electrical hazard of selective angiography.' *Can. med. Ass. J.* **87,** 286.

Brennand, R. (1969). 'Protective interface circuits for use with hyperbaric oxygen chambers.' In *The Induction and Hazards of a Hyperbaric Oxygen Environment*, p. 107. Ed. by G. S. Innes. Oxford: Pergamon.

Bruner, J. M. R. (1967). 'Hazards of electrical apparatus.' *Anesthesiology* **28,** 396.

Bulgin, D. (1953). 'Factors in the design of an operating theatre free from electrostatic risks.' *Br. J. appl. Phys.* **4,** 587.

Dalziel, C. F. and Massoglia, F. P. (1956). 'Let-go currents and voltages.' *Trans. Am. Inst. elect. Engrs* **75,** 49.

Denison, D. M., Ernsting, J. and Cresswell, A. W. (1966). 'Fire and hyperbaric oxygen.' *Lancet* **2,** 1405.

Dobbie, A. K. (1965). 'Why screened rooms in hospitals?' *Wld med. Electron.* **3,** 157.

— (1966). 'Electrical safety of patient monitoring equipment.' *Br. Hosp. J.* **76,** 1996.

— (1967a). 'Interference due to magnetic fields in hospitals.' *Proc. electrophysiol. Technol. Ass.* **13,** 120.

— (1967b). 'A special interference problem with chopper-type amplifiers.' *Wld med. Electron.* **5,** 124.

Forrest, J. S. (1953). 'Methods of increasing the electrical conductivity of surfaces.' *Br. J. appl. Phys.* **4,** 537.

Gentille, E. (1956). 'Electrocardiogram distortions due to a high skin resistance. A simple clinical method for measuring this resistance.' *Am. Heart J.* **51,** 906.

Hill, D. W. (1971). *Physics Applied to Anaesthesia,* 2nd edn. London: Butterworths.

— and Khandpur, R. S. (1969). 'The performance of transistorized ECG amplifiers.' *Wld med. Instrum.* **7,** 12.

Hopps, J. A. (1969). 'Shock hazards in operating rooms and patient-care areas.' *Anesthesiology* **31,** 142.

— and Roy, O. Z. (1963). 'Electrical hazards in cardiac diagnosis and treatment.' *Med. Electron. biol. Engng* **1,** 135.

Leadbitter, A. F. C. (1963). 'Screening against electrical interference.' *Wld med. Electron.* **2,** 17.

Macintosh, R., Mushin, W. W. and Epstein, H. G. (1963). *Physics for the Anaesthetist,* p. 326. 3rd edn. Oxford: Blackwell.

Mapleson, W. W. (1961). 'Device for protecting recording pens from interference from surgical diathermy.' *J. scient. Instrum.* **38,** 260.

Mundl, W. J. (1970). 'An E.E.G. preamplifier with transformer input.' *Med. biol. Engng* **8,** 323.

Murari, B. (1967). 'E.C.G. and E.E.G. pre-amplifiers.' *Wld med. Electron.* **5,** 264.

Nightingale, A. (1959). *Physics and Electronics in Physical Medicine.* London: Bell.

Quinton, A. (1953). 'Safety measures in operating theatres and the use of a radioactive thallium source to dissipate static electricity.' *Br. J. appl. Phys.* **4,** 592.

Said, K. and El-Shiribiny, A. (1962). 'Accidental repeated electrical shocks during anaesthesia.' *Acta anaesth. scand.* Suppl. **12,** 111.

REFERENCES

Segal, L. (1966). 'Fire suppression in hyperbaric chambers.' *Fire Journal* **60,** 17.

Scott, B. O. (1957). *The Principles and Practice of Diathermy.* London: Heinemann.

Weinberg, D. I. (1964). 'Grounding for electrical safety.' *Med. Electron. biol. Engng.* **2,** 435.

Chapter 10

Power Supplies

The operating power for most types of electronic equipment is obtained from the mains power supply, but portable equipment can be conveniently powered from dry batteries or accumulators. This imposes the need to change the batteries or recharge the accumulator, but does provide an additional safety factor in the form of isolation from the mains. Active circuits which are implanted inside the body ideally require a power supply which derives its energy from the body and does not need to be renewed. Some account will be given of possible approaches to this problem, whilst a discussion of batteries and rechargeable cells is given in Chapter 3. The almost universal use of transistorized apparatus has required d.c. supply voltages in the range 6–24 V with current drains which are often below 1 A but can attain several amperes. The circuit performance is generally dependent on the stability of the supply voltages, so that a great deal of effort has been put into the development of circuits which will stabilize the output voltage of the power supply against changes in the input d.c. or a.c. voltage or changes in the load.

Most stabilized power supplies provide a d.c. output, but there is a requirement for units which provide a stabilized a.c. output. When a number of instruments are to be used in a laboratory, it is feasible to provide a stabilized mains supply for the room as a first line of defence to improve their performance stability. This approach is helpful also when items involving substantial current drains have to be considered, such as lamps, heaters and motors.

STABILIZED A.C. VOLTAGE SUPPLIES

It is convenient to stabilize the mains supply to a laboratory requiring a supply of perhaps 15 A by means of a servo-operated a.c. stabilizer

(Collinge and Marsham, 1951; Long, 1952). The mains voltage supply to be stabilized is applied to a 'lamp bridge'. This is a Wheatstone bridge network with three resistive arms, the fourth being a filament lamp. The bridge is first set up to be in balance at the nominal value of the a.c. mains voltage. If the supply voltage to the bridge changes, the bridge becomes unbalanced, since a change of current through the lamp filament alters its resistance. Any imbalance voltage from the bridge output is amplified and applied to an a.c. servo-motor. The motor shaft rotates the control of a variable auto-transformer, adjusting the voltage tapping. The action of the auto-transformer is such as to raise or lower the value of the output voltage from the stabilizer as required to maintain it at the desired nominal value (*Figure 10.1*). An improved version of this arrangement is described by Ackland and Buckland (1964).

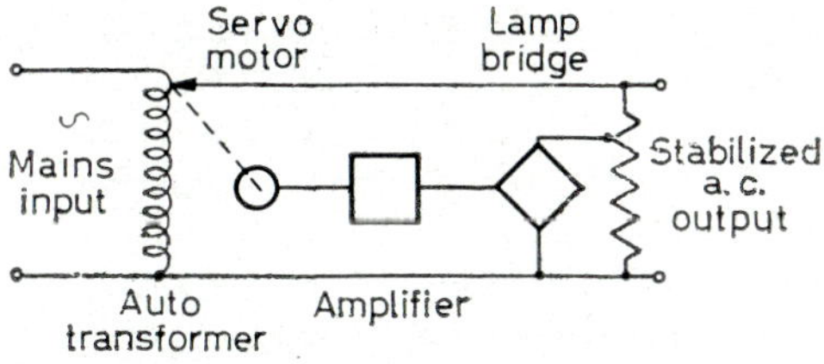

Figure 10.1. Schematic diagram of a servo-operated a.c. voltage stabilizer

A typical unit could supply a stabilized voltage of 240 V r.m.s. at up to 15 A. The maximum speed of voltage correction is 147 V/sec to within ±0·5 per cent accuracy.

When the stabilized a.c. power requirement is smaller, perhaps 150 or 250 W, a 'constant voltage transformer' is often used. This has a three-limbed core with a magnetic leakage path dividing the winding space (*Figure 10.2*). The upper winding space is wound with

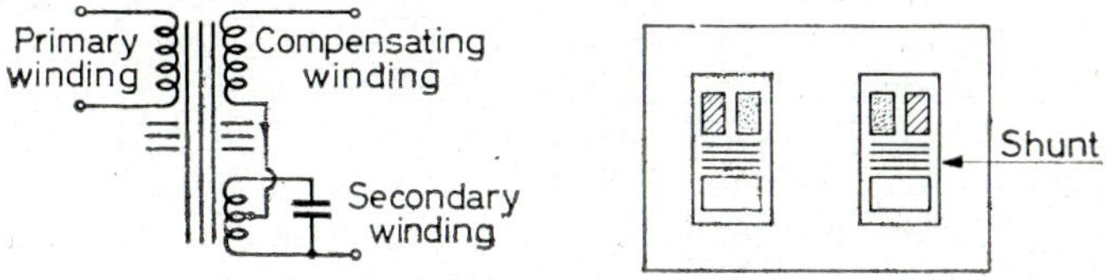

Figure 10.2. Construction of a constant voltage transformer

the primary winding and a compensating winding. The lower winding space is wound with a secondary winding across which is connected a capacitor. An increase in the mains voltage applied to the primary gives rise to an increased magnetic flux in the main magnetic circuit. As a result, the secondary voltage increases in proportion. The increasing flux produces an increase in the leakage reactance of the secondary winding and this tends to a value which resonates with the capacitor. As resonance is reached, the secondary current increases rapidly, saturating the lower part of the magnetic circuit. The flux due to the primary is directed through the magnetic shunt, and any further increase in the primary voltage produces little change in the secondary voltage. It increases very slowly, and the increase is offset by the voltage induced in the compensating winding which is connected in series opposition to the secondary winding. The transformer is operated with the secondary winding resonating, so that although the primary voltage may change, the combined output of the secondary and compensating windings stays constant. Typically, for an input variation of ± 15 per cent the output voltage is stabilized to within ± 1 per cent of the nominal value. Stabilization takes place within approximately one cycle of the supply frequency, and the efficiency of the device is better than 75 per cent at full load.

The stabilizing action of some types of constant voltage transformer is seriously impaired if the mains frequency departs from its nominal value. The simpler types may produce as much as 25 per cent distortion of the sine waveform at their output. In this case, readings taken with the usual rectifier type of a.c. voltmeter will be in error. These factors have affected the popularity of the constant voltage transformer.

RECTIFIERS

In the case of mains powered power supplies, it is necessary to employ some form of rectification as a first step in the process of producing a d.c. output. Basically the rectifier(s) select either positive or negative half cycles of the a.c. supply and feed them to a smoothing circuit. As has been explained in Chapter 8, a semiconductor *p–n* junction will function as a rectifier or one-way device. Silicon junction diodes are used in most cases, silicon-controlled rectifiers being employed when the output current is required to be several amperes.

The voltage–current characteristic of an ideal rectifying device is shown in *Figure 10.3a* and that of a practical rectifier in *Figure 10.3b*. In the latter case, the device exhibits an appreciable 'forward' and 'reverse' resistance. Ideally, the resistance offered to a forward flow of current should be infinitesimal, and that to a reverse flow of current should be infinite. The presence of the resistances

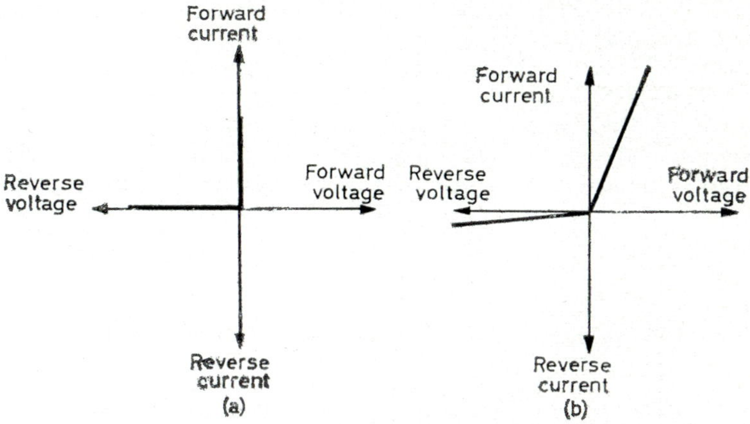

Figure 10.3. Characteristics of (a) an ideal rectifier and (b) a practical rectifier

dissipates power in the rectifier, and in order to keep the junction within safe limits the rectifier is normally mounted on a heat sink.

HALF WAVE POWER SUPPLY

Figure 10.4 shows the simplest type of power supply using half wave rectification. The output from the secondary winding of the mains transformer is applied to the diode and the load in series. The

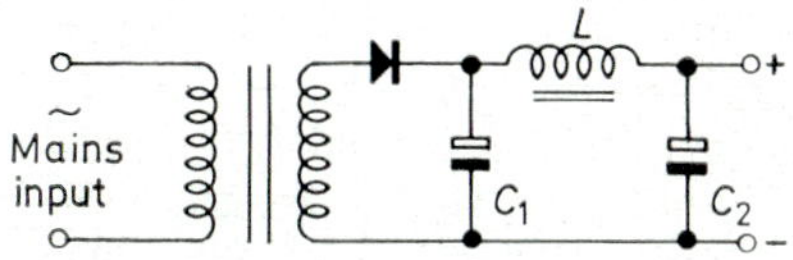

Figure 10.4. Half wave power supply

diode conducts only during the positive half cycles of the mains when its anode is positive with respect to its cathode. The waveforms of the circuit are illustrated in *Figure 10.5.*

The reservoir capacitor C_1 provides a source of current during the missing half cycles. The action is not perfect, and so the output voltage is not completely steady or 'smooth' but consists of a d.c level with a superimposed ripple. This is removed by the smoothing circuit, consisting of the inductor (choke) and the smoothing capacitor C_2. The reactance of the smoothing capacitor (200 Ω) is small at the ripple frequency (50 Hz in Europe, 60 Hz in America and Canada) in comparison with the reactance of the choke (6,000 Ω). Since the output voltage is taken from across the smoothing capacitor, the choke–capacitor combination acts as a voltage divider for the ripple, ensuring that the proportion of the ripple voltage tapped off to the output is small. Because the half wave rectifier conducts only on alternate half cycles, it is not efficient.

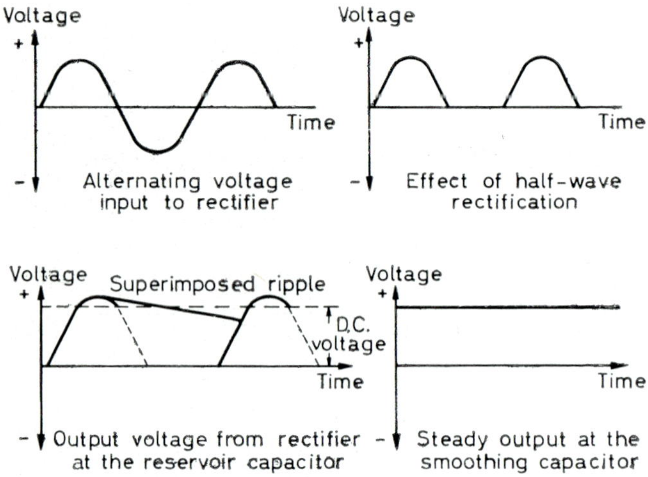

Figure 10.5. Waveforms in a half wave power supply

For purposes of comparison, consider the rectifier to be connected only to a resistive load and the components C_1, L and C_2 to be missing. In this case, across the load the amplitude of the ripple voltage is greater than that of the d.c. upon which it is s perimposed, since the ripple factor $v_{r.m.s.}/V_{d.c.}=1{\cdot}21$. The efficiency of rectification is given by $V^2_{d.c.}/v^2_{r.m.s.}=40$ per cent. The peak voltage developed across the rectifier during its non-conducting half cycles is known as the Peak Inverse Voltage (PIV) and is equal to the peak value of the a.c. applied to the rectifier. The half wave rectifier has a lower PIV than any other circuit, and hence a number of half wave rectifiers are used, connected in series, for high voltage applications such as the EHT supply for a cathode ray tube.

Because it is fed only on every other half cycle, the half wave circuit possesses a poor 'regulation' in that if a substantial current is drawn from it, the output voltage falls markedly. That is, the internal resistance of the circuit is relatively high. Regulation is defined as

$$\left(\frac{\text{no-load output voltage}-\text{full-load output voltage}}{\text{full-load output voltage}}\right)\times 100 \text{ per cent.}$$

Half wave rectification is generally used for the lower current applications, and the choke is often replaced by a wirewound resistor. When a negative voltage output is required, the diode polarity is reversed and the output is now taken from the anode instead of the cathode. It is important to ensure that if C_1 and C_2 are electrolytic capacitors, as is usually the case, their polarity has also been reversed.

FULL WAVE (BIPHASE) POWER SUPPLY

An improvement in efficiency can be obtained by using a full wave rectifier. In this case a centre-tapped secondary winding of the mains transformer feeds a pair of diodes. For a positive output voltage, the output is taken from the pair of cathodes joined together as in *Figure 10.6*. Antiphase signals appear at the ends of the secondary

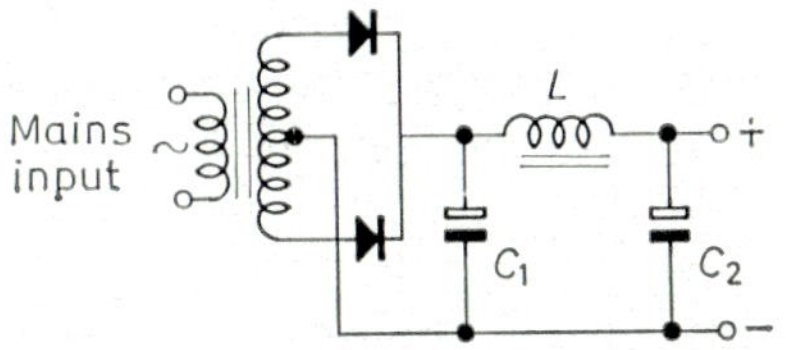

Figure 10.6. Biphase full wave rectifier circuit

winding, and the phases reverse after each half cycle of the mains supply. As a result, one diode will conduct with its anode positive relative to its cathode on one series of alternative half cycles, whilst the second will conduct on the other series of alternate half cycles. In this way all the half cycles are utilized (*Figure 10.7*), hence the term 'full wave'. Since the capacitors receive increments of charge twice per cycle, the full wave circuit has a better regulation than the half wave circuit. The efficiency of rectification is 80 per cent, i.e. double that of the half wave circuit, and the ripple factor is 0·5.

Full wave rectifiers of either the biphase or the bridge type are used in all d.c. power supplies which have to supply more than a few tens of milliamperes of current. At the voltage levels encountered in transistor power supplies, it is usual to employ high capacity (250 μF or more) electrolytic capacitors in the

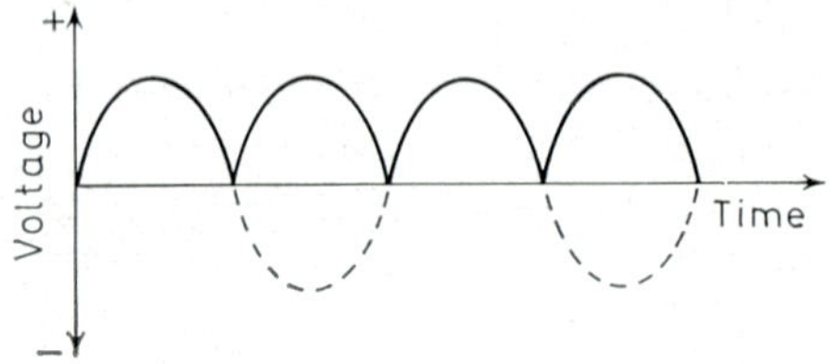

Figure 10.7. Full wave unsmoothed output waveform

smoothing circuit. The disadvantages of the biphase arrangement are that the peak inverse voltage (PIV) for each rectifier is now twice that in the half wave case. In addition, the use of the centre-tapped winding means that the voltage required to be developed across the secondary is twice that needed for the half wave circuit.

THE BRIDGE FULL WAVE RECTIFIER POWER SUPPLY

This circuit uses four diodes connected in a bridge arrangement (*Figure 10.8*) and does not require the mains transformer to have a centre-tapped secondary winding. During half the mains cycle,

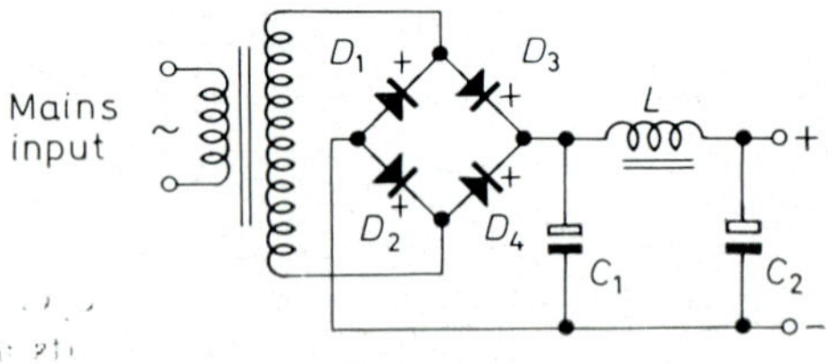

Figure 10.8. Bridge rectifier circuit

current flows from the secondary winding through D_3, the load and D_2, all in series. Diodes D_1 and D_4 will be reverse biased and will not pass current. During the next half cycle, diodes D_1 and D_4 will conduct while diodes D_3 and D_2 will be cut off. The voltage which has to be provided by the secondary winding is half that required in the biphase circuit, so that the risks of shock or insulation breakdown are reduced. The voltage is always applied to two diodes in series, so that diodes with a lower peak inverse voltage rating can be used. Since the output current must traverse two diodes, there is a slightly greater voltage drop than in the case of the biphase circuit. The PIV requirement for each diode is the same as in the half wave circuit, and the ripple factor and efficiency of rectification are the same as for the biphase circuit.

Small bridge type rectifiers are used as the rectifying element in a.c. voltmeters and ammeters of the moving coil type. These meters are commonly used with mains frequency signals, but are usable up to approximately 10 kHz (Dayal, 1964). They are also commonly encountered in complete instruments where the output from an a.c. amplifier has to be displayed on a panel meter.

With both full wave and half wave rectifier circuits, if the output is open circuit or if only a small current is drawn, the output voltage is equal to the peak value of the secondary winding voltage in the case of the half wave and bridge circuits or half of that in the case of the biphase circuit. This follows because the capacitors charge to the peak voltage passed by the rectifiers and will hold this throughout subsequent cycles if the load current is negligible. It is desirable that high value 'bleeder' resistors be placed across the reservoir and the smoothing capacitors so that these will not hold a dangerous charge when the circuit is switched OFF.

VOLTAGE DOUBLER POWER SUPPLY

Voltage doubler circuits are encountered in applications which call for a high voltage at a low current. Typical applications include the e.h.t. voltage supply for a photomultiplier or small cathode ray tube.

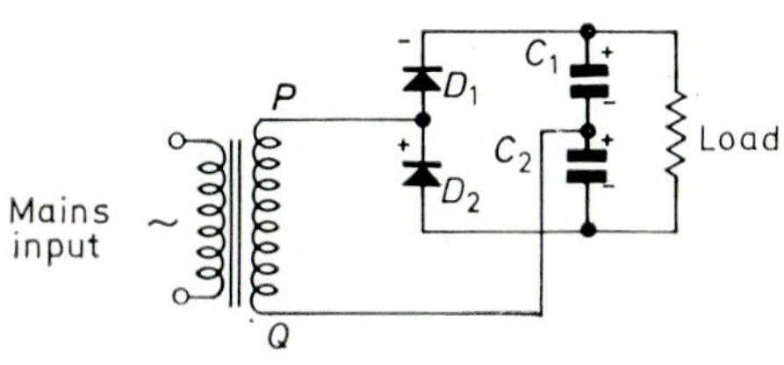

Figure 10.9. Voltage doubler circuit

In *Figure 10.9*, suppose that on one particular half-cycle of the mains the end P of the secondary winding is positive and the end Q is negative. Diode D_1 conducts, charging C_1 to the peak value of the secondary winding voltage. During the next half cycle, diode D_2 charges capacitor C_2. The voltages appearing across the capacitors add in series, so that the output voltage is double the peak voltage from the secondary winding. The regulation of the arrangement is poor, and the output voltage falls markedly with increasing load current.

SERIES VOLTAGE STABILIZERS

When the current requirement is low, a stabilized voltage can be taken from across a Zener diode. Variations in the supply voltage will alter the current through the Zener diode, but within limits this will not materially alter the voltage drop appearing across the diode. Higher load currents can be provided by using the Zener diode to provide the base bias for an emitter follower.

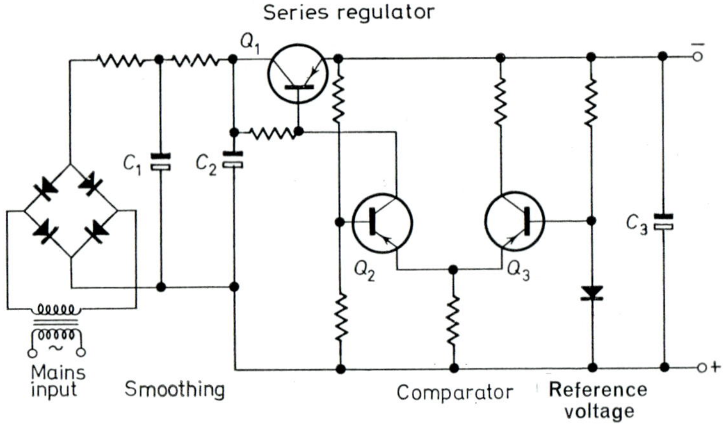

Figure 10.10. Series stabilizer constant voltage circuit

However, the arrangement most widely encountered in laboratory stabilized power supplies is the series stabilizer. Essentially, the output current from a full wave rectifier and smoothing circuit is passed through a variable control element and the load in series. A fraction of the output voltage supplied to the load is tapped off and compared in a comparator circuit with a reference voltage, usually obtained from a Zener diode. Any change in the output voltage is sensed and caused to alter the resistance of the series element (usually a power transistor) in such a way as to compensate for the change.

A simple form of this arrangement is illustrated in *Figure 10.10*. Transistors Q_2 and Q_3 form a differential amplifier which compares a fraction of the output voltage with that developed across the Zener diode D_5. If the output voltage rises (goes more negative), Q_2 draws more current, causing the base of Q_1 to go more positive and thus Q_1 to pass less current, thereby compensating for the output voltage change. Attree and Topliss (1962) advocate the use of silicon-controlled rectifiers to supply a series stabilizer circuit. The SCRs are arranged to adjust the unstabilized supply and thus reduce the dissipation in the series element at low output voltages.

Series Stabilizer Short-circuit Protection

Transistor series stabilizer circuits can be damaged very quickly if an accidental overload current is allowed to flow. The series element is overloaded as it passes maximal current in an effort to alleviate the effects of the short-circuit. Even fast-acting fuses are not satisfactory and electronic protection circuits are needed.

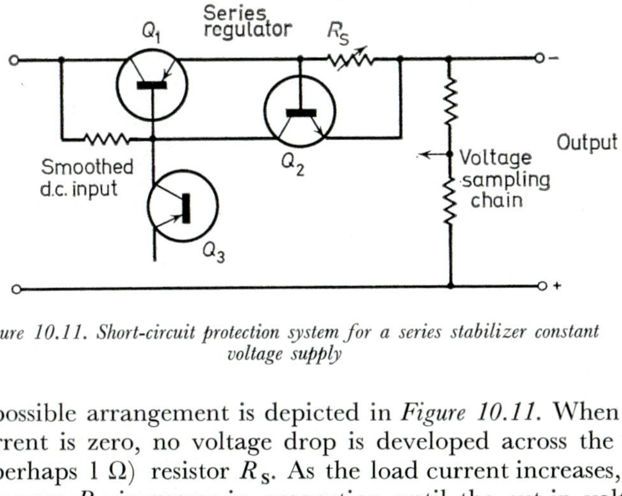

Figure 10.11. Short-circuit protection system for a series stabilizer constant voltage supply

One possible arrangement is depicted in *Figure 10.11*. When the load current is zero, no voltage drop is developed across the low value (perhaps 1 Ω) resistor R_S. As the load current increases, the voltage across R_S increases in proportion until the cut-in voltage for Q_2 is reached, when Q_2 starts to conduct. By suitably adjusting the value of R_S, it can be arranged that when the load current approaches a dangerous value as far as Q_1 is concerned, Q_2 either draws enough current to save Q_1 or cuts it off so that the output voltage falls to zero. If Q_1 does not cut off completely, the effect will be that the output voltage will fall markedly with increasing load above a predetermined value of the load current.

Another possible system is that of *Figure 10.12*. At some value of the load current, the voltage drop across R_2 becomes sufficient to fire the SCR and thus protect the series element. R_1 prevents the firing

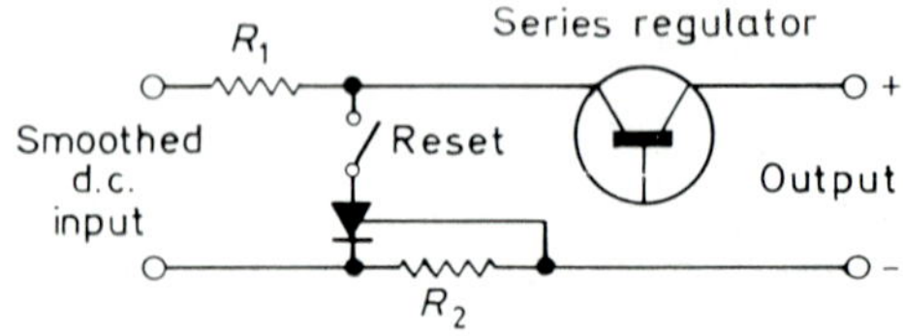

Figure 10.12. SCR short-circuit protection for a series stabilizer constant voltage supply

of the SCR from shorting the rectifiers. However, removal of the output short-circuit will still leave the SCR conducting. Opening the RESET switch will cut off the SCR and allow normal operation to be resumed if the short-circuit has been removed.

Cooper (1960) describes a short-circuit protection arrangement.

INTEGRATED CIRCUIT STABILIZED VOLTAGE POWER SUPPLIES

Integrated circuit operational amplifiers normally require both a positive and a negative voltage supply line, since the output of the amplifier under quiescent conditions may be required to be set at 0 V. Typical values would be ± 15 V.

The advent of monolithic techniques allows a dual polarity regulator circuit complete with Zener diode reference voltage to be laid down on a single chip. The output current drain is limited to about 300 mA because of the small size of the chip, but additional power transistors can be added externally to act as series elements when the output current has to be increased to 2 A. The stabilizer can be made to be little affected by changes in the ambient temperature by making the layout of the chip thermally symmetrical. As indicated in *Figure 10.13*, the circuit elements which dissipate an appreciable amount of power are mounted at each end of the chip, so that a longitudinal axis of thermal symmetry exists along the chip. Resistors, diodes and transistors are mounted symmetrically on either side of this axis, so that the temperature distribution will be as nearly as possible equal for each of a pair of components.

The temperature coefficient for the output voltages is 2·2 mV per degree centigrade and the chip dimensions are 80×114 mils (2×2·43 mm since 1 mil=0·001 in). As Davis (1971) points out, this is a sophisticated regulator since it provides for pre-adjusted output voltages to within ±1 per cent, internal frequency compensation, current limiting and shut-down when the temperature of the output transistor junctions exceeds a safe value.

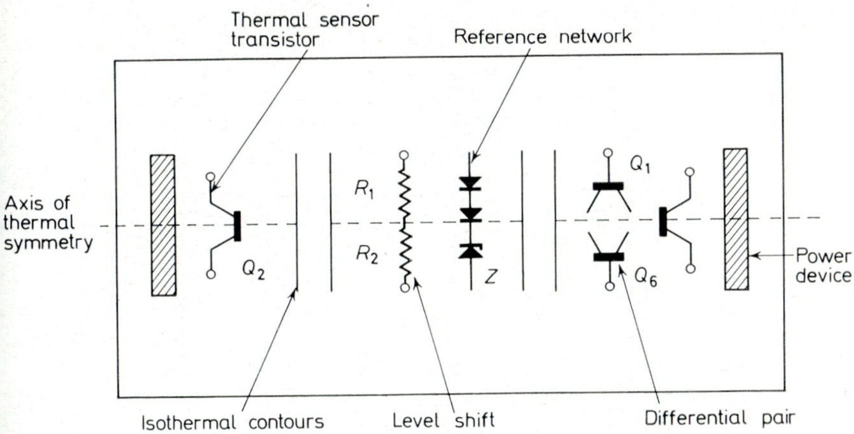

Figure 10.13. The distribution of components on an integrated circuit power supply chip with regard to the axis of thermal symmetry

(Reproduced after Davis, 1971, by courtesy of I.E.E.E.)

The circuit of the dual regulator is given in *Figure 10.14.* A temperature-independent reference voltage is produced by cancelling the sum of the negative temperature coefficients of two base–emitter junctions (Q_3 and Q_4) in *Figure 10.15* with the positive temperature coefficient of a Zener diode Z. The noise voltage appearing across this compound structure is minimized by increasing the current through it. The positive regulated output voltage is established by using a negative feedback amplifier which level shifts the reference voltage to +15 V (with resistors R_1 and R_2) and provides a low output impedance. By connecting the input of a unity gain inverting feedback amplifier directly to the positive output as shown in *Figure 10.16*, it is arranged that the negative output voltage will follow any small changes that may occur in the stabilized positive voltage, but in a complementary manner. The circuit is provided with four additional terminals to which can be attached two

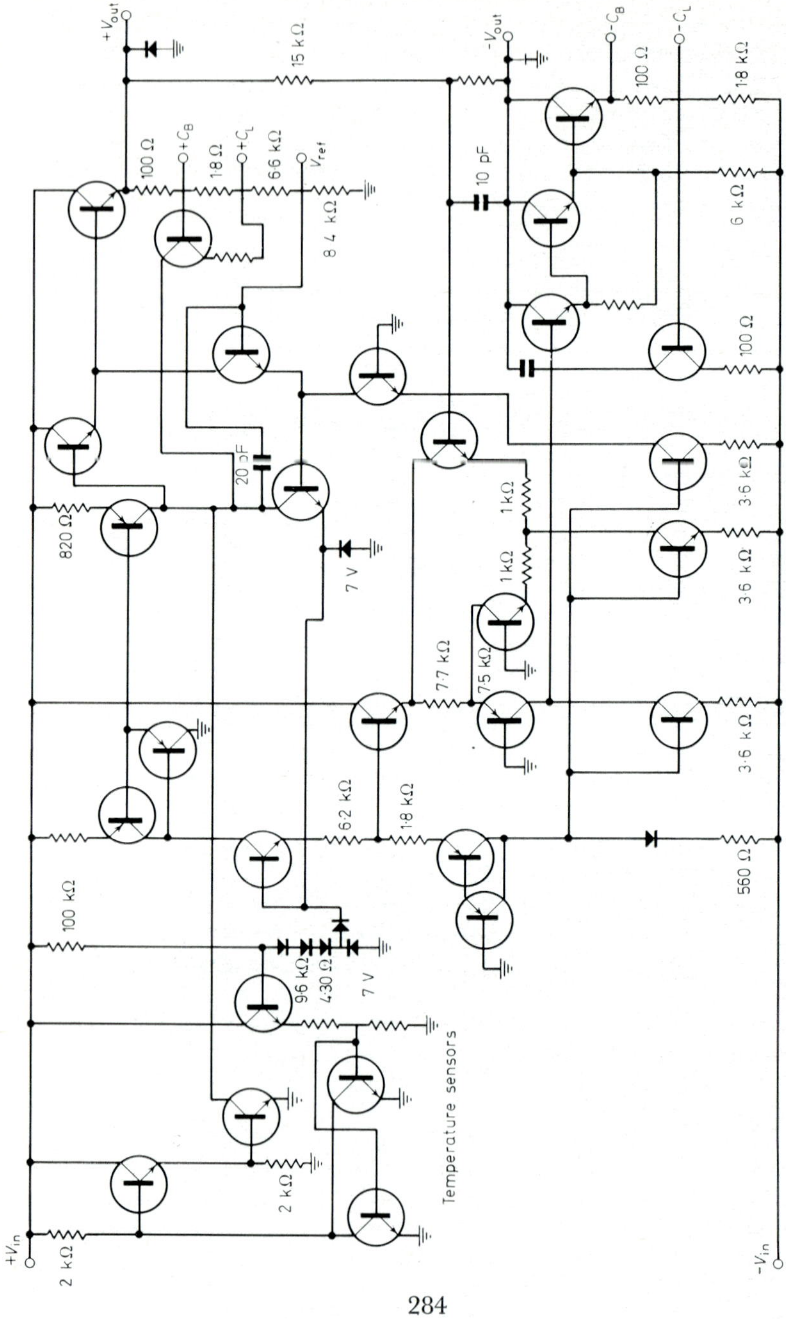

Figure 10.14. Dual polarity integrated circuit power supply
(Reproduced after Davis, 1971, by courtesy of I.E.E.E.)

external *n–p–n* power transistors. This increases the current that may be drawn from the stabilizer to ± 10 A. In manufacture, the output voltages are adjusted during the wafer probing operation by adding

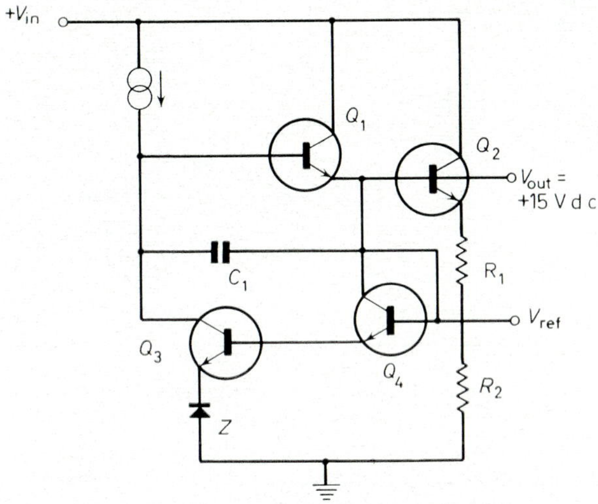

Figure 10.15. Basic positive voltage regulator circuit

(Reproduced after Davis, 1971, by courtesy of I.E.E.E.)

incremental resistance to the d.c. level shifting resistors. Fusable metal links placed across these resistors are selectively disconnected to achieve the ± 1 per cent output voltage tolerance.

Changes in the load condition of an integrated circuit voltage regulator give rise to a change in the power dissipation which produces not only a uniform change in the surface temperatures, but also a change in the thermal gradient across the surface of the dice. The arrangement of *Figure 10.15* will compensate only for the uniform thermal changes. As has been previously mentioned, changes occurring in the thermal gradients are overcome by placing groups of circuit components on predicted isothermal contours.

Davis (1971) points out that current-limiting by itself does not guarantee a complete protection against external fault conditions for an integrated circuit regulator. Hence this circuit includes a junction temperature-limiting system to ensure protection against excessive power dissipation. Temperature-sensing transistors are placed close to the positive and negative series regulators in order

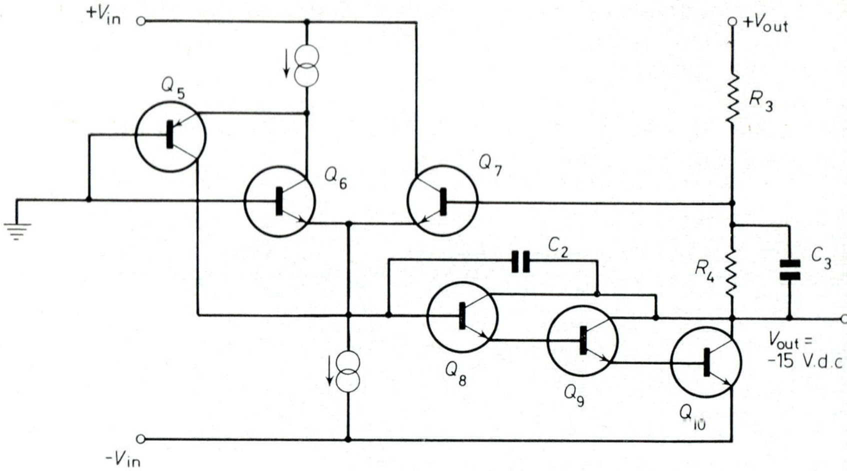

Figure 10.16. Basic negative voltage regulator circuit
(Reproduced after Davis, 1971, by courtesy of I.E.E.E.)

to provide an accurate junction temperature measurement for these devices. Using the circuit of *Figure 10.17*, the base drive to the positive series regulator is removed for the duration of the excessive junction temperature occurrence in either power device. The high gain

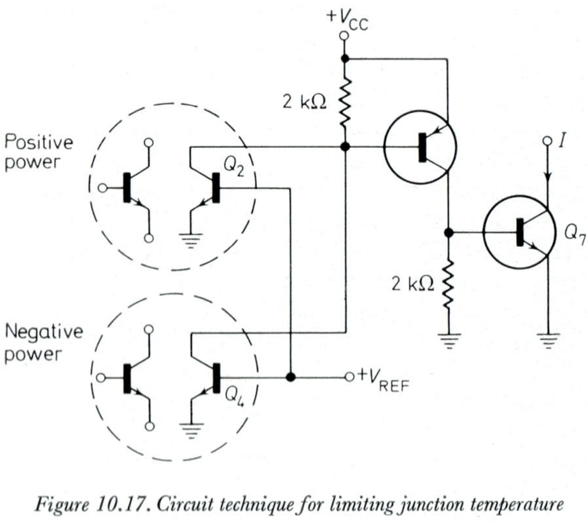

Figure 10.17. Circuit technique for limiting junction temperature
(Reproduced after Davis, 1971, by courtesy of I.E.E.E.)

of this cascaded non-linear amplifier causes both output voltages to fall to zero within 2° C of +185° C. When the basic integrated circuit stabilizer was connected to a 120 Ω load, the periodic shut-down of the output produced by the temperature sensing gave rise to a square wave output (thermal oscillation), the OFF time being 200 μs and the ON time 700 μs.

CONSTANT CURRENT POWER SUPPLIES

The stabilized power units so far described have been designed to have a low value of internal impedance. As a result, even though the output current may vary over quite a wide range, the output voltage remains almost constant. On the other hand, for some types of stimulation and for supplying current-operated devices such as electromagnets, there is a need for a power supply which delivers a constant current even though the resistance of the load alters within limits. For example, the coil resistance of an electromagnet will increase as the coil heats up. This implies that a constant current power supply must possess a high value of internal impedance so that any changes occurring in the load will be insignificant.

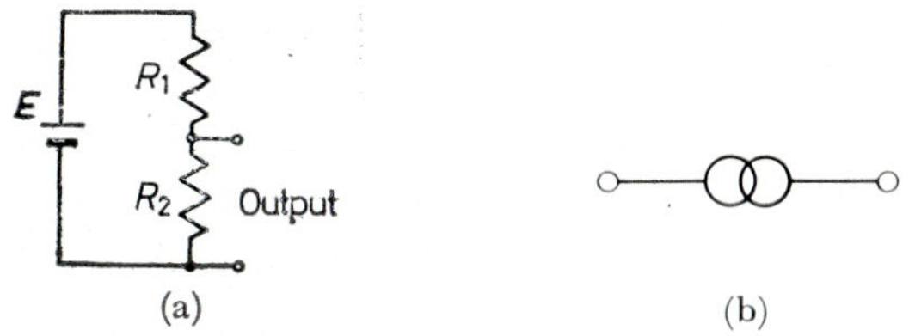

Figure 10.18. (a) Simple resistive constant current circuit. (b) Circuit symbol for a constant current circuit

In *Figure 10.18*, if R_1 is much greater than R_2, the circuit current will be determined almost entirely by the value of R_1. Changes in the value of the load resistance R_2 will have a negligible effect on the current, which stays constant. If R_2=1,000 Ω and changes by 10 per cent, then if R_1 is low, the circuit current will also change by about 10 per cent. If R_1 is increased to 100,000 Ω, the change in resistance of 100 Ω in R_2 is now slightly less than 0·1 per cent of the total resistance. Hence the circuit current will only be altered by this small amount. If the circuit current was 1 mA with R_1 small, the voltage to supply the circuit will have to be slightly greater than 1 V. However, for the same current with R_1=100,000 Ω, the supply voltage will have to be slightly greater than 100 V.

The drawback to this simple resistive system lies in the fact that a very high value of the supply voltage is required if more than a small current is to be made available. The power dissipated in the series resistor also becomes excessive.

One way of making a constant current circuit for currents of a few milliamperes is to utilize the fact that a field effect transistor has a relatively high value of dynamic resistance, that is, the drain current is almost independent of the drain-to-source voltage. Thus, if the load is placed in the source circuit of the field effect transistor (*Figure 10.19*), the load resistance will cause little variation

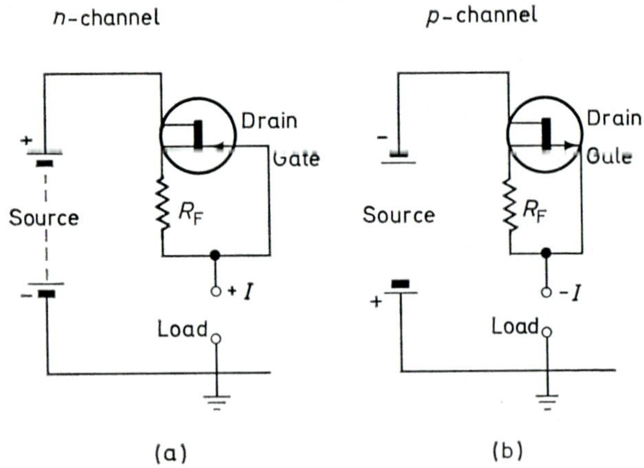

Figure 10.19. Field effect transistor constant current circuit: (a) n-channel; (b) p-channel

in the drain current. The feedback resistor R_F further stabilizes the drain current. If the load resistance should increase, the drain-to-source current will decrease slightly. However, this will reduce the voltage drop across R_F and hence the bias. The effect will be to make the drain current increase and compensate for the initial change. Both *n*-channel (*Figure 10.19a*) and *p*-channel (*Figure 10.19b*) FETs can be used, but not enhancement FETs since these require a bias voltage to form the channel which allows drain–source current to flow.

Walker (1962) describes a constant current circuit with a current stability of better than 0·1 per cent. It can supply from 0·05 to 1 A with a maximum voltage of 40 V. *Figure 10.20* shows a block diagram of the arrangement. The output current is sampled by sensing the voltage drop appearing across R_S and comparing this with a reference voltage R_{ref}. If a difference exists, a correction is made to the current passing through the series regulator in order to maintain a constant current through R_S and hence the load impedance.

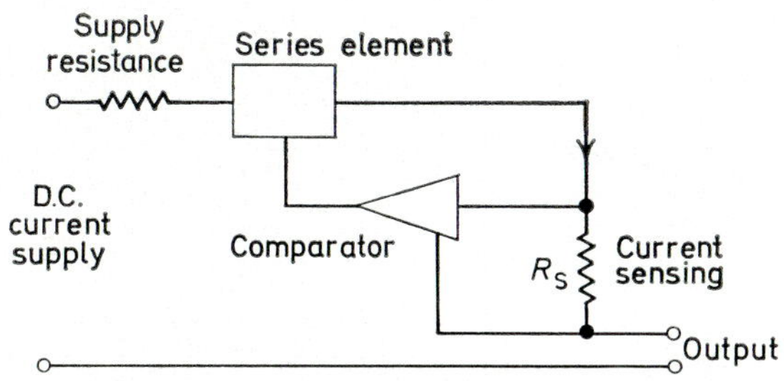

Figure 10.20. Block diagram of the closed loop of a stabilized constant current power supply
(Reproduced after Walker, 1962, by courtesy of the Editor of *Electronic Engineering*)

The outline circuit is given in *Figure 10.21.* The mains supply voltage is rectified by a bridge arrangement followed by a choke input filter in order to obtain a good regulation (8 per cent). This figure of regulation limits the collector voltage swing of the series transistors over the range of load currents allowed. The series regulator consists of three power transistors, each with emitter current equalizing resistors, followed by the current sampling network connected to the negative output terminal. A separate 90 V d.c. supply is dropped to 24 V by two 12 V power Zener diodes D_1 and D_2 in series to provide a constant voltage supply for the sensing differential amplifier. The amplifier consists of a long-tailed pair differential amplifier Q_1 and Q_2 comparing the sampled voltage across R_S with the reference voltage from D_3. Two common collector stages Q_3 and Q_4 follow, the second compounded with the series regulators Q_5, Q_6 and Q_7.

The complete circuit incorporates an overvoltage limiting circuit which is triggered by the output voltage rising above 40 V. This could arise due to the load being disconnected if increased to such a value as to cause the voltage to exceed 40 V and cause the unit to go into an unstabilized condition. For a capacitive or resistive–capacitive load, the capacitive component must be discharged before switching off to prevent discharge back into the supply. For an inductive or resistive–inductive load, the inductive component must be reduced to zero by progressively reducing a shunt resistance across the load before switching off in order to prevent damage to

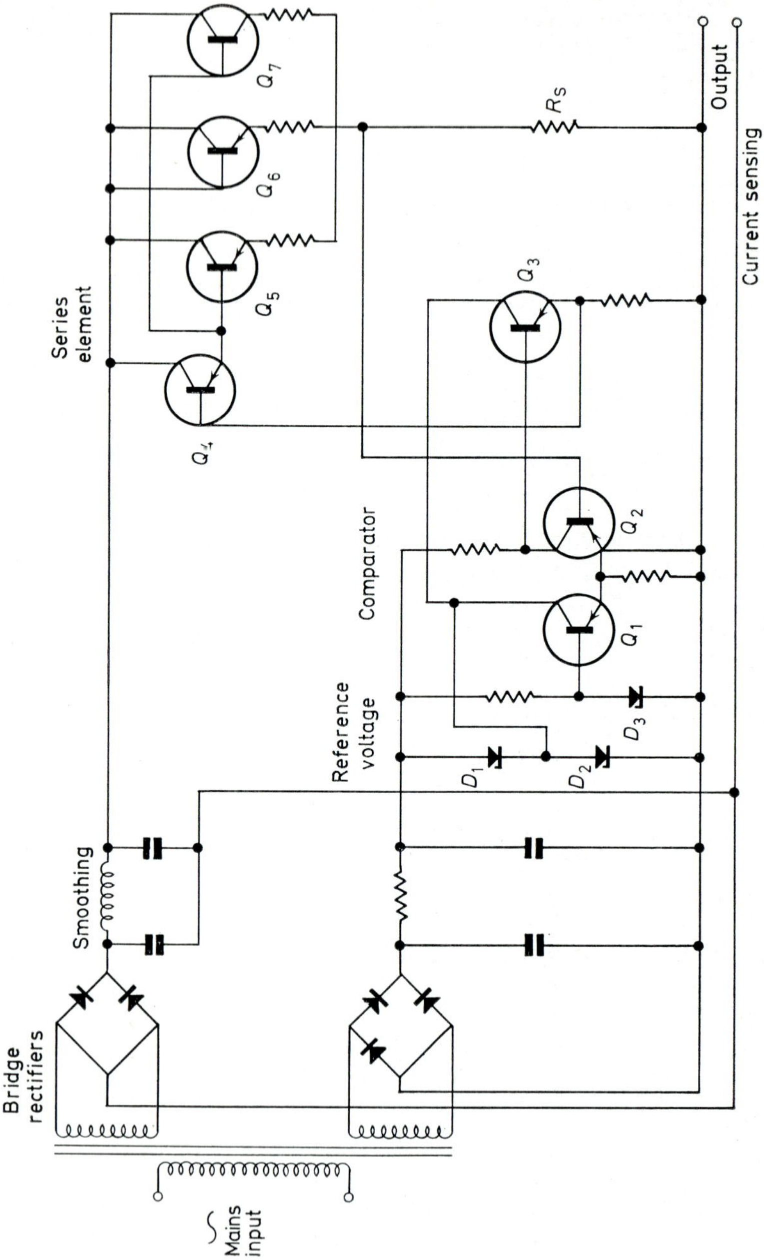

Figure 10.21. Outline circuit of a stabilized current power unit
(Reproduced after Walker, 1962, by courtesy of the Editor of *Electronic Engineering*)

the supply from voltage transients. Lovick (1962) describes a constant current supply with a maximum output of 1 A into a 7·5 Ω load.

D.C. TO D.C. CONVERTERS

In medical electronics there is a requirement to provide 1·35 V or 5–6 V to supply transistor circuits from nuclear power sources. A typical application occurs with the use of a nuclear source to power an implanted cardiac pacemaker. The life of the nuclear cell is expected to be 10 years compared with the 2 years achievable with conventional mercury cells. Basically a plutonium-238 source is used to provide heat to a bismuth telluride alloy semiconductor thermopile. This produces an output voltage of approximately 0·4 V d.c. By means of transistor switches, this is interrupted at regular intervals and either stepped up in a transformer or the voltage multiplied to give the required circuit supply voltage.

Wirewound components such as transformers are always suspect from the viewpoint of reliability. Poirier, Cochrun and Riccio (1971) describe a suitable transformerless d.c.-to-d.c. converter. It can provide a dual polarity output of ±1·35 V. The conventional approach using transformers and solid state diodes was not feasible on the grounds of weight, size and the large junction voltages associated with diodes. For these reasons, bipolar transistors were used since saturation voltages of less than 50 mV can be obtained with currents of a few milliamperes. Germanium transistors are employed in an astable multivibrator circuit followed by a quadrupler that can deliver 1·35 V with an input as low as 0·35 V. With this level of input, the use of germanium transistors is mandatory in the clock circuit because of their turn-on voltages.

THE CONVERSION OF BODY MOTION TO ELECTRICITY

Myers *et al.* (1964) have described a cardiac pacemaker which was powered from a piezoelectric source consisting of two sheets of ceramic bimorph placed on either side of a dog's aorta. The expansion and contraction of the aorta bent the sheets of ceramic, each 32 × 38 mm, which were placed in a hinged clamp and encapsulated in silicone rubber. The output from the crystals was rectified in a voltage doubler and fed to the pacemaker circuit.

REFERENCES

Ackland, R. G. and Buckland, N. M. (1964). 'An improved control system for a.c. voltage stabilizers.' *Electron. Engng* **36,** 480.

Attree, V. H. and Topliss, R. J. (1962). 'A variable-voltage stabilized supply.' *Electron. Engng* **34,** 176.

Collinge, B. and Marsham, T. N. (1951). 'An a.c. stabilizer.' *J. scient. Instrum.* **32,** 374.

Cooper, E. G. (1960). *Mullard Reference Manual of Transistor Circuits*, 1st edn., p. 299. London: Mullard Ltd.

Davis, W. F. (1971). 'A five-terminal complementary tracking ± 15 V ± 300 mA monolithic voltage regulator.' In *Proceedings of I.E.E.E. International Solid State Circuits Conference*, Philadelphia.

Dayal, M. (1964). 'Rectifier diode operation at kilocycle frequencies.' *Mullard Tech. Comm.* **8,** 66.

Long, J. V. P. (1952). 'A simple electro-mechanical stabilizer.' *Electron. Engng* **24,** 26.

Lovick, F. W. (1962). 'Current stabilized transistor power supplies.' *Electron. Engng* **34,** 332.

Myers, G., Parsonnet, V., Zuker, I. R. and Lotman, H. (1964). 'Biologically energized cardiac pacemakers.' *Am. J. med. Electron.* **3,** 233.

Poirier, N., Cochrun, B. L. and Riccio, M. J. (1971). 'A unique hybrid transformerless DC-to-DC converter for long-term nuclear power sources.' In *Proceedings of I.E.E.E. International Solid State Circuits Conference*, Philadelphia.

Walker, D. E. (1962). 'A stabilized constant current power unit.' *Electron. Engng* **34,** 406.

Chapter 11

Switching Circuits

THE ASTABLE MULTIVIBRATOR

The term 'multivibrator' applies to a class of pulse generating circuits. Multivibrators may be of the astable, monostable or bistable type.

Basically, each circuit has two states of operation, the circuit being in one at any given time. An astable multivibrator continuously switches from one state to the other and thereby generates a continuous succession of pulses. A monostable multivibrator, also known as a univibrator, changes state and thus generates an output pulse only when it is commanded to do so by the application of a suitable trigger pulse. Having changed state, it then returns to its original stable state and awaits the next trigger pulse. In contrast, a bistable circuit stays in either of its two stable states until the receipt of a trigger pulse causes it to change over. Unlike the monostable circuit, it then remains in the other state until the next trigger pulse causes it to revert. The three configurations have much in common. The differences between them occur in the method adopted for coupling together the two halves of each circuit.

Figure 11.1 shows the circuit of an astable or free-running multivibrator. It is seen to consist of a two-stage R–C coupled amplifier, having the output of the second stage fed back to the input of the first stage. The output is thus in phase with the input and oscillation results. Since the whole of the output is fed back, the oscillations are markedly non-sinusoidal. The waveform approximates to a square wave and is rich in harmonics, hence the term 'multivibrator'. In these switching circuits the transistors are either hard on or hard off.

When the supply voltage is applied to the circuit, noise on the supply will produce small random voltage changes at the transistor bases. Suppose that at some particular time the base of Q_1 is going slightly negative. The collector current of Q_1 increases and the collector voltage of Q_1 falls. Coupling via C_1 makes the base of Q_2 go more positive. This reduces the current through Q_2 and the collector voltage of Q_2 increases. A negative-going pulse is fed via C_2 back to the base of Q_1, reinforcing the original voltage change.

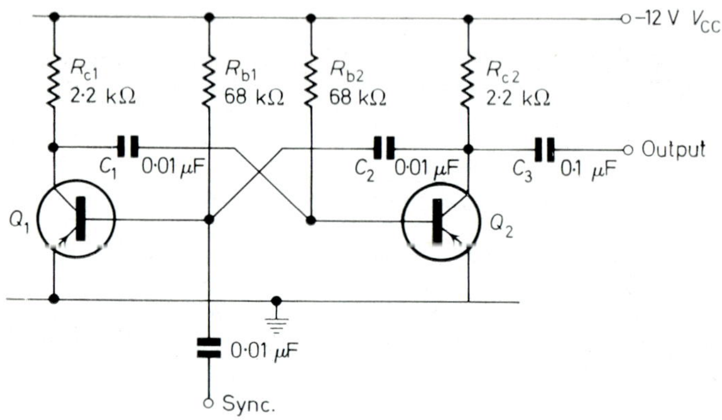

Figure 11.1. Astable multivibrator circuit

The process is cumulative or regenerative in action, Q_1 being turned hard on and Q_2 becoming cut off. When Q_2 is cut off, amplification ceases, but Q_2 does not stay cut off indefinitely, since the base of Q_2 is returned to its emitter via R_{b2}. C_1 discharges through R_{b2} and Q_1 with a time constant $R_{b2}C_1$. Once C_1 has fully discharged and just started to charge negatively on the right-hand side, Q_2 will start to conduct again and the cycle repeats with Q_1 being cut off and Q_2 turned hard on. The switching-on time for each transistor is short, since both base and collector current is supplied via a resistive path and the positive feedback signal from each collector to the other base arrives via a loop which includes the gain of both transistors.

Figure 11.2 illustrates the various collector and base waveforms. The free-running frequency of the circuit given in *Figure 11.1* is approximately 1,000 Hz. When the time constants $R_{b1}C_2$ and $R_{b2}C_1$ are made equal, the collector waveforms will be symmetrical. That is to say that the 'Mark–Space' ratio is unity (equal ON and OFF times). Under these conditions, the free-running frequency is given approximately by $f = 1/(1{\cdot}4\ C_1R_{b2})$ Hz. This is the Pulse Repetition

Frequency or PRF. When it is required to alter the PRF, either C_1 and C_2 or R_{b1} and R_{b2} can be varied. It is usual to have C_1 and C_2 switched in steps as a coarse control, with a double ganged potentiometer for R_{b1} and R_{b2} as a fine control. By making $R_{b1}C_2$ and $R_{b2}C_1$ unequal, an asymmetrical output waveform can be generated.

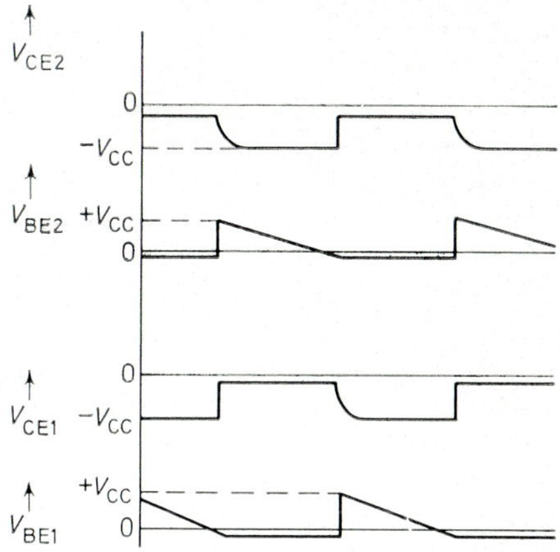

Figure 11.2. Waveforms of a transistor astable multivibrator

The limit in practice is about 20 to 1 for the ratio of the OFF to ON times. The maximum value of R_{b1} and R_{b2} is limited to *hfe* R_{c1} and *hfe* R_{c2} respectively where *hfe* is the minimum d.c. current gain for the particular transistor type measured at the working saturation point. The minimum values of R_{b1} and R_{b2} must be such that the collector voltages can complete their full excursion during the pulse period. Assuming that $R_{b1}C_2=R_{b2}C_1$, the half period of the cycle lasts for a time equal to $0{\cdot}7\ C_1R_{b2}$. At least four time constants must be allowed for the collector swing to be 98 per cent completed. Therefore $T_1=0{\cdot}7\ R_{b2}C_1 \geqslant 4\ R_{c2}C_2$. Since $C_1=C_2$, $R_{b1} \geqslant 5{\cdot}7\ R_{c2}$. Thus the minimum values of R_{b1} and R_{b2} are $5{\cdot}7\ R_{c1}$ and $5{\cdot}7\ R_{c2}$ respectively for $C_1=C_2$.

It is usually more convenient to apply synchronizing pulses to one of the bases, that is, to synchronize the multivibrator by making the controlled transistor non-conducting. Astable multivibrator circuits are commonly used to provide the primary timing element for stimulating and other circuits. However, with the simple circuit described, the pulse repetition frequency depends on both the value of the supply voltage and the transistor characteristics. It is thus temperature-dependent and in this configuration does not make a stable frequency source. Fortunately, it is easily possible to lock or synchronize a free-running multivibrator to a stable signal such as that from a crystal-controlled oscillator. The synchronizing action follows, since if a negative-going pulse is applied to the base of the *p–n–p* transistor which is cut off, the change-over starts ahead of its normal time in the free-running state. In this way a series of multivibrators can be used to divide down a standard frequency. For example, the output from a 100 kHz crystal oscillator can be applied to a 10 kHz free-running multivibrator. The multivibrator locks on to the crystal-controlled sinewave and produces an exact 10 kHz square wave output. This can be fed in turn to synchronize a 1 kHz multivibrator, the output of which, when differentiated, can be used to produce 1 ms timing marks for calibrating the time-base of a cathode ray tube oscilloscope.

The switching action of the simple multivibrator circuit is not so rapid as in the case of a valve circuit. This is because of 'hole storage effects' which occur when a transistor which has been switched hard on (saturated) comes out of saturation. This results in a delay of a few microseconds before the collector voltage moves to its new value. The pulse repetition frequency of the simple circuit is subject to a considerable dependence upon the ambient temperature. Ristic (1964) has described a series emitter type of multivibrator. This has not only a better thermal stability but better rise and fall times than the conventional circuit. It is stated to oscillate over the range 0·01 to 250 Hz.

It is possible to simplify the circuitry of an astable multivibrator by using two transistors of opposite polarity, i.e. a *p–n–p* type with an *n–p–n* type. In this case, the pulse generated when one switches off is of the correct polarity to switch the other on. This arrangement has been employed in implantable cardiac pacemakers (Davies and Sowton, 1964).

The Generation of Large Space-to-mark Ratios by a Multivibrator

Cliff (1969) describes the circuit shown in *Figure 11.3* for the production of a pulse having a large space-to-mark ratio. The addition of a transistor and a diode to the basic astable multivibrator allows a large space-to-mark ratio without requiring the power supply to provide vastly different currents during the mark and space periods. The limitation in the basic astable circuit is the fact that the larger timing capacitor must discharge through a collector load resistor during the shorter time interval. When Q_2 goes OFF, D_3 is reverse biased and Q_3 acts as an emitter follower to charge C_2. This results in the waveform at Q_2 collector rising much more rapidly and C_2 charging in a shorter time. Without D_3 and Q_3 the maximum space-to-mark ratio obtainable was 20/1, and with them 1,500/1

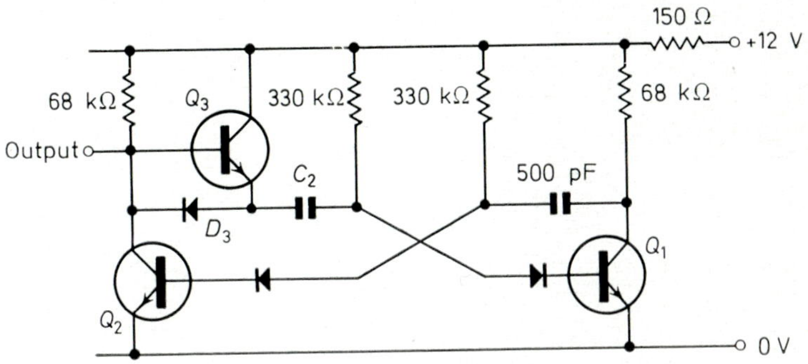

Figure 11.3. Large space-to-mark astable multivibrator
(Reproduced after Cliff, 1969, by courtesy of the Editor of *Wireless World*)

was possible. The pulse width at the collector of Q_2 was 100 μs wide. Another circuit to produce small mark-to-space ratios is that of Tesic (1967).

THE MONOSTABLE MULTIVIBRATOR

This circuit is also known as a 'one-shot' multivibrator or univibrator. It has one stable and one unstable state. In the United Kingdom the circuit is also known as a 'flip-flop', since the application of a trigger pulse flips the circuit over into its unstable state and the circuit flops back after a predetermined interval.

A typical transistor monostable circuit is shown in *Figure 11.4*. Whereas in the astable circuit the couplings between the stages were both via capacitors, in the monostable circuit one is via a capacitor and the other is via a d.c. path. Q_1 is normally ON and Q_2 OFF. The application of a positive-going trigger pulse to the base of Q_1 causes Q_1 to stop conducting and Q_2 to switch on. The charge on C_3 leaks away via R_3 and the circuit reverts to its original condition. The time for which the circuit is in its unstable state is given by $T=0{\cdot}7\ R_3C_3$.

The monostable multivibrator is a commonly encountered circuit, particularly for the production of time delays and pulse shaping.

A pulse repetition frequency might be generated by an astable multivibrator. The square wave output is differentiated and passed through a diode to select the positive-going pulses which are used to

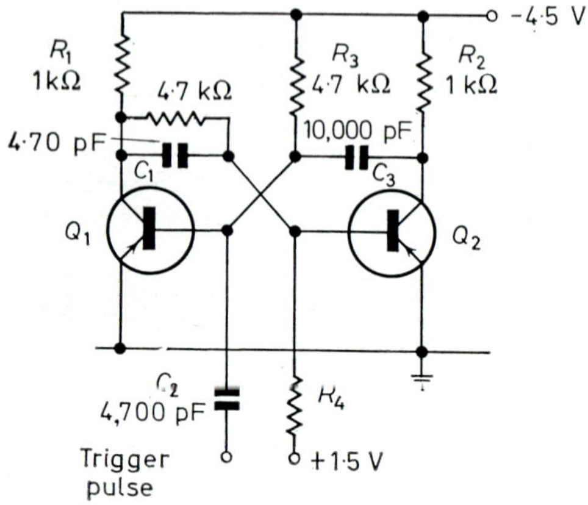

Figure 11.4. Monostable multivibrator circuit

trigger a monostable circuit. This produces pulses of a required width at the repetition frequency.

THE BISTABLE MULTIVIBRATOR

The bistable circuit, also known as a binary or Eccles–Jordan circuit, can be regarded as a d.c. coupled multivibrator (*Figure 11.5*). The ON state must be stable for either transistor, and this is accomplished by the use of the 1·5 V supply which holds the other transistor in the OFF state. The states can be reversed by the application of a negative-going pulse to the base of the OFF transistor or a positive-going pulse to the base of the ON transistor. When Q_1 is conducting, its collector voltage will be low, and this in conjunction with the bias supply holds Q_2 cut off. When a positive-going pulse of short duration is applied to both bases, the collector current of Q_2 cannot be altered since it is zero, but that of Q_1 is reduced. The collector of Q_1 thus goes more negative and carries the base of Q_2 with it, bringing Q_2 into conduction. The cumulative action causes Q_1 to become cut off and leaves Q_2 conducting. The new state is held until the receipt of a second input trigger pulse, when the circuit reverts to its original state. The bistable thus forms a 'scale of two', since each collector only produces half as many output pulses as trigger pulses applied to the bases. An idealized description of the switching action is shown in *Figure 11.6*.

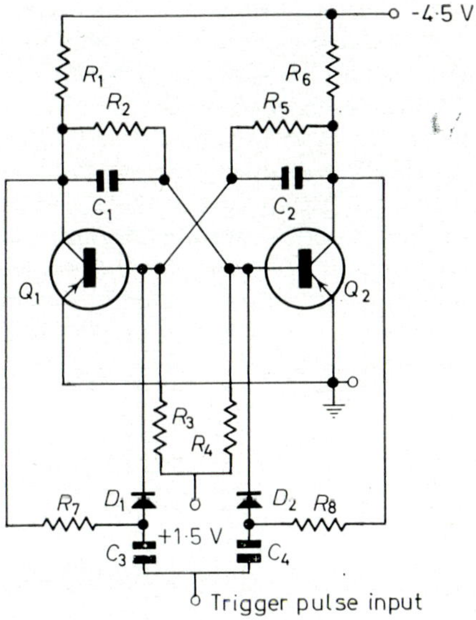

Figure 11.5. Bistable circuit

Bistable circuits are encountered in large numbers in frequency meters, in digital computers, and in scaling circuits used to measure the activity of radio-isotopes. When the trigger pulses are applied

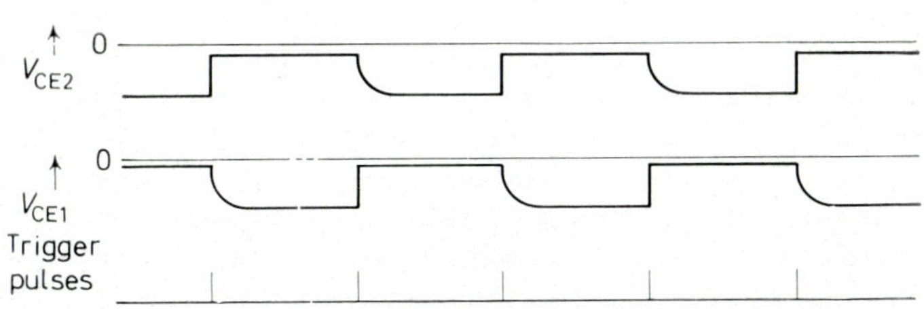

Figure 11.6. Idealized switching waveforms of a bistable circuit

simultaneously to both bases, they must have a duration which is short compared with the change-over time of the circuit. The small capacitors C_1 and C_2 in *Figure 11.5* assist the action by transferring the leading edge of the trigger pulse to the bases without attenuation.

Transistors Q_1 and Q_2, together with resistors R_1, R_2, R_3, R_4, R_5 and R_6 and capacitors C_1 and C_2, constitute a conventional bistable circuit. A problem arises if the narrow trigger pulse should become differentiated, since the resulting negative-going pip could trip the bistable back to its initial state so that the change-over action was not completed. Reliable binary counting is obtained by means of the 'steering' diodes D_1 and D_2 together with R_7, R_8 and C_3, C_4. The diodes D_1 and D_2 are controlled by the transistor collector voltages. When Q_1 is hard on, D_1 is arranged to be just conducting, Q_2 is off and D_2 is not conducting due to the negative value of Q_2 collector voltage. The next positive trigger pulse is fed to the base of Q_1, switching Q_1 off and Q_2 on. The time constant $C_3R_7 = C_4R_8$ is made sufficiently long to give the bistable time to complete its change-over before the next positive input pulse is fed to the base of Q_2. It is also possible to make a simple, direct coupled bistable from a complementary pair of transistors.

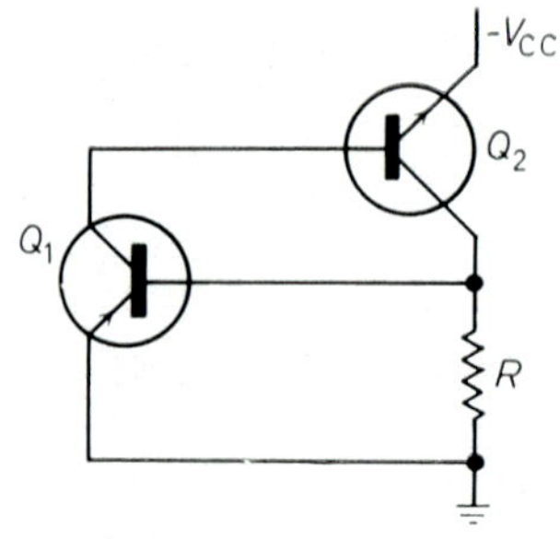

Figure 11.7. Basic complementary pair bistable circuit

Figure 11.7 shows the basic complementary pair bistable circuit. In this configuration, the collector current of Q_2 is also the base current of Q_2. If the collector current of Q_1 increases, its collector voltage goes more positive (*p–n–p* transistor). This has the effect of decreasing the collector current of Q_2, and thus the collector voltage of Q_2 goes more negative. This is in the correct sense to apply positive feedback to the base of Q_1, and this regenerative action results in a rapid switch-on for both transistors. Similar considerations apply when the collector current is reduced in either transistor, both then becoming rapidly switched off. Thus the circuit has two stable states with both transistors either ON or OFF.

The time for which astable or monostable multivibrators dwell in the transient state is dependent to some extent upon changes in the ambient temperature. This is partly due to a change in base–emitter voltage V_{BE}, as this defines the value of the voltage which must be applied to the base to switch the transistor, and to the fact that the leakage current I_{CO} is temperature-dependent and adds to the timing current which flows. At low temperatures the drop in h_{fe} could mean that the transistors are not fully saturated in the ON position. It is best to work with low leakage current silicon transistors and to check that full saturation is possible over the required working temperature range.

THE SCHMITT TRIGGER CIRCUIT

The regenerative multivibrator circuits so far described have basically required input current trigger pulses to cause them to switch. This implies that they have comparatively low input impedances.

The Schmitt trigger circuit changes state when a given voltage level is reached at its input, the input impedance being high until the circuit switches ON. The basic circuit is given in *Figure 11.8.*

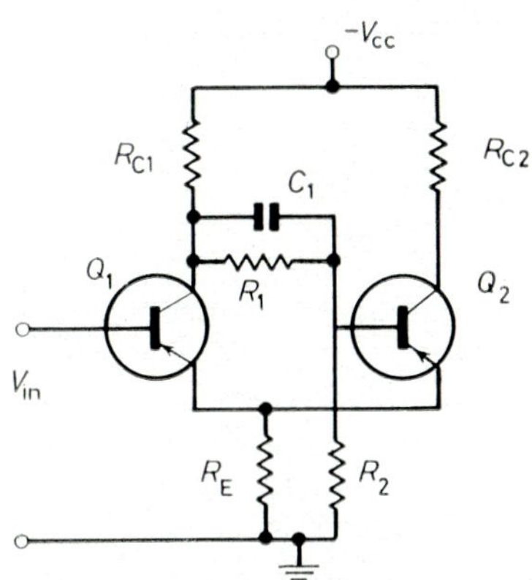

Figure 11.8. Basic Schmitt trigger circuit

Q_2 is normally ON and its emitter voltage is $-V_2$. Q_1 remains OFF until such time as its base is made more negative than $-V_1$. When Q_1 turns ON, its collector voltage goes positive and this rise in voltage is applied via the speed-up capacitor C_1 to the base of Q_2, which becomes switched OFF. Q_2 stays switched OFF since the voltage applied to its base is more positive than that applied to its emitter. This follows because the potential divider R_1R_2 is now fed from the collector voltage of the saturated transistor Q_1 rather than from the supply voltage $-V_{CC}$. The circuit stays in its new state until the input voltage is made less negative than V_2, when it will revert to its initial condition. *Figure 11.9* depicts the idealized waveforms from a Schmitt trigger circuit.

It is necessary for $-V_1$ to be more negative than $-V_2$. If this were not so, the circuit would change back to its initial state immediately after triggering had occurred, and switching would occur continuously as long as the input voltage was between $-V_1$ and $-V_2$.

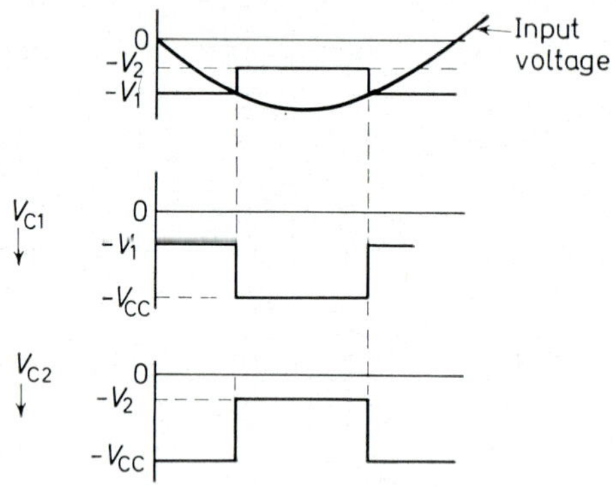

Figure 11.9. Switching action of a Schmitt trigger

Schmitt trigger circuits are commonly used, for example, to trigger a timebase on a certain portion of a repetitive waveform, or to provide a variable threshold when it is required to count only pulses greater than a certain amplitude. Hampshire and Petersen (1967) analyse the action of a Schmitt trigger circuit.

THE BLOCKING OSCILLATOR

In the regenerative switching circuits previously described, the necessary positive feedback has been obtained via capacitive or resistive networks. It is possible, however, to produce monostable or astable regenerative circuits by means of transformer coupling.

The circuit of *Figure 11.10* consists of a transistor having inductive coupling via the transformer from the collector to the base and an R–C timing network in the emitter circuit. On applying the supply voltage, the collector current starts to increase. Insufficient positive feedback is applied to the base to cause the transistor to be driven hard ON at the commencement of the first cycle of oscillation.

When saturation occurs, the collector voltage becomes constant and the load current continues to increase at a constant rate through the inductive branch of the load. The emitter current is almost constant and is determined by the feedback voltage from the transformer and the resistance in the emitter circuit.

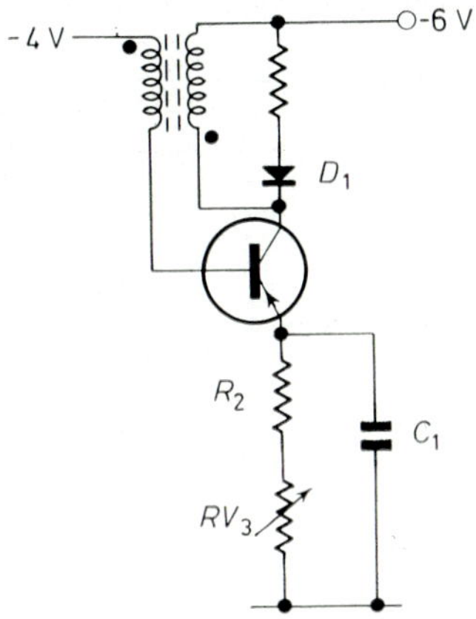

Figure 11.10. Blocking oscillator circuit

After a time, the emitter current is no longer sufficient to maintain the rate of increase of the collector current, and the feedback voltage produced by the transformer falls. This results in the transistor coming out of saturation, and the feedback from the transformer causes it to switch OFF rapidly. The rapid switching ON and OFF results in a sharp output pulse being generated at the collector. The reset time that must elapse before the circuit can produce another pulse is the time required for capacitor C_1 to discharge to such a voltage that the transistor can again conduct. This time is a function of the value of RV_3, which acts as a repetition rate control.

In order to produce an accurately defined ON time for the circuit, the transformer core is made from an alloy such as Permalloy-F, which has a very rectangular hysteresis loop. The field strength in the core rises very rapidly with the magnetizing force until the core saturates and the inductance falls sharply. The ON time of the blocking oscillator is largely determined by the characteristics of the core, since this governs the amount of feedback.

COMPLETE PULSE GENERATOR SYSTEMS

An Electrocardiogram Waveform Generator

The idea of using an astable multivibrator to generate the basic heart rate and to use this to trigger monostable delay circuits and pulse shaping circuits in order to simulate the various components of an electrocardiogram is well illustrated by de Sa and Molyneux (1964). Monostable circuits are employed to generate the *P–R* and *R–T* delays and to set the width of the *P*, *R* and *T* waves as illustrated in *Figure 11.11.* A more sophisticated simulator is that of

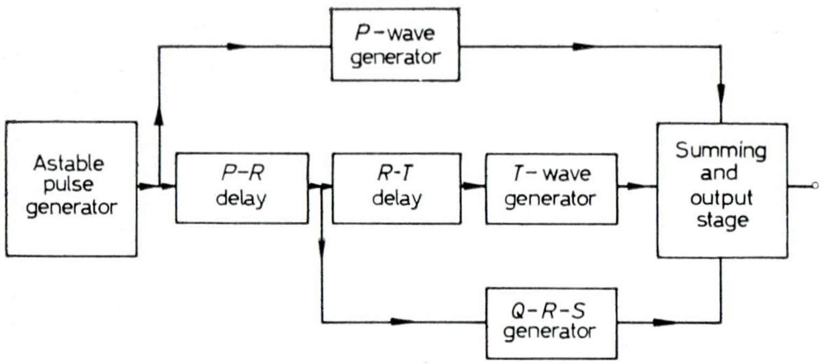

Figure 11.11. Schematic diagram of an ECG waveform generator

Maurer (1970), which can generate arrhythmias and respond to cardiac pacing.

Physiological Stimulation

Physiological stimulators are essentially complete pulse generator systems in which the pulse repetition rate, pulse width and pulse amplitude are normally all variable. The pulse repetition rate is determined by the frequency of an astable multivibrator which triggers a monostable circuit to set the pulse width. The trigger pulses for the monostable can be obtained by differentiating the square wave output from the astable and selecting the positive or negative spikes by means of a suitable polarity diode to match the polarity of the monostable input. Provision may also be made for generating a biphasic output consisting of pairs of positive and negative pulses of equal amplitudes and widths (Petrohilos *et al.*, 1963). For the measurement of refractory periods, pairs of similar polarity pulses may be required, the separation between the two pulses forming each pair being variable. The output stage of the stimulator may possess a low output impedance and provide an essentially constant voltage stimulus, or it may possess a high output impedance and provide an essentially constant current stimulus.

In the constant voltage case an emitter follower output is provided, whilst in the constant current case the output is arranged to be in series with a device having a high value of slope resistance such as a field effect transistor. Bignall (1963) describes a transistorized constant current output unit which can be added to a constant voltage stimulator.

Bakema and Koopmans (1968) describe a simple, rugged, transistorized, constant voltage stimulator for use by students. Three outputs are available: a d.c. voltage, single pulses and repetitive pulses. In each case the amplitude is adjustable from 20 mV to 24 V. For the pulses the width is variable from 0·5 to 120 ms, and for continuous pulse stimulation the rate can vary from 0·25 to 100 pulses per second. The rise and fall times of the stimulus are less than 10 μs. Three coarse amplitude ranges are provided, with a fine adjustment on each. Depending on the range, the unit is designed to work into loads of 100, 500 or 2,500 Ω. It will withstand short-circuiting of the output and can also provide a trigger pulse for triggering the timebase of an oscilloscope. A trigger pulse is available just prior to each stimulus pulse.

A transistorized stimulator for students' use, provided with a constant current output stage, is described by Meyer (1967). Ross and Brust (1968) give details of a transistorized high current, long pulse stimulator for the massive stimulation of isolated skeletal muscles.

An interesting approach to stimulator design is that of Hertzler and Kaminski (1968). They use a four-layer diode oscillator to generate stimulus repetition rates in the range 0·1 to 140 pulses per second. Integrated circuit flip-flops are used to provide a delay which can be varied from 1 to 13 ms, between the production of a trigger pulse and the delivery of the stimulus pulse, which can be varied in width from 0·05 to 80 ms. A pair of high voltage transistors in the output stage provide pulse amplitudes adjustable from 0·04 to 67·5 V.

Dual channel stimulators are those of Hinschelwood and Seabridge (1967) and Lewis (1967).

Stimulus Isolation

The output from a stimulator is normally single-ended with respect to earth, whilst the evoked potential generated as a response to the stimulus is picked up by means of a differential input amplifier. Thus the stimulus represents a massive common mode input signal for the amplifier. In spite of the common mode rejection ratio of the amplifier, sufficient of the stimulus may appear at the amplifier output to swamp the response signal. Under these circumstances, it is necessary to take considerable precautions to ensure that the stimulus pulse is well isolated from earth so that it does not appear as a differential input for the amplifier.

In mains powered stimulators, one source of coupling to earth is the capacity across the mains transformer. Several forms of isolation have been used. Catton and Farlier (1965) employed a radio frequency output stage for the stimulator so that the output was taken from a demodulator in the secondary of the low capacity r.f. transformer. A beam of modulated light can also be used for isolation purposes. The photon-coupler comprises a gallium arsenide diode which emits in the infra-red at about 990 nm. The light intensity is controlled by the forward input current. The receiver is a silicon *p–i–n* photodiode. The d.c. current transfer from input diode to output diode is approximately 0·002. The stray coupling impedance consists of 2 pF of capacitance in parallel with $10^{11}\ \Omega$ of leakage. A transistor amplifier is used to follow the photon coupler in order to achieve an overall current gain of about unity. Suitable arrangements are those of Baird (1967) and Ross and Bassett (1967).

OPERATIONAL AMPLIFIER MULTIVIBRATOR

Referring to *Figure 11.12* (Clayton, 1969), the two astable states between which the circuit switches are those in which the amplifier output is either positively or negatively saturated. The output voltage is thus a square wave with its period set by the time constant CR and the feedback ratio which is determined by the potential divider R_1+R_2.

Consider a time t^* in the cycle and suppose that the negative input signal applied to the negative input of the amplifier is sufficient to produce saturation. The feedback fraction $\beta=R_1/(R_1+R_2)$, so that the input is $\beta V^-_{o,max}$. As capacitor C charges through R, the potential at input B goes more negative. When the potential difference between inputs A and B is almost zero, the amplifier comes out of saturation. The positive feedback from the output to input A drives the amplifier into positive saturation. The time constant CR ensures that the potential at input B remains almost constant during this transition. Capacitor C now charges positively through R and the amplifier again comes out of saturation when the potential at B reaches $\beta V^+_{o,max}$.

$$t_1=CR\log_e\frac{(V^+_{o,max}-\beta V^-_{o,max})}{[V^+_{o,max}\,(1-\beta)]}$$

and

$$t_2 = CR \log_e \frac{(V^-_{o,max} - \beta V^+_{o,max})}{[V^-_{o,max}(1-\beta)]}$$

If $V^-_{o,max} = V^+_{o,max}$, the total period $t = t_1 + t_2 = 2CR \log_e [1 + 2(R_1/R_2)]$.

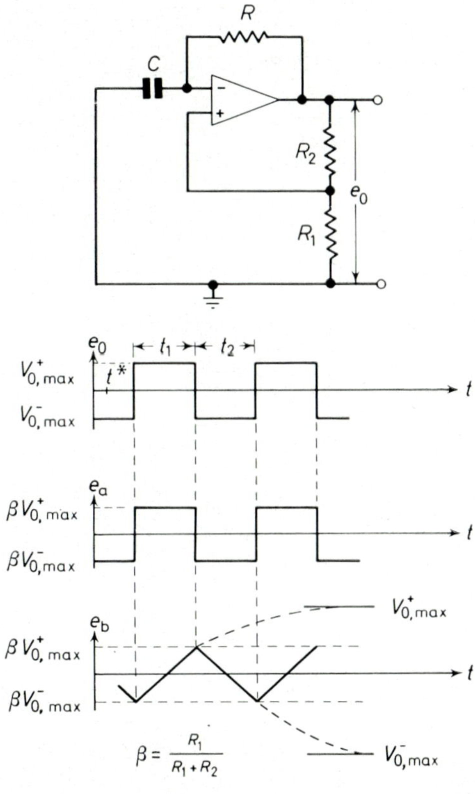

Figure 11.12. The circuit and waveforms of an operating amplifier astable multivibrator

(Reproduced after Clayton, 1969, by courtesy of the Editor of *Wireless World*)

Clayton shows that it is possible to have a non-symmetrical output waveform by the use of separate timing resistors R_3 and R_4 (*Figure 11.13*). The appropriate timing resistor for each period is selected by the diodes D_1 and D_2. The free-running frequency of the multivibrator can be locked or synchronized to be a multiple of the frequency of a synchronizing signal which is fed into the sync input.

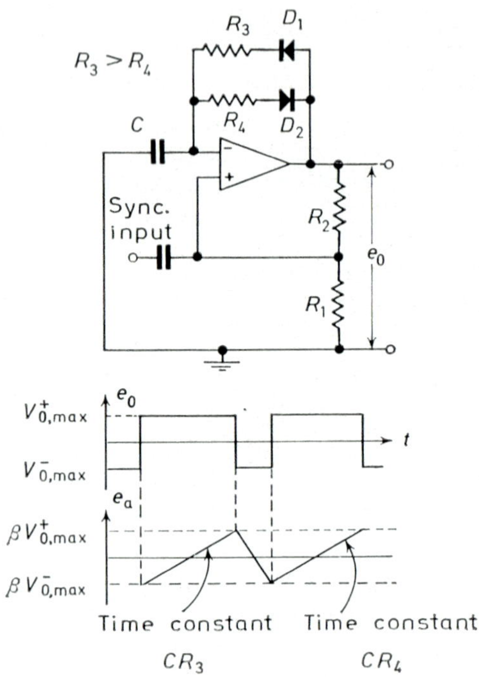

Figure 11.13. The circuit and waveforms of an operational amplifier asymmetrical multivibrator

(Reproduced after Clayton, 1969, by courtesy of the Editor of *Wireless World*)

This technique provides a useful method for dividing down the frequency of a standard crystal-controlled oscillator, perhaps in multiples of ten.

Operational Amplifier Monostable Multivibrator

Monostable or 'one-shot' action may be obtained by connecting a diode D_1 in parallel with the timing capacitor of the astable circuit, thus preventing the inverting input B from going positive (*Figure 11.14*). In the stable state, the amplifier output is at positive saturation, input B is clamped to earth via D_1 and input A is positive with respect to earth by $\beta V^{+}_{o,max}$. If input A is reduced to earth potential by the application of a negative pulse of sufficient amplitude, the circuit switches to its unstable state with a negative

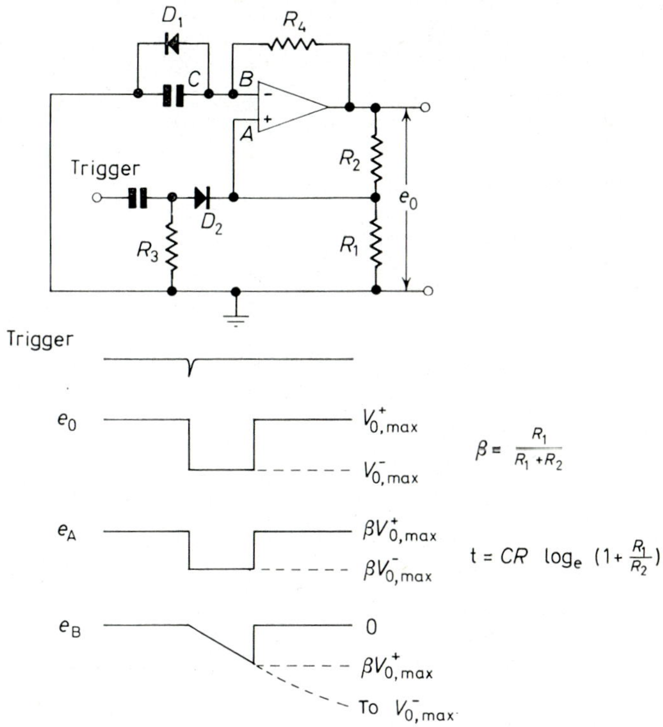

Figure 11.14. The circuit and waveforms of an operational amplifier monostable multivibrator

(Reproduced after Clayton, 1969, by courtesy of the Editor of *Wireless World*)

saturated output. Input A is then at a potential of $V^{-}_{o,max}$ with respect to earth, the potential at input B falls exponentially as C charges through R, and diode D_1 is reverse biased and non-conducting. The circuit reverts to the stable state when the potential at input B reaches $\beta V^{-}_{o,max}$. The pulse width generated is given by $t = CR \log_e (1 + R_1/R_2)$.

Operational Amplifier Bistable

The circuit now has two stable states corresponding to positive or negative saturation of the operational amplifier. A triggering pulse of the correct polarity applied to the inverting input terminal of the amplifier causes a regenerative change of state (*Figure 11.15*).

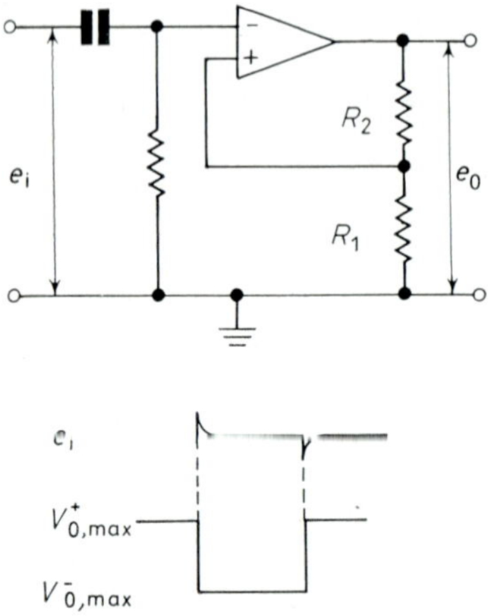

Figure 11.15. The circuit and waveforms of an operational amplifier bistable

(Reproduced after Clayton, 1969, by courtesy of the Editor of *Wireless World*)

VOLTAGE-CONTROLLED MULTIVIBRATOR

The astable multivibrators so far described have been free-running at a pulse repetition rate determined by the circuit time constants. A useful extention is the use of an external voltage supply to affect the charging time of the timing capacitors and thus make the free-running frequency controllable by the magnitude of the control voltage.

A voltage-controlled multivibrator is described by Jones (1967) and the basic circuit is given in *Figure 11.16*. Transistors Q_1 and Q_2 correspond with those used in a conventional multivibrator, Q_3 and Q_4 are emitter followers, and Q_5 and Q_6 produce a constant charging current for the timing capacitors C_1 and C_2. Jones points out that at low frequencies the circuit operates as a conventional multivibrator except that Q_3 and Q_4 ensure that the charging rate of C_1 and C_2 is linear and not exponential. At high repetition rates, the voltages developed across R_3 and R_4 due to the high charging currents reduce the amplitude of the voltage changes across the capacitors. The combination of a high charging current and low voltage drop permits a high upper limit to the repetition rate.

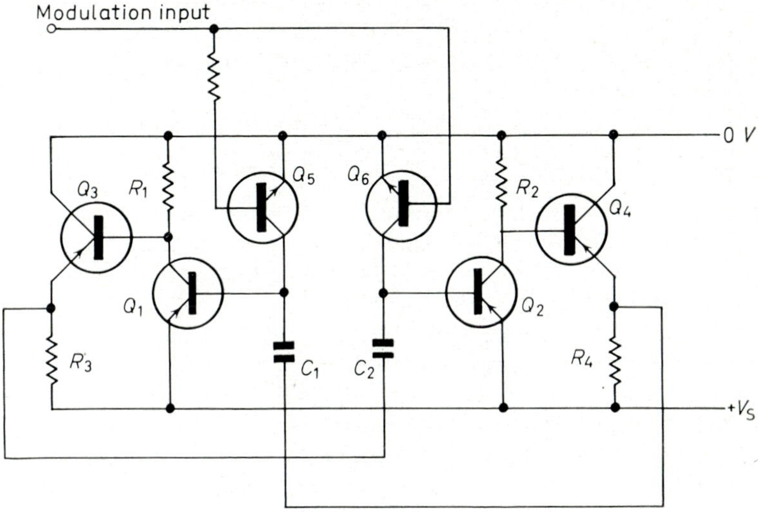

Figure 11.16. Voltage-controlled multivibrator circuit
(Reproduced after Jones, 1967, by courtesy of the Editor of *Electronic Engineering*)

Jones quotes the following relationship for the circuit frequency:

$$2CR_E.f = \frac{(I_C.R_E)/V_S}{1-(I_C.R_E)/V_S}$$

where C is the timing capacitor in farads. (It is assumed that $C=C_1=C_2$.) R_E is the emitter resistor in ohms, f is the repetition frequency in Hz, I_C is the charging current of the timing capacitors in amperes, and V_S is the circuit supply voltage. In this simple form, both the repetition rate and the mark-to-space ratio are sensitive to small changes in transistor characteristics and component values. Jones describes a stabilizing circuit to overcome these problems and also to linearize the frequency versus control voltage relationship. In this form the frequency range was 20 Hz to 35 kHz.

Another form of high-performance voltage-to-frequency converter is that of Bombi (1970). The error in the output frequency for an input in the range 1 mV to 10 V is less than $\pm 3\times 10^{-4}$ of the full scale, and the temperature coefficient of the conversion factor is

—250 parts in 10^6 per degree centigrade over the ambient temperature range -10 to $+50°$ C. Two integrated circuit operational amplifiers are used in a modified relaxation oscillator arrangement.

REFERENCES

Baird, I. (1967). 'A new stimulus isolator for biological applications.' *Med. biol. Engng* **5,** 295.

Bakema, H. and Koopmans, J. J. C. (1968). 'A transistorized constant voltage stimulator for use in combination with mechanical recording.' *Med. biol. Engng* **6,** 199.

Bignall, K. E. (1963). 'A transistorized constant current converter.' *Electroenceph. clin. Neurophysiol.* **15,** 702.

Bombi, F. (1970). 'High performance voltage-to-frequency converter with improved linearity.' *Electron. Engng* **42,** 61.

Catton, W. T. and Farlier, R. G. (1965). 'An R.F. stimulus isolation unit for use in electrophysiology.' *Electron. Engng* **37,** 828.

Clayton, G. B. (1969). 'Operational amplifiers: voltage comparators and multivibrators.' *Wireless Wld* **75,** 384.

Cliff, K. D. (1969). 'Large space–mark ratio multivibrator.' *Wireless Wld* **75,** 184.

Davies, J. G. and Sowton, G. E. (1964). 'Cardiac pacemakers.' *Physics Med. Biol.* **9,** 257.

de Sa, A. and Molyneux, L. (1964). 'An E.C.G. waveform generator.' *Wld med. Electron.* **2,** 174.

Hampshire, D. W. H. and Petersen, D. (1967). 'An analysis of the action of a Schmitt trigger circuit.' *Electron. Engng* **39,** 38.

Hertzler, E. C. and Kaminski, R. J. (1968). 'Compact stimulator using integrated circuits and battery power.' *J. appl. Physiol.* **24,** 249.

Hinschelwood, J. W. and Seabridge, A. G. (1967). 'A dual channel stimulator.' *Electron. Engng* **39,** 16.

Jones, R. J. P. (1967). 'A wide frequency range voltage controlled multivibrator.' *Electron. Engng* **39,** 14.

Lewis, A. F. (1967). 'Constant voltage double pulse generators for use in electrophysiology.' *Electron. Engng* **39,** 252.

Maurer, D. D. (1970). 'A cardiac response demonstrator useful in teaching pacemaker function.' *Med. Res. Engng* **9,** 15.

Meyer, A. A. (1967). 'A transistorized stimulator for students' use with constant-current output for use in physiology.' *Med. biol. Engng* **5,** 61.

Petrohilos, H. G., Simpson, R., Welford, N. T. and Valenstein, E. S. (1963). 'A design for a reliable and inexpensive biphasic stimulator.' *Electroenceph. clin. Neurophysiol.* **15,** 1042.

REFERENCES

Ristic, V. M. (1964). 'A new type of free-running multivibrator.' *Electron. Engng* **36,** 232.

Ross, S. M. and Bassett, A. L. (1967). 'Stimulus isolation employing a light-activated coupler.' *J. appl. Physiol.* **22,** 820.

— and Brust, M. (1968). 'A transistorized high-current long-pulse amplifier for massive stimulation of isolated skeletal muscle.' *J. appl. Physiol.* **24,** 583.

Tesic, S. (1967). 'Multivibrator with very small mark to space ratio.' *Electron. Engng* **39,** 671.

Chapter 12

Noise

A practical limit is set to the degree of amplification which can be applied to a signal of interest by the presence of 'noise' in that signal and the degradation of the signal by noise arising from the active devices through which it is passed. The 'noise level' at the output corresponds to the magnitude of the random movement of the base line of the recording, which is due to spontaneous fluctuations occurring in the system. When the signal amplitude is so small that the output noise level is not exceeded, it will be unrecognizable at the output unless special techniques are employed, since the unwanted random noise will be amplified to a greater level than the signal. On a cathode ray tube oscilloscope screen, noise appears as a series of random voltage spikes, often referred to characteristically as 'grass'. If the random noise level is amplified sufficiently to be audible via a loudspeaker a hissing sound is heard, hence the term 'noise'. From a knowledge of the amplifier gain, the noise level at the input can be expressed in terms of an input signal amplitude—for example, so many microvolts r.m.s. measured over some stated bandwidth.

Noise is a random phenomenon which can be represented as a superimposition of alternating currents or voltages of different frequencies. The average value of random noise, taken over a long time, is zero. Hence its magnitude must be represented by its r.m.s. value. The noise generated in a circuit element may be represented by a voltage generator in series with it of output $\sqrt{(\overline{v^2})}$ where v is the instantaneous voltage and $(\overline{v^2})$ is the average value of v^2. Similarly, the noise may be represented by a current generator of output $\sqrt{(\overline{i^2})}$ in parallel with the circuit element.

Any signal which is to be recorded in a recognizable form must have an amplitude which is several times greater than the amplitude of the noise if it is to be clearly recorded by ordinary techniques. The signal-to-noise ratio is defined as the ratio of the total signal power to the actual noise power in the waveform considered. This is usually expressed in decibels so that s.n.r. (db) $= 10 \log$ (total signal power/total noise power). The s.n.r. can be increased either by increasing the signal power while keeping the noise power constant or by decreasing the total noise power.

Noise signals can be divided into two main classes. First, there is 'source noise' which depends on both the impedance and the temperature of the source producing the signal to be measured. This noise is inherent in the signal from that source and is the lowest level to which the noise in the recording can be reduced. It is not affected by any subsequent method of amplification. The other category of noise is that which is subsequently introduced by the amplification system, and depends upon the system chosen.

SOURCE NOISE (THERMAL NOISE)

Thermal noise occurs in any circuit component having electrical resistance. It arises from the fact that electricity is carried by discrete particles (electrons or positive holes) which move about in a random fashion due to thermal excitation. Any motion of a charged particle gives rise to an electric current, and the sum of the r.m.s. values of these currents produces the thermal noise. This noise increases with temperature, and occurs whether external electrical excitation is present or not. The source noise cannot be entirely eliminated, but it can be reduced by operating at very low temperatures. For example, the semiconductor infra-red photocell of a scanning device for recording the distribution of the infra-red radiation emitted by a human body (thermography) is operated at liquid nitrogen temperature. For ordinary temperatures, the noise power P in watts produced by a signal source is given by $P = \boldsymbol{k} T \triangle f = \frac{1}{4}(\overline{v^2})/R = \frac{1}{4}(\overline{i^2})R$ where $\boldsymbol{k}$ = Boltzmann's constant $= 1{\cdot}38 \times 10^{-23}$ erg.sec., T = the absolute temperature, R = the source resistance to which the circuit is supposedly matched, and $\triangle f$ = the frequency bandwidth considered.

It is seen that the noise per cycle is independent of the frequency. The spectrum of the noise is flat, and the noise is said to be 'white'. That is, all frequencies are equally represented in it. It is seen that noise power is proportional to the bandwidth considered. The amount of noise present in a narrow band amplifier will be much smaller than in a broad band amplifier operating under identical conditions.

Consider the noise produced by a resistive source matched to an amplifier capable of passing a frequency band of from 0 to 5 kHz. The noise power entering the amplifier at 290° K (17° C) is $P=1{\cdot}38\times10^{-23}\times290\times5{,}000=20\times10^{-18}=2\times10^{-17}$ watts. Since $\overline{(v^2)}=4RP$, if $R=1$ MΩ, $\overline{(v^2)}=4\times10^6\times2\times10^{-17}=80\times10^{-12}$, so that $v=9\ \mu$V.

The r.m.s. noise produced by a resistor of value R ohms in a bandwidth of B Hz at 17° C is given by $v_{\text{r.m.s.}}=126\sqrt{(RB)}$. Resistors made from carbon particles generate spontaneous voltage fluctuations which appear as noise when a constant signal current flows. The fluctuations arise from variations in the contact resistance between the particles. As mentioned in Chapter 4, wirewound or preferably metal oxide film resistors should be employed in low noise applications.

Thermal or Johnson noise occurs in any resistance and in theory is not a function of current. 'White noise' covering all frequencies is generated. In fact, the noise power is independent of the value of the resistance, since $P=\boldsymbol{k}T\triangle b$. In practical resistors the passage of d.c. as well as signal currents will increase the noise. Rheinfelder (1964) states that this is due to a non-linear function of resistance and applied voltage, internal arcing and other defects. He mentions that differences in noise as great as 25 db have been observed between a standard carbon resistor and a high quality deposited carbon resistor when d.c. current was present.

AMPLIFIER NOISE

When a signal source is connected to the input of an amplifier, both input signal and noise will be amplified equally over the bandwidth considered, but in addition, noise generated within the amplifier will be added. Thus the signal becomes degraded during its passage through the amplifier, and the signal-to-noise ratio at the output will be worse than that obtaining at the input. The amount of degradation which results can be defined in terms of the Noise Figure (n.f.). The noise figure is defined as

$$\text{n.f.} = \frac{\text{signal-to-noise ratio at the input}}{\text{signal-to-noise ratio at the output}}$$

where both ratios are defined for the same frequency bandwidth $\triangle f$ at a specified frequency f and the noise factor is expressed in db. N.F. is often defined for a bandwidth of 1 Hz at a frequency of 1 kHz. This is the Spot Noise Figure. Clearly this is applicable to an amplifier which must respond only to a narrow band of frequencies, such as the filter circuits of an EEG wave analyser.

The case also arises of an amplifier which must respond to a wide band of frequencies as in the case of a high fidelity audio amplifier. Here the Broadband Noise Figure $\overline{\text{n.f.}}$ is used. $\overline{\text{N.F.}}$ is quoted by some transistor manufacturers as an averaged noise figure over a passband with 10 and 10,000 Hz as the half-power (3 db) frequencies. In most applications, the gain of the first stage of an amplifier is sufficiently high to allow the noise figures of the remaining stages to be neglected.

Both noise voltage and power depend on the frequency, so that the thermal noise will be reduced if the bandwidth can be reduced. Thus the 9 μV noise level quoted for the 1 MΩ source over the bandwidth 0–5 kHz would be reduced to 0·09 μV if only the band 0–50 Hz were considered.

SHOT NOISE

In addition to thermal noise (arising from fluctuations in the motion of the current carriers), many elements in a circuit produce noise due to random fluctuations in the number of their current carriers. When the carriers are situated in an electric field, the fluctuations in their numbers produce current fluctuations which are called 'shot noise'. This type of noise, like thermal noise, is inevitable since it depends upon a fundamental effect.

In junction diodes and transistors, shot noise is generated whenever a carrier crosses the space-charge region between *p*-type and *n*-type material. Some of these crossings arise from the action of the external current, but others occur whether there is a current flowing through the device or not. Shot noise is the most important noise component in transistors above a few kHz. It is proportional to the current flowing. If the shot noise is considered to be produced by a voltage generator in series with a resistor r_{n}, then $\overline{(v^2)} = 2 \times e \times i \times r_{\text{n}}^2 \times f$.

FLICKER OR MODULATION NOISE

Flicker noise arises in junction diodes, transistors and carbon resistors. The fluctuations occurring with this type of noise are larger than those due to thermal or shot noise.

Flicker noise in semiconductor devices arises from two main surface effects. These are as follows.

(1) A fluctuation occurring in the number of majority carriers

trapped at certain states, called 'slow' states, on the surface of the material. The number of trapped carriers varies with the electrical or thermal gradients in the surface layer. These fluctuations in surface charge influence the generation and recombination of electrons and holes at other states (called 'fast' states) at the surface. The fluctuations arising from both types of state modulate the conductivity of the material, giving rise to a noise component called 'surface' noise. The variation of this noise with frequency is governed by the slow states and is approximately in inverse proportion to the frequency, so that it is important mainly at low frequencies. It is also known as excess noise or $1/f$ noise. Flicker noise has not the 'fundamental' quality of thermal and shot noise. Because it is due to recombination effects at the semiconductor surface, it can be controlled to some extent by suitable treatment of the surface. Surface noise increases rapidly with current and is not important in forward biased junctions.

(2) Leakage due to the presence of a thin conducting film in parallel with a *p–n* junction. This effect is negligible with a forward or reverse bias of a few volts, but it can be quite large with a high reverse voltage. A low frequency noise component obeying the $1/f$ law arises from spontaneous fluctuations in the leakage current. Improved manufacturing techniques, such as the silicon planar construction, have led to the production of low noise bipolar transistors. A useful account of noise in transistors is that of Simpson and Richards (1962).

NOISE CHARACTERISTICS OF BIPOLAR TRANSISTORS

The general noise characteristic of a junction transistor is shown in *Figure 12.1*. OA represents the Flicker Noise Region, where the noise

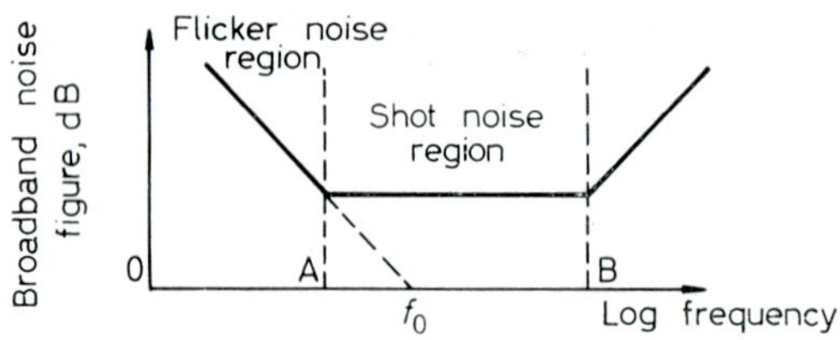

Figure 12.1. The general noise characteristic of a junction transistor

figure varies approximately as $1/f$. For the 2N929 low noise silicon transistor, the frequency f_0 is approximately 4 kHz. From A to B the noise is independent of the frequency, and this is known as the White Noise Region. Above B (approximately 1 MHz for the 2N929), the noise developed is still due to shot and thermal phenomena, and is constant as the frequency increases. However, the noise figure increases beyond B because of the decrease in gain of the transistor at the high frequencies. This has the effect of reducing the signal-to-noise ratio at the output.

The noise figure for a bipolar transistor depends on both the collector current and the value of the source resistance. To obtain a low noise figure, a low value of collector current should be employed. Silicon planar transistors are now available having high current gains at collector currents of the order of a few micro-amperes. For example, Murari (1969) used a type BFX36 low noise double transistor as the first stage of a preamplifier. This is a silicon planar type. For the EEG version of the circuit, the collector current of this transistor was 8 μA, whilst for the ECG version it was 1 μA.

Figure 12.2 shows the relationship between noise figure, source resistance and collector current for an I.T.T. type BFY19 silicon planar transistor. For a given collector current, there is an optimum

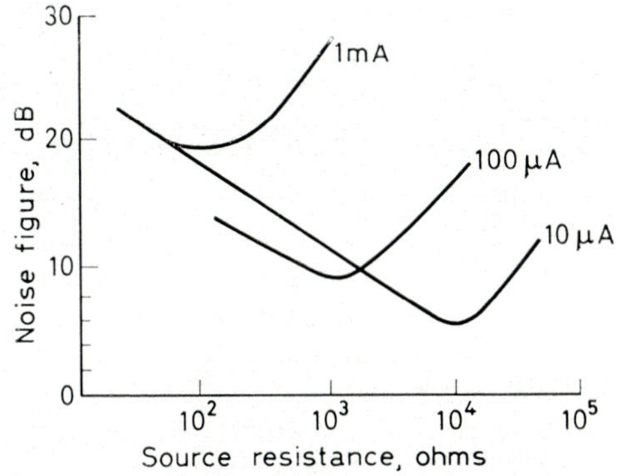

Figure 12.2. The relationship between the noise figure, source resistance and collector current for a silicon planar transistor

source resistance for the lowest noise. This does not change much over the frequency range 300 Hz to 100 kHz. Normally an amplifier is 'matched' to the resistance of the signal source when its input resistance is the same as that of the source. By mismatching the source resistance and the input resistance, it should be possible to find a minimum value for the noise figure. However, Rheinfelder (1964) points out that mismatching does not result in any worthwhile improvement if the matched noise figure is 8 db or more. With selection of transistors and circuit conditions, noise figures of the order of 2 db can be achieved.

An example of a special low noise transistor is the Type 2N929 *n–p–n* silicon planar transistor by Texas Instruments Ltd. By excluding all contaminants from the crystal surface, room temperature leakage currents are kept to near the theoretical minimum values. Because the number of surface recombination centres is low, careful control of the diffusion process results in high values of h_{fe} which are high even at very low current levels. With a collector-to-emitter voltage of 5 V and a collector current of 10 μA, the minimum value of h_{fe} is 40 and the maximum is 120. If the source (generator) resistance is 10 kΩ, the broadband noise figure measured with an amplifier having a frequency response which is 3 db down at 10 Hz and 10 kHz is a maximum of 4 db. It is interesting to note that a noise figure of 4 db at 1 kHz is quoted for the Ferranti general purpose plastic encapsulated silicon planar *n–p–n* transistors types ZTZ107, 108 and 109 with $V_{CE}=5$ V and $I_C=10$ μA.

NOISE CHARACTERISTICS OF SILICON PLANAR FIELD EFFECT TRANSISTORS

Noise sources in a field effect transistor can be represented by noise current generators in the gate-to-source junction and the source-to-drain junction. In practice the noise produced by the reverse biased gate-to-source junction is small in planar devices and can be neglected. At low frequencies the contribution from the source-to-drain junction represents $1/f$ noise, but at the higher frequencies where $1/f$ can be neglected, it is mainly dependent upon the transconductance of the FET and approaches a constant value. FETs are capable of low noise figures: for example, the Fairchild types 2N3277 and 2N3278, operated from a 1 MΩ source, give a noise figure of 2 db at 1 kHz. These are *p*-channel devices. The low noise *n*-channel epitaxial planar silicon FET type BC264L is quoted as having a minimum average noise figure of 0·5 db and a typical value of 2 db with $V_{DS}=15$ V, $V_{GS}=0$, with a source resistance of 1 MΩ and a bandwidth of 5 Hz at 1 kHz.

Klaasen (1970) has investigated the geometrical dependence of $1/f$ noise in MOST transistors by comparing devices with different geometries laid down on one source. When measured at the same bias voltage, the equivalent noise voltage is proportional to the oxide thickness and inversely proportional to the active gate area.

THE NOISE FIGURE FOR A COMPLETE SYSTEM

Consider a complete system (perhaps an amplifier or receiver) composed of several stages connected in series. Let the noise figures for the various stages be F_1, F_2 . . . F_n and the corresponding power gains be G_1, G_2 . . . G_n. If it can be assumed that the noise power contributed by any stage is independent of that produced by all the other stages, then

$$F_{total}=F_1+(F_2-1)/G_1+(F_3-1)/G_1G_2 \ldots (F_n-1)/G_1G_2 \ldots G_n$$

It can be seen that to obtain a low overall noise figure, the first stage must be designed to produce a small noise figure and to have a high power gain. This makes the first and second terms of the expression small.

REFERENCES

Klaasen, F. M. (1970). 'On the geometrical dependence of 1/f noise in MOS transistors.' *Philips Res. Rep.* **25,** 171.

Murari, B. (1967). 'ECG and EEG pre-amplifiers.' *Wld med. Electron.* **5,** 264.

Rheinfelder, W. A. (1964). *Design of Low-noise Transistor Input Circuits.* London: Iliffe.

Simpson, J. H. and Richards, R. S. (1962). *Physical Principles of Junction Transistors.* Oxford University Press.

Chapter 13

Electrometers

The term 'electrometer' is used in electronic practice to describe a d.c. voltmeter (or millivoltmeter) having a very high value of input resistance. Electrometers can thus be used to measure the voltage present on a capacitor, or the e.m.f. of a voltage source which has a high value of internal resistance. A typical application would be the measurement of the millivoltage output from a pH-sensitive glass electrode, or for recording d.c. electrophysiological signals from a micro-electrode (Kennard, 1958). The resistance at the tip of a micropipette filled with 3M KCl is typically 10 to 200 MΩ.

Electrometers are also widely used to measure the ionization current developed in an ionization chamber by the presence of radioactivity. Thus, if a current of 10^{-12} A is passed through a 10^{10} Ω resistor, the resulting voltage drop of 10 mV can be measured by means of an electrometer.

THE USE OF AN INSULATED GATE FIELD EFFECT TRANSISTOR AS AN ELECTROMETER

The IGFET or MOSFET unipolar transistor is becoming widely used in electrometer circuits. In new instruments its only rival is the capacitive (vibrating reed) modulator. The once almost universally used electrometer valve has been supplanted, except perhaps where there is a possibility of radiation damage to semiconductor devices. In addition to its small size, the IGFET has been shown to have the required degree of stability and is capable directly of a millivolt sensitivity.

The simplest type of semiconductor electrometer circuit is the source follower of *Figure 13.1* (Pacák, 1969). For the measurement of voltages up to about ±1 V, the signal may be connected directly to the input terminals with respect to the polarity if a centre zero meter is used. The 1 V range can be subdivided down to the lowest range of the meter, perhaps 0·2 V f.s.d. The range resistors are

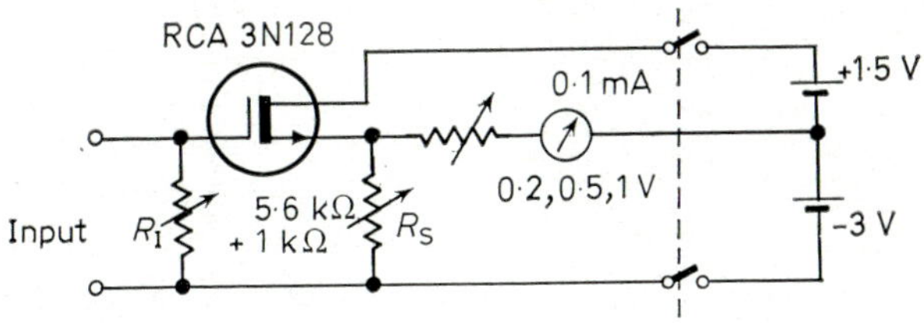

Figure 13.1. Simple IGFET emitter follower circuit
(Reproduced from Pacák, 1969, by courtesy of the Editor of *Electronic Engineering*)

adjusted to give the correct calibration since the gain of the follower is slightly less than unity when loaded by the meter. For the measurement of higher input voltages, a high megohm resistive divider is used at the input. Without this, the direct voltage range is 1 mV to 1 V. R_S acts as a zero adjustment. For current measurements the input resistor R_I acts as a shunt, so that $V_{in}=I.R._{in}$ and currents from 10^{-11} A upwards can be measured. Since this circuit is not symmetrical, temperature changes are likely to produce drifts, and steps must be taken to hold the temperature of the circuit components as uniform as possible. The accuracy attainable with the simple arrangement of *Figure 13.1* is about 5 per cent. The drawback to the simplicity and economy of the source follower occurs in its limited range, its non-linearity and the effect of the input capacitance.

A better circuit is shown in *Figure 13.2* (Pacák, 1969). Here the source follower input stage is followed by Q_2, a common emitter stage with a gain of about 50, and an emitter follower output stage to drive the meter. The common resistor R_{E2} eliminates the need to provide for clamping of the emitter of Q_2. By making R_{E3} a little smaller than R_{C2}, positive feedback occurs, increasing the forward gain of the circuit to about 200 and improving the performance of the circuit. Since the circuit is still asymmetrical, drift will occur due to temperature and supply voltage variations. The circuit originally had a positive temperature coefficient. This has been compensated by means of the copper wire resistor R_{Cu} in parallel with R_T, which is chosen to have a zero temperature coefficient. Resistor R_U compensates for the fall in battery voltage with life. The neon diode protects the IGFET against input voltages which could break it down. Resistor R_C provides a symmetrical load for the batteries and minimizes the effect of supply voltage changes.

Components R_F and C_F are chosen to ensure circuit stability even when R_I is small or the positive feedback tends to become critical. An input voltage range of about ±5 V can be handled, with a maximum sensitivity range of 50 mV.

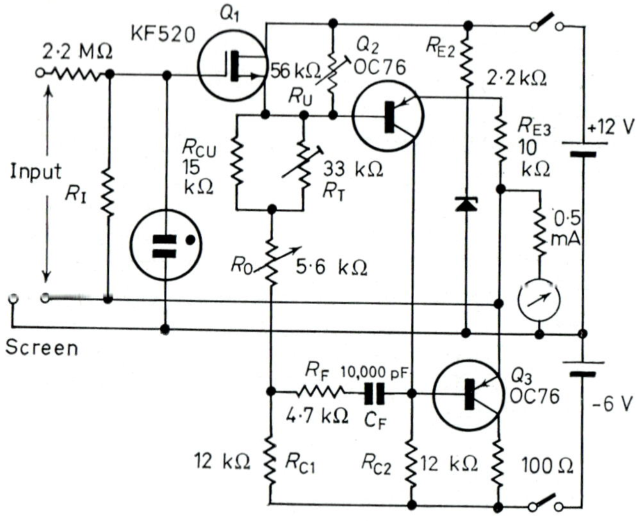

Figure 13.2. An economic feedback IGFET electrometer with a loop gain of about 200 increased by the small positive feedback loop between Q_2 and Q_3 and including compensation for temperature and supply voltage changes.

(Reproduced from Pacák, 1969, by courtesy of the Editor of *Electronic Engineering*)

A more sophisticated circuit is that of *Figure 13.3* (Pacák, 1969). A balanced IGFET input stage is employed, followed by an operational amplifier A_1 having a closed loop gain of 100. A further gain factor of 100 is available from A_2, giving a full-scale output of 10 V on all input ranges from 1 mV to 10 V or 1 mA to 10^{-14} A. Amplifier A_2 also provides an active filter for noise reduction, its time constant being defined by C_T and R_T. A series stabilizer is used for the circuit supply, and this is fitted with a temperature compensation resistor R_{Cu}. The input signal is connected to the circuit via a polythene insulation screened cable. The screen is connected by switch S_1 to the circuit's 0 V line when current is to be measured or to the lower end of R_I for voltage measurements. Pacák has used a PTFE insulated switch to select values for R_I of 990 Ω to 10^{12} Ω, making possible current ranges from about

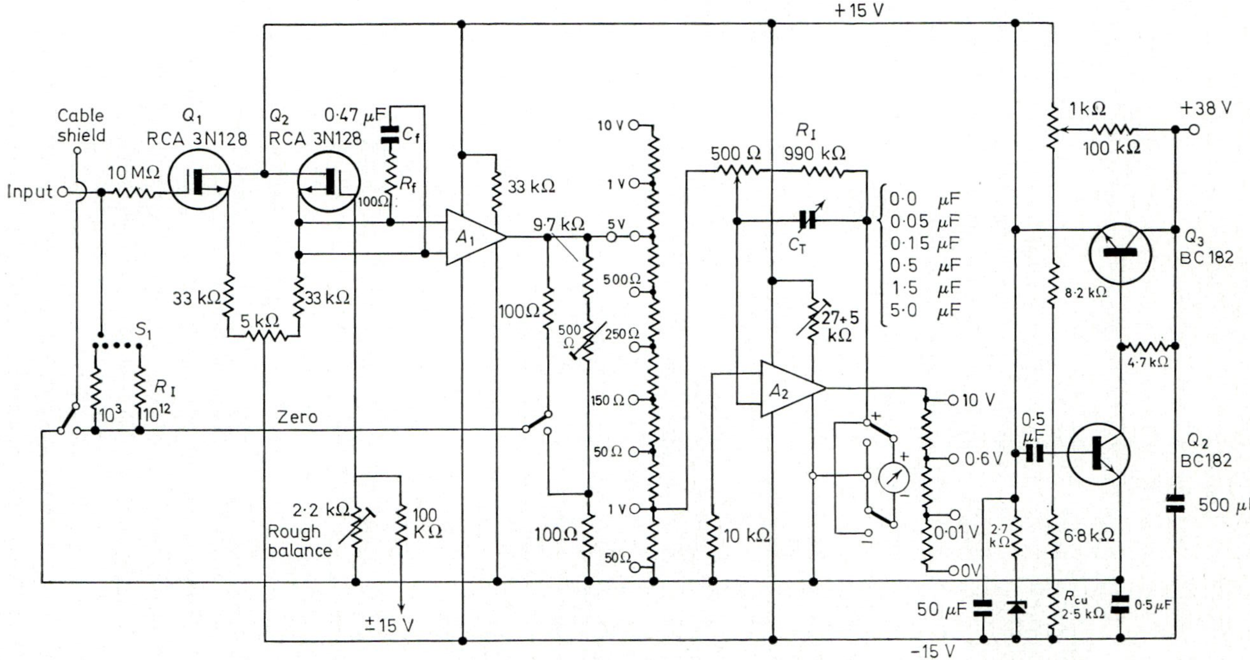

Figure 13.3. A symmetrical input stage IGFET electrometer having two values of closed loop amplification (1 and 1,000), giving a measurement range of 1 mV to 10 V f.s.d. or 1 mA to 10^{-14} A f.s.d. Additional amplification is available to give a 10 V output on all ranges. An adjustable single time constant noise filter is available

(Reproduced from Pacák, 1969, by courtesy of the Editor of *Electronic Engineering*)

1 mA to 10^{-14} A. The circuit gave a one hour stability of about 10^{-4} V or 10^{-15} A with a noise level of about one-tenth of these values.

THE CAPACITATIVE MODULATOR

Capacitative modulators or vibrating reed electrometers are generally used as laboratory instruments when currents of the order of 10^{-15} A have to be measured, typically in connection with ionization chamber measurements of radioactivity. They are also used in some blood pH meters.

Figure 13.4 illustrates the principle of the capacitative modulator, originally described by Pavlensky, Swank and Grenchick (1947).

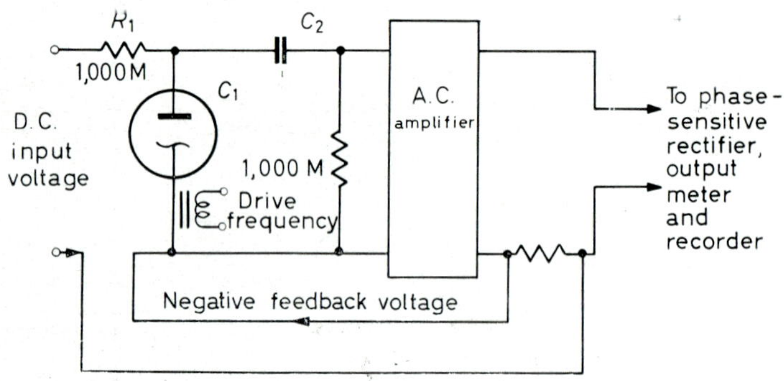

Figure 13.4. Schematic diagram of a vibrating reed electrometer

The d.c. input voltage to be measured (usually as the result of a current flowing through a high value resistor) is applied to the fixed plate of capacitor C_1. The other plate is energized by means of a drive coil so that it vibrates at a frequency which may be the power line frequency of 50 or 60 Hz or higher (e.g. 400, or 2,000 Hz). The vibration produces an alternating component of voltage across C_1, and this is passed by C_2 and amplified by means of an R–C coupled amplifier. The resulting a.c. output is converted back to d.c., using a phase-sensitive rectifier so that account is taken of the polarity of the original d.c. input signal.

The capacitance of a parallel plate capacitor is given by $C=(kA/4\pi d)\times 1{\cdot}11\times 10^{-6}$ μF where k is the dielectric constant of the medium between the plates, A is the area of the plates in cm^2, and d is the plate separation in cm. The charge stored on the capacitor is given by $Q=VC$ where Q is in coulombs, V is the voltage across the plates, and C is the capacitance in farads.

Since the lower plate vibrates sinusoidally with time about a mean position, $d_t=d_o+d_1 \sin 2\pi ft$ where d_t is the instantaneous separation of the plates at time t, d_o is the plate separation when no drive is applied, and d_1 is the maximum amplitude of vibration of the plate. The time constant R_1C_1 is chosen to be sufficiently long that Q remains practically constant over a period of one cycle of the drive frequency. The voltage developed across the vibrating capacitor C_1 is $V=Q/C_1=Q4\pi d_t/kA=Q4\pi d_o/kA+Q4\pi d_1 \sin 2\pi ft/kA$. For a given drive amplitude and plate spacing the ratio d_1/d_o is a constant, so that the alternating component, which is subsequently converted back to a d.c. output voltage, is proportional to V_1 which is the original input voltage. Because the ratio (d_1/d_o) must be a constant, the plates of C_1 are optically worked for flatness, polished and sealed in an inert gas atmosphere.

A typical vibrating reed electrometer would have switched full-scale voltage sensitivities of 3 mV, 30 mV, 300 mV and 1 V. Switched input resistors of 10^8, 10^{10} and 10^{12} Ω allow maximum current sensitivities of 3×10^{-11}, 3×10^{-13} and 3×10^{-15} A to be measured.

A LOW INPUT CAPACITANCE ELECTROMETER FOR USE WITH MICRO-ELECTRODES

Holmer (1970) describes the design of an interesting dual FET electrometer for use with micro-electrodes having a tip diameter of about 500 nm. When filled with 3M KCl, the resistance is about 50 MΩ. The input resistance of the electrometer should be at least 1,000 times greater and the input current should be less than 10^{-11} A. The range of the electrometer should be ±1 V with a d.c. drift of less than 0·5 mV per day. Since the electrometer will be required to respond to action potentials as well as to d.c. changes, Holmer recommends that the amplifier rise time should be 10 μs or less for a step voltage change applied in series with 10 MΩ to the input.

The basic input stage to the circuit is a source follower (*Figure 13.5*) where Q_1 is an n-channel FET operating with a constant current generator as a source resistance. The constant current generator is shown in detail in *Figure 13.6*, where D_2 is a Zener diode which determines the current through Q_3. The diode D_4 is included for temperature compensation. The circuit still has a high value of input capacitance between gate and drain, and this gives an unacceptably long time constant. This is reduced by bootstrapping so that the drain potential is forced to follow input potential changes. The bootstrapping principle is illustrated in *Figure 13.7*, where a battery is used to couple the source (which follows the input voltage) and the drain. In *Figure 13.9*, the battery voltage has been replaced by the voltage drop developed across R_2 when a constant current from Q_4, D_1, D_3 and R_2 is passed through it. By this means,

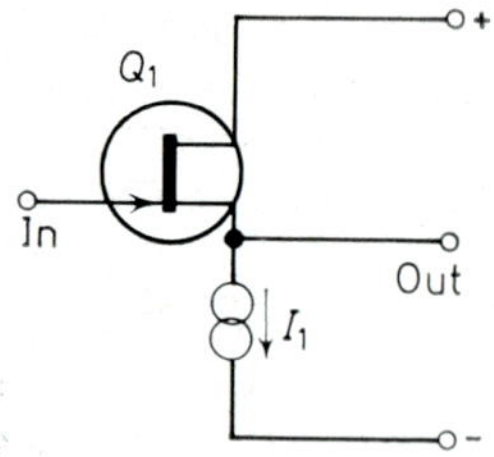

Figure 13.5

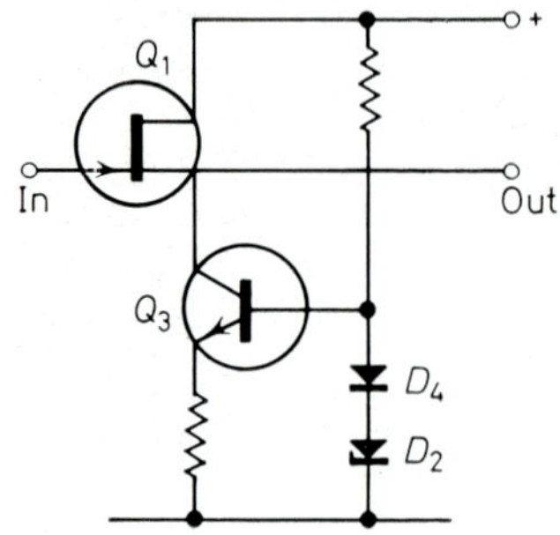

Figure 13.6

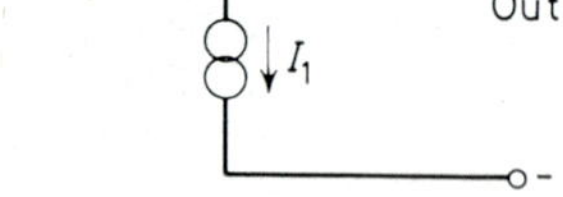

Figure 13.7

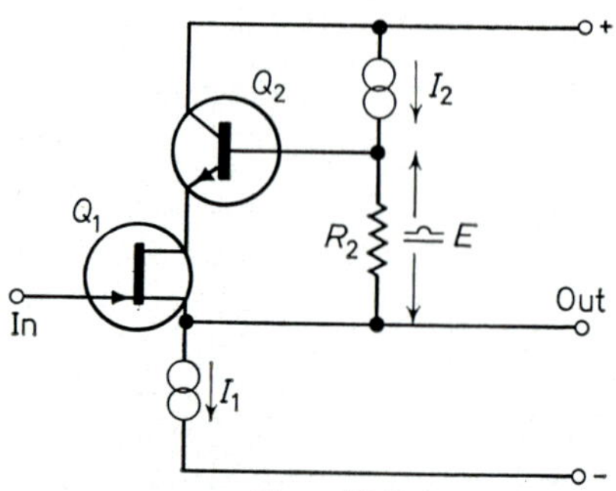

Figure 13.8

Figures 13.5 to 13.8. Development of an electrometer follower
(Reproduced from Holmer, 1970, by courtesy of the Editor of *Medical and Biological Engineering*)

Holmer reports that a rise time of 5 μs can be attained with a 10 MΩ resistor in series with the input. In the final form of the circuit (*Figure 13.9*), temperature drift is minimized by using a dual FET as a balanced source follower. The 150 pF capacitor is connected between the output and the inverting input of A_1.

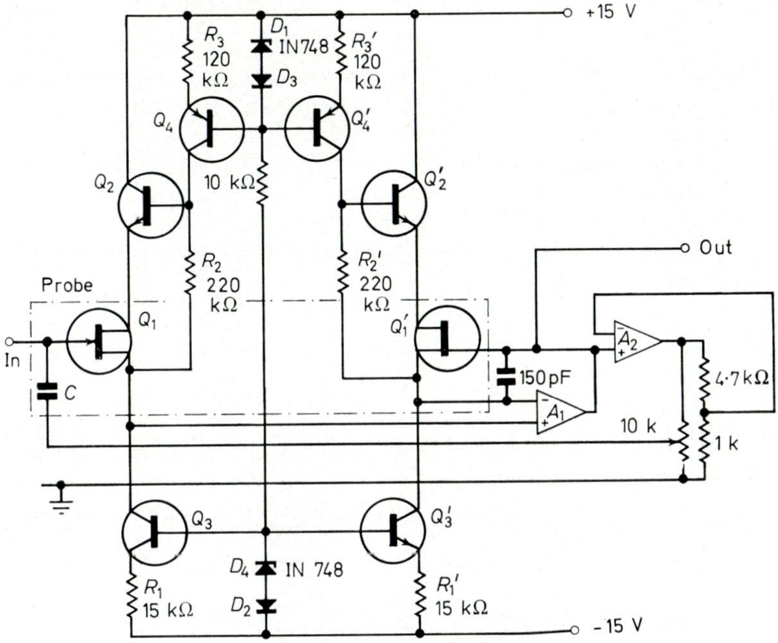

Q_1, Q_1', dual FET 2N5198 Siliconix
Q_2, Q_2', Q_4, Q_4', 2N2484 Texas
A_1, A_2, type D–5 BY DDC

Figure 13.9. Low input capacitance FET electrometer for use in electrophysiology

(Reproduced from Holmer, 1970, by courtesy of the Editor of *Medical and Biological Engineering*)

Holmer points out that in electrophysiology, a low input capacitance follower does not eliminate all capacitance losses because the capacitance existing between the micro-electrode and the surrounding non-earthed solution can invalidate the measurements. This capacitance can be neutralized by the use of positive feedback. This is accomplished by feeding a suitable fraction of the output signal back to the gate of Q_1 via the capacitance C. A_2 has a gain of about 5 times. Two separate amplifiers were used as the circuit was also designed for application as a constant current generator where as large an input signal swing as possible is required. Holmer states that the circuit has a voltage gain of 0·99, an input resistance of greater than 10^{12} Ω, an output impedance of 2 kΩ and a bandwidth of d.c. to 0·9 MHz.

HIGH INPUT IMPEDANCE A.C. BIPOLAR TRANSISTOR CIRCUITS

The application of suitable feedback techniques to a bipolar transistor amplifier enables input impedance values of 250–500 MΩ to be realized. Typically, a value of 250 MΩ can be realized over a frequency band of 1 Hz to 40 kHz. A circuit with this performance has been described by Bell and Venning (1963). The voltage gain was unity and the noise level about 0·5 mV peak to peak. These authors also describe a method suitable for the measurement of input impedances of this order.

REFERENCES

Bell, A. G. and Venning, B. H. (1963). 'High input resistance transistor amplifiers.' *J. scient. Instrum.* **40,** 239.

Holmer, N-G. (1970). 'An electrometer amplifier for electrophysiology with low input capacitance.' *Med. biol. Engng* **8,** 509.

Kennard, D. W. (1958). 'Glass micro-capillary electrodes used for measuring potential in living tissues.' In *Electronic Apparatus for Biological Research,* p. 534. Ed. by P. E. K. Donaldson. London: Butterworths.

Pacák, M. (1969). 'Simple MOSFET electrometer circuits.' *Electron. Engng* **41,** September, p. 24.

Pavlensky, H., Swank, R. K. and Grenchick, R. (1947). 'Design of dynamic condenser electrometer.' *Rev. scient. Instrum.* **18,** 298.

Chapter 14

Digital Techniques

Most circuitry employed in medical electronics applications is concerned with the amplification and processing of signals which originate in an analogue form. The signals are continuous functions, usually of time, and can be regarded in terms of their fundamental and harmonic frequencies. In the time domain, the signal amplitude is a continuous function of time. On the other hand, in the frequency domain the signal is seen as being composed of a number of frequency components, each having its own amplitude. Previous chapters have dealt with analogue filters and amplifiers.

The advent of compact digital computers has focused attention on the digital manipulation of the primary analogue signals after they have been converted into a digital form. To do this, the continuous analogue signal is sampled at a predetermined rate by means of an analogue-to-digital converter (ADC). The ADC outputs in a coded form the value of the amplitude of the analogue signal at the time of sampling. Thus if an ECG is sampled 300 times per second by an ADC of suitable speed, the output from the ADC in one second will consist of 300 values of the amplitude of the ECG waveform occurring over that second.

Using combinations of pulse circuits such as logic gates and flip-flops (bistables), it is possible to carry out arithmetical manipulations upon the series of digital values such as addition and subtraction, multiplication and division. In a digital computer, the series of instructions giving the manipulations to be performed is contained in the particular program chosen for the computer. Much of this work is based upon the use of binary arithmetic, i.e. working to the power of two. Here only two states are required for the active circuit devices, binary nought corresponding to a transistor being cut off and binary one to its being switched on.

Switching circuits also lend themselves to logic circuits, that is, circuits which test whether a predetermined set of conditions has been obeyed and can route the path of signals accordingly. Digital circuits are widely used in counting operations and feature, for example, in arrhythmia monitors for storing the number of ectopic beats of various types occurring within a stated time interval. The pattern of noughts and ones corresponding with the digital representation of a number can be stored on a series of flip-flops or magnetic cores. This, together with the availability of integrated circuit logic modules, has opened the way for a universal use of digital techniques.

DECIMAL, BINARY AND OTHER NUMBER SYSTEMS

The conventional decimal numbering system utilizes ten digits: 0, 1, 2, 3, 4, 5, 6, 7, 8 and 9. The number of digits used is known as the base or radix, i.e. ten for the decimal system and two for the binary system. Each term in a particular number is associated with the radix raised to a power depending on the position of the term in the number. Thus the decimal number five is in the zero order position, whilst decimal 45 has a four in the first order position and a five in the zero order position. The build-up can be seen from decimal $9=9\times10^0$, decimal $99=9\times10^1+9\times10^0$, decimal $999=9\times10^2+9\times10^1+9\times10^0$. The space to both the left and the right of a number is understood to be filled with zeros, i.e. decimal $9=00{\cdot}90$.

The simplest number system is the binary system with just two values, 0 and 1. Binary digits are referred to as 'bits', a ten-bit number having ten binary digits. An example of a six-bit binary number might be 42 with the bit pattern 101010, i.e. $2^5+2^3+2^1=32+8+2=42$. Since the binary pattern $111=2^2+2^1+2^0=7$, it is possible to express a binary number in the octal system by grouping successive binary bits in groups of threes. For example, 11000 in binary$=16+8=24$ in decimal. In octal this is $11{,}000=24$.

To convert a binary number into an octal number, divide the binary number into groups of three, commencing with the 2^0 digit. Each group of three is then written down as its decimal equivalent. Thus, $1101110_2=001,\ 101,\ 110_2=156_8$.

THE REPRESENTATION OF A NUMBER LESS THAN UNITY

Quantities smaller than unity are represented by placing a dot or point before the fractional part of the number. The point shows where the power to which the radix is raised becomes negative. In the decimal system, reference is made to the decimal point, and in the binary system to the binary point. For example,

$$0{\cdot}35_{10}=(3\times10^{-1})+(5\times10^{-2}).$$
$$1{\cdot}43_{2}=(1\times2^{0})+(4\times2^{-1})+(3\times2^{-2}).$$

BINARY DECIMAL CODES

When the decimal number 12 is expressed as 1100, this is an example of a pure binary code. A decimal code is the most convenient for humans, whilst a binary system is the most convenient for logic devices. By coding decimal numbers in binary form, numbering systems can be obtained which are acceptable to both human operators and machines. Any decimal number (0–9) can be represented by a group of four binary digits. In the 8421 binary-coded-decimal (BCD) code, the least significant digit has a value of 2^0 (= 1) and the most significant digit has a value of 2^3 (= 8) (Table 14.1).

Table 14.1

Decimal number	*Pure binary*	*8421 code*
0	0000	0000
1	0001	0001
2	0010	0010
3	0011	0011
4	0100	0100
5	0101	0101
6	0110	0110
7	0111	0111
8	1000	1000
9	1001	1001

So far the 8421 code is similar to pure binary. After a count of decimal 9, the 8421 BCD values change by a factor equivalent to decimal 10. The first four bits of the 8421 code cover decimal digits in the range 0 to 9, whilst the next four bits cover the decimal numbers 10, 20, 30 . . . 80, 90. Hence eight bits cover from decimal 0 to 99 (Table 14.2).

Table 14.2

Decimal number	*8421 BCD*							
	80	40	20	10	8	4	2	1
9	0	0	0	0	1	0	0	1
10	0	0	0	1	0	0	0	0
11	0	0	0	1	0	0	0	1
69	0	1	1	0	1	0	0	1
85	1	0	0	0	0	1	0	1

PARITY CHECKS

Once analogue information has been converted into digital form it can be subjected to a substantial amount of processing and can be stored on magnetic tape or paper tape. Whenever the information is being transferred from one place to another, there is always the possibility of reading or copying a bit pattern incorrectly. As a check on the validity of the numbers, it is usual to make use of a parity bit. This is an extra bit for each group of the code. If even parity is used, the parity bit is zero if the total sum of the ones in the group is even and it is unity if the sum of the ones is odd (Table 14.3).

Table 14.3

Decimal number	*Parity bit—even parity*	*8421 BCD code*
0	0	0000
1	1	0001
2	1	0010
3	0	0011
4	1	0100

A number of digital computers use a seven-bit International Standards Organization (I.S.O.) code to represent numbers. This is punched as a series of eight characters (seven+parity bit) in the form of holes for binary noughts and blanks for binary ones on one inch wide paper tape. When the computer reads the paper tape, it checks for even parity. If this is not found, the tape reader is stopped and attention is drawn to the fact.

ANALOGUE-TO-DIGITAL CONVERTERS

Shaft Position Encoders

It is often required to convert the angular position of a shaft into a digital form, an example being the need to digitize the output from a potentiometric pen recorder or from a spirometer. A suitable shaft in the mechanism can then be fitted with an encoding disk. The disk (*Figure 14.1*) is opaque except for transparent segments arranged in the form of a set of concentric tracks on its face. A radial light source illuminates the tracks, whilst a photocell is placed behind each track. The pattern of the tracks is such that a unique pattern of signals appears for each position of the shaft. The signals from each photocell appear simultaneously to give a parallel output.

Particularly with optical types of ADC, it is possible to obtain an ambiguous output. This may occur if the device is not correctly aligned. The use of a cyclic binary or Gray conversion code then greatly reduces the risk of ambiguity compared with that found when a straight binary code is employed. The Gray code is built up from a simple 0 and 1 combination which is progressively reflected as the magnitude of the system increases. The first two numbers in the Gray code are 0000 and 0001, representing nought and one.

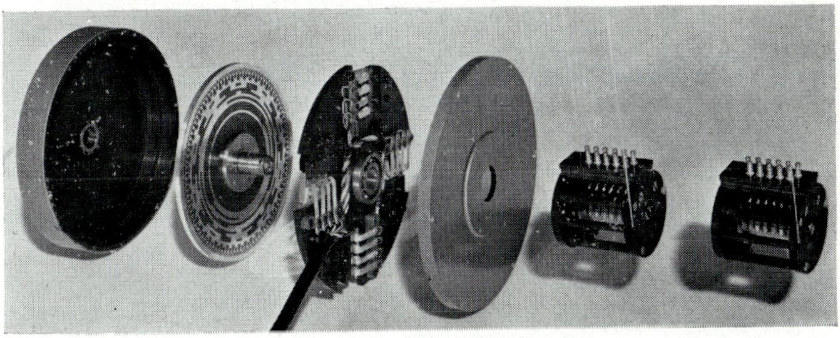

Figure 14.1. Optical encoder disk
(By courtesy of Rank Precision Industries Ltd.)

The next two numbers are obtained by reflecting the combination and adding a one in the next higher digit. The reflection process can be seen by considering successive pairs of numbers in the right-hand column of the Gray code (Table 14.4).

Table 14.4

Decimal	*Gray code*	*Decimal*	*Gray code*
0	0000	8	1100
1	0001	9	1101
2	0011	10	1111
3	0010	11	1110
4	0110	12	1010
5	0111	13	1011
6	0101	14	1001
7	0100	15	1000

The advantages of the cyclic binary code over the pure binary code in this application are shown in *Figure 14.2*, taken from Hartley (1962). For a slight misalignment of the photocells, the pure binary code output might take the values 10000=16, 10001=17, 10011=19,

10111=23, 11111=31. For the same range of misalignment, the use of the cyclic binary code restricts the output to 11000=16 or 11001=17, the ambiguity having now been reduced to the value of the least significant digit.

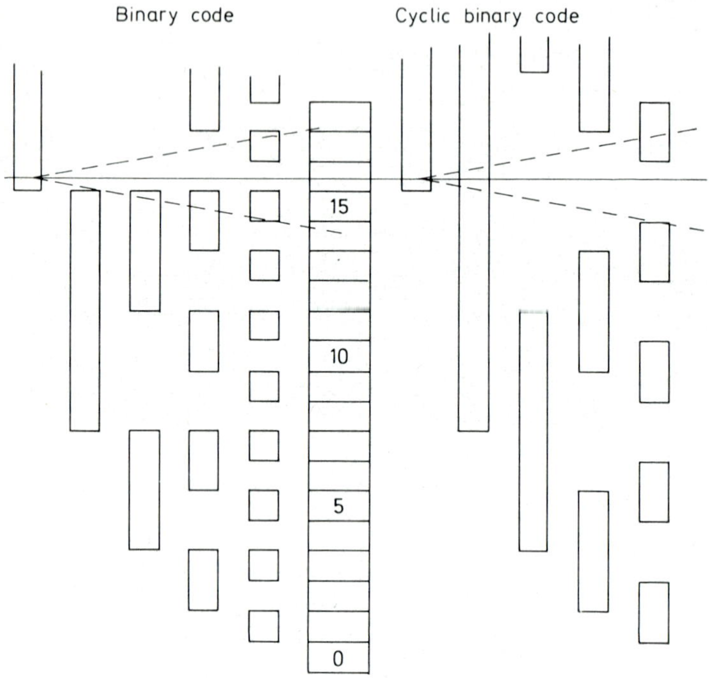

Figure 14.2. Effect of a slight misalignment of the photocells of an optical encoder on the output in pure binary code and in a cyclic binary code

(Reproduced after Hartley, 1962, by courtesy of Methuen & Co. Ltd.)

Solid State Circuitry Analogue-to-digital Converters

Fast analogue-to-digital converters are being used in an increasing range of digital computer systems and instruments such as signal averagers and digital voltmeters. One simple type of converter employs a voltage-controlled oscillator, the deviation of the oscillator frequency from its centre frequency being proportional to the amplitude of the input voltage. During a fixed time interval, a count is kept of the number of zero crossings made by the output signal from the oscillator. The count is proportional to the value of the input voltage plus a constant. This technique has been employed in average response computers.

In a ramp type ADC, a ramp is started at some definite voltage level and stopped when the ramp voltage is coincident with the input voltage. The time between the starting and stopping of the ramp is proportional to the amplitude of the input voltage plus a constant. A schematic diagram of the arrangement is shown in *Figure 14.3.*

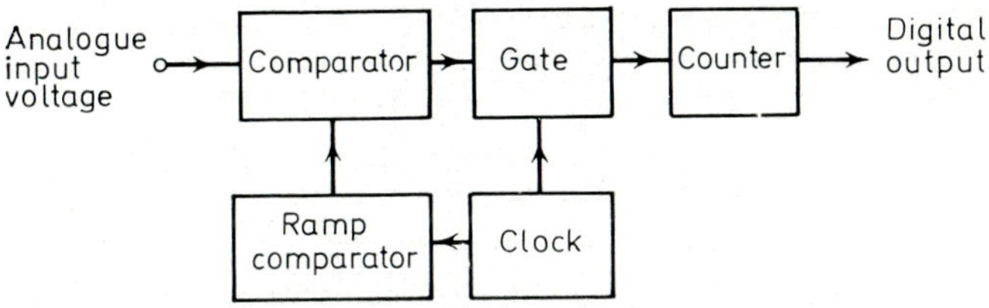

Figure 14.3. Block diagram of a ramp type analogue-to-digital converter

Successive approximation or weighing type converters are widely used. The input voltage is successively compared with a set of known voltages, each of which is related to its neighbours by a factor of two. Starting with the highest known voltage, each is compared with the input. If the input is less, the standard is removed and replaced with the next lowest. If the standard is greater, it is left in position. When the smallest reference voltage has been compared, the sum of the reference voltages left in place will give the binary equivalent of the input. An advantage of this arrangement is that an n-bit number can be determined in n-trials.

Figure 14.4 is the block diagram of an Analog Devices H series ADC which is available in either an eight-bit or a ten-bit configuration. The complete converter is mounted within a single 51 mm × 102 mm × 10 mm (2 in × 4 in × 0·4 in) package. The eight-bit version requires the following power supplies: +15 V d.c. ±2 per cent at 40 mA, −15 V d.c. ±2 per cent at 30 mA, and +5 V d.c. ±5 per cent at 320 mA. The full-scale input range for the analogue signal is 0 to 10 V (8 kΩ input resistance), 0 to −10 V (5 kΩ), or ±10 V (6·6 kΩ). The conversion time is 12 μs maximum for a Convert Command pulse width less than 0·6 μs.

The converter contains its own internal timing clock, which has a nominal frequency of 750 kHz (square wave). When it is desired to start a conversion of the analogue signal, a positive pulse having a minimum width of 50 ns is applied to the converter. This sets the status signal to the 'logic one' level and starts the clock and the conversion process. It also resets the previous output word to zero.

The decision as to which is the most significant bit (MSB) is made on the second positive edge of the clock following the fall of the Convert Command. The MSB is available as an output as well as its logical inversion ($\overline{\text{MSB}}$). Subsequent bit decisions are made on successive positive edges of each clock cycle. In addition to outputting

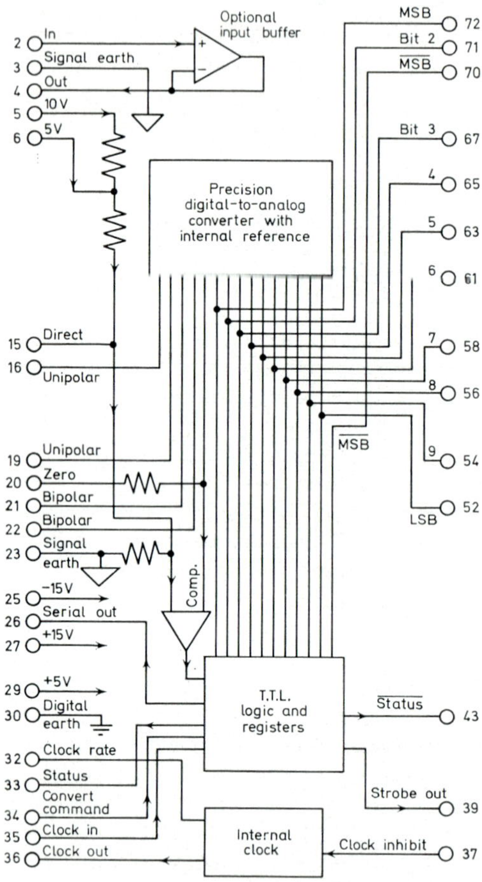

Figure 14.4. Block diagram of a commercial eight-bit analogue-to-digital converter

(By courtesy of Analog Devices)

a logical 0 or logical 1 level as appropriate for each bit position one after the other (serial output), the complete bit pattern is available as a parallel output when the status level returns to logical 0 level.

Figure 14.5 gives the timing diagram for the converter. Offset and Gain trimming adjustments are provided for obtaining an accurate output. With a unipolar output converter, the analogue input voltage is first adjusted to have a value giving one least significant bit away

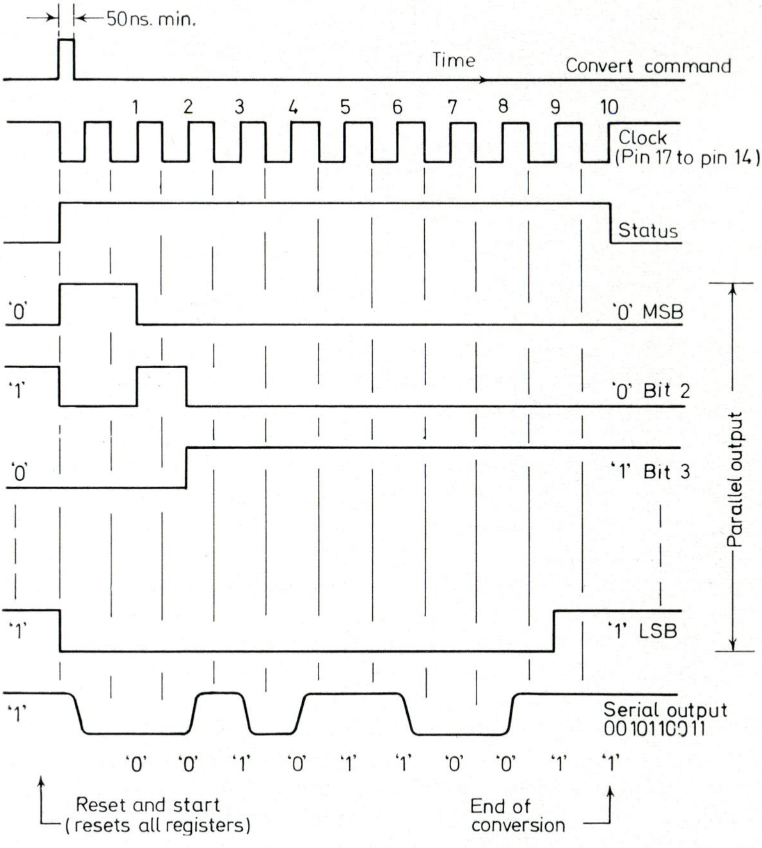

Figure 14.5. Timing diagram of the analogue-to-digital converter featured in Figure 14.4. Previous code=010 . . . 1; new code=001 . . . 1

(By courtesy of Analog Devices)

from 0 V. The Offset control is then adjusted until the proper digital code (00000001) appears at the output. The input voltage is then set to a value of (full scale—one least significant bit) and the Gain control adjusted until the correct full-scale code (11111111) appears at the output.

DIGITAL VOLTMETERS

Another version of a successive approximation ADC is illustrated in *Figure 14.6.* The single reference voltage used has a value equal to half the full-scale voltage range of the converter. For the first comparison, the input signal is compared directly with the reference.

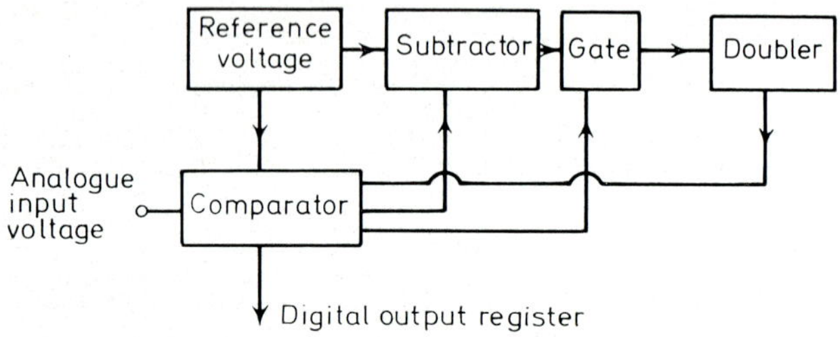

Figure 14.6. Block diagram of a single reference voltage successive approximation ADC

If the input is greater than or equal to the reference, the latter is subtracted from the input signal. Simultaneously, the most significant bit of the digital output is set to 1. Any voltage difference between the reference and the input is now doubled and the doubled value compared with the reference. If, however, at the first comparison the reference voltage exceeded the input signal, the most significant bit is set to 0 and no subtraction occurs. The input is now doubled and the comparison made again. This process is repeated until the number of bits required for the output has been determined.

Suppose that the output is to consist of five binary bits. This is equivalent to 31 V (16+8+4+2+1). Let the reference voltage be 16 V and the input analogue voltage be 26 V. At the first comparison the difference is +10 V, so the most significant bit is set to 1. The difference is doubled to give 20 V. On subtracting the reference, the difference is +4 V; this is doubled to 8 V, and the next bit is also set to 1. On attempting to subtract the reference, the difference is −8 V, so the third bit becomes 0. Doubling gives 16 V and a zero difference from the reference, so that the fourth bit becomes 1 and the fifth bit 0. The bit pattern stored in the output register is thus 11010, which is the binary equivalent of 26 as required. A six-bit converter would have a full-scale capability of 63 V and a reference voltage of 32 V.

Successive Approximation Digital Voltmeters

In one version of this digital voltmeter, a set of standard reference voltages derived from a Weston cadmium mercury cell is provided against which the input analogue signal amplitude is automatically compared. When equality is achieved, the value of the reference voltage needed for balance is output to a display unit in the case of a digital voltmeter.

In practice, the input signal is compared with the reference voltage by means of a bank of precision resistors. Each resistor is sequentially connected to the reference through bistable controlled switching transistors. In this way the proportion of the reference voltage applied to the summing junction of a balance detection amplifier is increased by discrete and known increments of opposite polarity to the input voltage until the input voltage is just equalized. Resistors introducing too great a proportion of the reference voltage are automatically rejected by command of the balance amplifier. The conversion process is complete when all the resistors have been successfully interrogated. When this occurs, the input signal will be balanced by the reference voltage to within a specified limit as determined by the amplitude of the input voltage, typically 10 μV for the range 0 to 0·29999 V.

The binary representation of the input voltage is now held on 19 bistable circuits, 18 for quantity and one for polarity. When the converter is used as part of a digital voltmeter, the outputs from the quantity bistables are taken via 36 lines to five decoding matrices. These drive five numerical display units giving a five-digit decimal display of the input voltage. A sixth display is used to show the algebraic sign of the voltage.

The internal reference supply consists of a +6 V or −6 V source derived from Zener diodes placed in a temperature-controlled oven feeding a drift-corrected d.c. amplifier. According to the polarity of the input signal, one or other of these supplies is switched to the bank of reference resistors. The balance amplifier is a high gain, low drift d.c. amplifier. The maximum resolution of the system is one part in 30,000.

Ramp Type Digital Voltmeters

In this type of digital voltmeter, a ramp voltage is generated which decreases linearly with time. From a voltage comparator circuit, a signal is produced when the ramp voltage passes through the unknown input voltage. A second comparator generates a signal when the ramp passes through zero. The period of time elapsing between the two comparator signals is then proportional to the value of the input voltage. The period is measured by counting pulses derived from a precision oscillator, typically having a frequency of

500 kHz, throughout the time interval. By introducing the correct scaling factor, a display of the accumulated count will directly indicate the value of the input voltage. The accuracy of this arrangement is set, not by the stability of the oscillator, but by the linearity of the ramp generator. The polarity of the input voltage can be either positive or negative if the ramp is allowed to run right through zero. The polarity of the input signal is detected from the order in which the signals from the comparators occur. An accuracy of 0·1 per cent is readily obtainable. The ramp voltage may run from greater than +2 V to less than −2 V, giving a basic ±2 V range for the instrument. Resistive potential divider circuits are provided to handle inputs up to 2 kV d.c. A block diagram of the arrangement is given in *Figure 14.3.*

Integrating Type Digital Voltmeters

This type of digital voltmeter usually employs a d.c. operational amplifier which is provided with resistive input and capacitive feedback elements. In one type of instrument, the input voltage is connected to the input resistor of the amplifier for a fixed period. The output of the amplifier, which initially starts at zero, rises or falls during that period with a slope dependent upon the value of the input voltage, and thus finishes at a level which depends upon the mean value of the input voltage. A reference voltage of opposite polarity to the input voltage is then connected to the same input resistor. The amplifier output voltage now returns towards zero with a slope dependent upon the value of the reference voltage. The time taken to return to zero depends upon the value of the input voltage and is measured with a timer as in the ramp type of digital voltmeter. Integrating digital voltmeters are particularly suitable for rapidly measuring the mean level of signals which have a large hum content. In this case the integration period is chosen to be an integral number of cycles of the hum. Integrating digital voltmeters cannot, however, make spot measurements of a voltage, unlike instruments of the ramp type.

Digital voltmeters of various types are being increasingly used as output devices in a wide range of medical instrumentation, a typical example occurring in blood–gas electrode systems.

THE USE OF A SAMPLE AND HOLD CIRCUIT

Ambiguities can arise if the input analogue signal to an analogue-to-digital converter changes during the conversion period. The fact that the value of the analogue signal is no longer precisely defined in regard to time introduces an error which has the same overall effect as a decrease in the sampling rate or an increase in the spacing of the samples by an interval equal to the uncertainty in the time.

When a change in the analogue signal is likely during the conversion period, it is usual to employ a 'sample and hold circuit'. This follows (tracks) the analogue signal and stores on a capacitor the analogue value. The stored value is presented to the converter. The sample and hold circuit must store the value to a better accuracy than the accuracy of the converter during the conversion period. A working rule quoted by Macy (1965) is that the storage time of the sample and hold circuit (or of the converter if used alone) must be short enough to ensure that the input signal at its maximum rate of change cannot vary by more than half of the conversion accuracy during this time.

ALIASING

Essentially the process of 'digitizing' is concerned with the conversion of continuous data into a series of discrete numbers. An important parameter in this process is the choice of sampling rate. In order not to lose information concerning the higher frequency components of the analogue input signal, it is necessary to have a sufficiently high rate of sampling. On the other hand, high input data rates can lead to core store overloading problems in a digital computer, and the sheer weight of data manipulations can prove troublesome. In practice the sampling rate should be the lowest which will avoid aliasing errors with the particular input signal concerned.

Figure 14.7 shows how, by not sampling at a sufficiently high rate, two quite different frequency signals can produce the same set of digitized samples. This is known as aliasing. If t seconds is the interval between successive samples, then the sampling rate is $1/t$ per second.

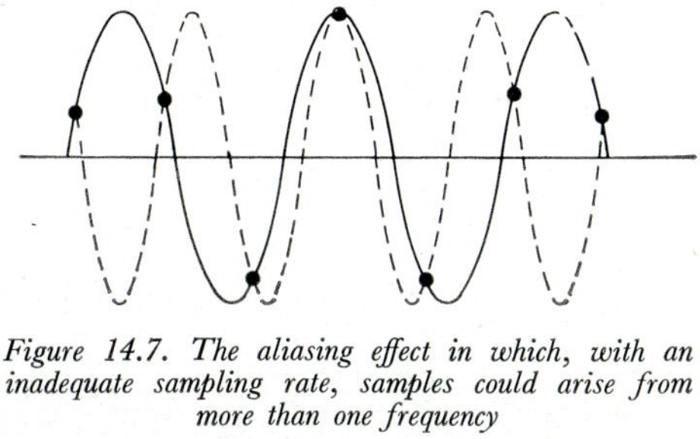

Figure 14.7. The aliasing effect in which, with an inadequate sampling rate, samples could arise from more than one frequency

Only data in the frequency range 0 to $\frac{1}{2}$ $(1/t)$ Hz are useful, since frequencies higher than this will be folded into the range 0–$\frac{1}{2}$ $(1/t)$ and will be confused with data in this range.

The effect of sampling is to introduce extra frequency components centred on harmonics of the sampling frequency. These will not overlap if the sampling frequency is equal to or greater than twice the bandwidth of the input signal. In practice this sampling theorem never applies exactly, as band-limited signals do not exist physically. However, it does apply to a very good approximation when the analogue input signal has been passed through a good low pass filter. It is then necessary to sample at a rate which is higher than the nominal cut-off frequency of the anti-aliasing filter. How much higher will depend upon the characteristics of the filter, the spectrum of the signal and the accuracy required. The frequency corresponding to twice the sampling rate is known as the Nyquist rate. In deciding on the sampling rate, consideration must be given to the roll-off characteristic of the low pass filter used as, if this is not very severe, considerable amplitudes of frequencies above the cut-off frequency may be present. If the roll-off is very severe, the filter may introduce analogue errors into the signal such as those arising from phase shift.

The low pass anti-aliasing filter cut-off frequency is the 3 db frequency. If folding is troublesome because of the filter roll-off, a sampling rate of three or four times the filter cut-off frequency should be chosen, depending on the rate of roll-off and the necessary dynamic range.

For equally spaced data, two frequencies f_1 and f_2 are aliases of one another if sinusoids of these frequencies cannot be distinguished in terms of their equally spaced values. This arises when $f_1 = 2m\, f_s + f_2$ where f_s is the sampling frequency and m is an integer.

ACCURACY OF CONVERSION

If sufficient digits are not provided, the effect is to introduce a recognizable number of 'steps' into the sampled waveform and thus to produce distortion (*Figure 14.8*).

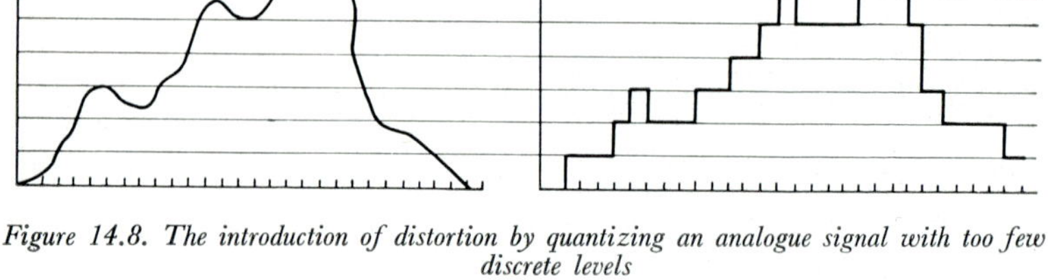

Figure 14.8. The introduction of distortion by quantizing an analogue signal with too few discrete levels

DIGITAL-TO-ANALOGUE CONVERTERS

A digital-to-analogue converter (DAC) is required at the output of a digital computer to produce an analogue (graphical) output. The converter is fed with a set of parallel inputs representing the output in binary code from the computer. In *Figure 14.9* five input resistors are provided. The summing amplifier sums the input signals. The height of each pulse in the set is equal, so that weighting factors are set by the values of the input resistors to the summing amplifier.

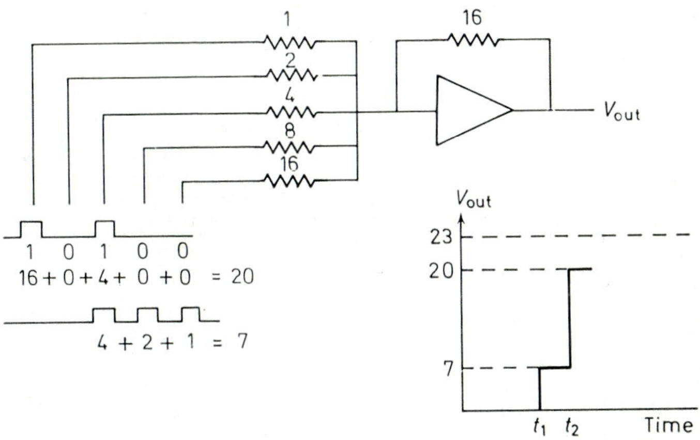

Figure 14.9. Schematic diagram of a simple digital-to-analogue converter

Thus the input signals are multiplied by constants of 1, 2, 4, 8 and 16 corresponding to their position in the binary scale. Supposing that at a time t_1 the binary input to the converter is 10100, the corresponding analogue output will be $1\times16+0\times8+1\times4+0\times2+0\times1=20$. When the binary input signals are presented to the converter with sufficient accuracy, the analogue output becomes a good approximation to a smooth curve. For an accurate conversion, the generation of the input pulses must be precise.

A good example of the use of digital-to-analogue converters occurs in the employment of a digital computer to calculate isodose curves in radiation therapy planning. The co-ordinates calculated for each point on the plot are fed on paper tape into an X and a Y converter to produce corresponding analogue outputs to actuate an X–Y recorder.

When a digital computer is used to perform operations such as filtering on an analogue signal, it is very desirable to employ a digital-to-analogue converter in order to be able to compare the processed and raw input signals. This provides a quick check on the validity of the processing.

Figure 14.10 gives the block diagram of an Analog Devices type DAC-10H digital-to-voltage converter. Essentially the device consists of (1) internal reference and control circuitry, (2) switched binary weighted constant current sources, and (3) an integrated circuit buffer amplifier. The input consists of a ten-bit binary

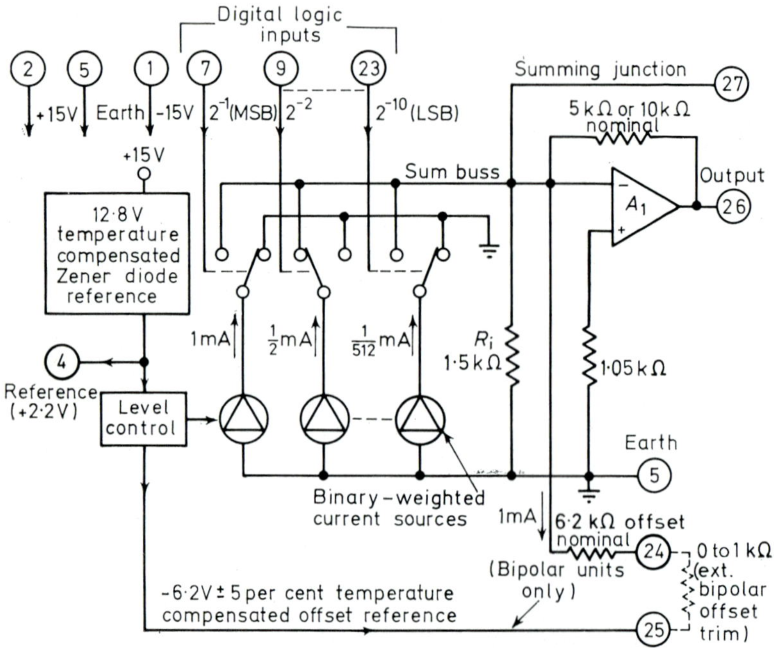

Figure 14.10. Block diagram of a commercial digital-to-analogue converter

(By courtesy of Analog Devices)

pattern of 0's and l's corresponding to the digital value of the input number. The '1' and '0' are not numbers; they are states represented by different voltage levels. The logical '0' level is taken as less than 0·8 V and the logical '1' level as greater than 2·4 V.

Each bit of the input pattern switches the corresponding binary weighted current source in the following manner: a logical '0' level switches the current source concerned to earth, and a logical

'1' level switches the source to the summing busbar. In this way the total summed current is the analogue equivalent of the input digital number. It is converted to a corresponding output voltage by an inverting operational amplifier. The weighted currents have the same algebraic sign, that is, they are unipolar. Bipolar operation can be accomplished by adding a half full-scale offset current of opposite polarity to that of the weighted current sources driving the summing busbar. The offset current is supplied from an internal reference voltage via an internal resistor. The gain can be changed by adjusting the value of the amplifier's feedback resistor. An external offset trim adjustment is needed for bipolar models, but unipolar models are supplied by the manufacturer with an absolute accuracy of $\pm 0{\cdot}05$ per cent for the specified full-scale output voltages.

When a digital input-to-current output device is required, a version is available which does not have the output voltage conversion amplifier. The current output can be terminated in either a resistor or the inverting node of an external operational amplifier. Terminating, feedback and bipolar offset resistors are included inside the device and have temperature coefficients which are matched to the gain and current source weighting resistors. In order to obtain the specified overall value of the temperature coefficient for the device, these internal rather than external resistors should be used for offset and scaling adjustments. The values of the internal feedback and bipolar offset resistors are set at less than their corresponding nominal values in order to facilitate the use of external series trim resistors for the adjustment of gain and the bipolar zero offset. The device has a fast settling time of 0·05 per cent in 300 ns. Settling time is defined as the time interval required for the output to settle to within one least significant bit (LSB) of the final value. The accuracy of the conversion is defined as the theoretical value of the equivalent analogue output $\pm\frac{1}{2}$ LSB.

The DAC-10H converter is mounted in a case 51 mm $\times$ 51 mm $\times$ 10 mm (2 in $\times$ 2 in $\times$ 0·4 in). The construction utilizes a silicon monolithic integrated circuit and hybrid thick film construction on a ceramic substrate. The high speed logic-operated switches and associated circuitry are monolithic integrated circuits on a single chip. The integrated circuits also contain the matched components for temperature compensation. In some cases the temperature drift can be as low as ± 5 p.p.m. per degree Centigrade. The switches, in conjunction with the reference circuitry and weighted resistor network, produce the required set of binary weighted currents. The MSB provides a current of 1 mA, which is equal to half the nominal full-scale current, while each successive bit provides half as much current. The unipolar output current of 0 to 2 mA can be converted to a voltage output of 0 to −10 V by the operational amplifier.

TRADITIONAL LOGIC

The processes of traditional logic can be illustrated by considering the categorization of groups of people. A population is divided into arbitrary groups and it is assumed that every person falls into one or more of the chosen categories. If he does not, then he is assumed not to exist.

Taking a particular case, a man can be considered as an engineer (E) or as a non-engineer ($\overline{\text{E}}$). The bar over the E indicates a logical inversion or negation. This is known as the logical NOT function. Thus $\overline{\text{E}}$=NOT E. A man who is not medically qualified but who is an engineer can be described as $\overline{\text{M}}$.E. The dot (.) between $\overline{\text{M}}$ and E refers to the logical AND function, or connection. The AND function is also known as the logical product function that is, $\overline{\text{M}}$.E is a man who is not a doctor AND is an engineer. For each selected group of people there are two possible classifications, for example, doctors and non-doctors or engineers and non-engineers. Considering the groups M and E, the following combinations are possible: M.E., M.$\overline{\text{E}}$, $\overline{\text{M}}$.E. and $\overline{\text{M}}$.$\overline{\text{E}}$.

The Laws of Logic

Using the binary notation a function is said to be true—that is, it exists—if it has the logical value '1'. If it is untrue or does not exist, then it has the logical value '0'. Considering some function A, the following laws can be shown to apply: $A+0=A$, $A.0=0$, $A+1=1$, $A.1=A$, $A+A=A$, $A.A=A$, $A+\overline{A}=1$, $A.\overline{A}=0$.

Whenever equality(=) signs are used in logical equations, they refer to logical equality. This may not have the same meaning as conventional arithmetical equality. Whereas (.) refers to the logical AND function, + refers to the logical OR function. Thus N=M.E is the number of people who are both medically qualified and engineers.

ELECTRICAL ANALOGUES OF THE LOGICAL 'AND' AND 'OR' FUNCTIONS

Consider two switches S_1 and S_2 connected in series (*Figure 14.11a*) and in parallel (*Figure 14.11b*). Let S represent the state of a switch closed and $\bar{S}$ represent an open switch. In the series case, if any one switch is open there is no output and this corresponds to $S.\bar{S}=0$. If both switches are closed, then $S.S=S$, since S is assumed to correspond to the voltage level of logical one. When the switches are

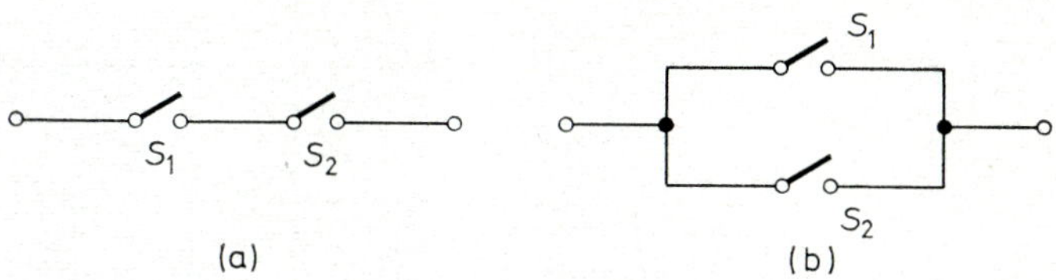

Figure 14.11. Switches connected (a) in series to represent the logical AND function and (b) in parallel to represent the logical OR function

in parallel, only one switch need be closed to secure an ouput, i.e. $S+\bar{S}=S$. Hence it is possible to simulate logical conditions in terms of a pattern of open and closed switches. In practice, conducting diodes or transistors are used in place of switches. A useful introduction to switching logic is that of Kaye (1968).

De Morgan's Theorem

In simplifying the various possible arrangements of switches to satisfy a particular logical function, use is often made of De Morgan's theorem, which states that $\overline{A+B+C}=\bar{A}.\bar{B}.\bar{C}$ and $\overline{A.B.C}=\bar{A}+\bar{B}+\bar{C}$.

Other relationships are the Commutative law $A+B=B+A$ and $A.B=B.A$; the Associative law $A+B+C=(A+B)+C=A+(B+C)$ and $A.B.C.=(A.B).C=A.(B.C)$; and the Distributive law $A+(B.C.D)=(A+B).(A+C).(A+D)$ and $A(B+C+D)=A.B+A.C+A.D$.

Representation of Logical Networks

The logical action of three common 'gate' circuits—NOT, AND and OR—is shown in Figure *14.12*. The term 'gate' is of agricultural origin, since if a gate is open, livestock can pass freely through it. When a logical gate is open, information can flow freely, but not when the gate is closed or inhibited.

Universal Logical Elements

The NOT, AND and OR gates can only perform their own function. This is in contrast to the NOR and NAND gates.

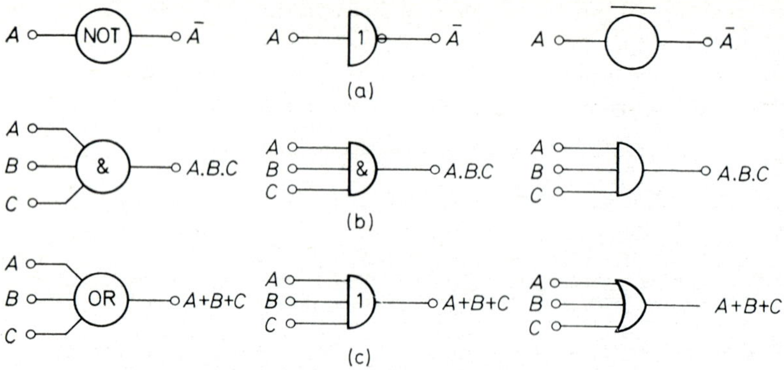

Figure 14.12. The logical action of NOT, AND and OR gates. (a) Old British Standard B.S.530, Supplement No. 5 (1962). (b) British Standard B.S.3939, Section 21. (c) American Standards A.S.A. Y32 14 of 1962

The NOR function is an inverted or negated OR function (NOT OR) so that NOR=$\overline{\text{OR}}$. The generation of the NOR function using an OR and a NOT gate is shown in *Figure 14.13.* The 'truth table' for this arrangement is shown in Table 14.5.

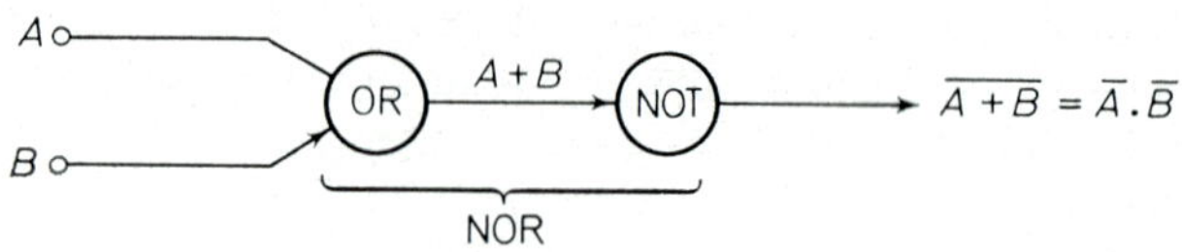

Figure 14.13. Generation of the NOR function using an OR and a NOT gate

Table 14.5

Inputs *A*	*B*	*A+B*	*Output* $\overline{A+B}$
0	0	0	1
0	1	1	0
1	1	1	0
1	1	1	0

The truth table lists the output obtained for all possible combinations of the inputs. The output is zero if a '1' appears at either or both inputs. The output is '1' only when both inputs are zero.

Because of this a NOR gate with a single input acts as a NOT gate (*Figure 14.14*). A pair of NOR gates can also generate an OR function (*Figure 14.15*). Three NOR gates can generate an AND function (*Figure 14.16*), which is an example of De Morgan's theorem.

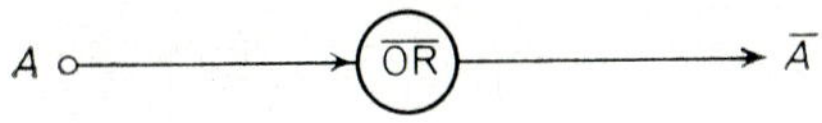

Figure 14.14. A NOR gate with a single input acts as a NOT gate

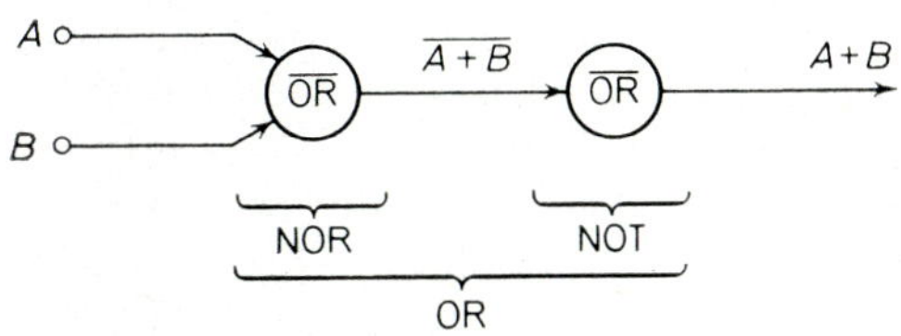

Figure 14.15. A pair of NOR gates generating an OR function

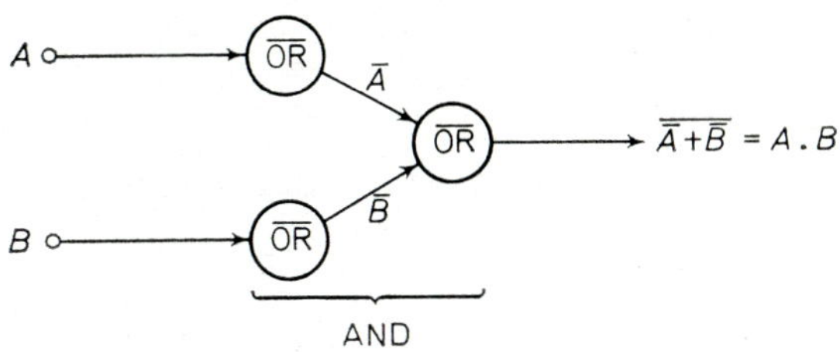

Figure 14.16. The use of three NOR gates to generate an AND function

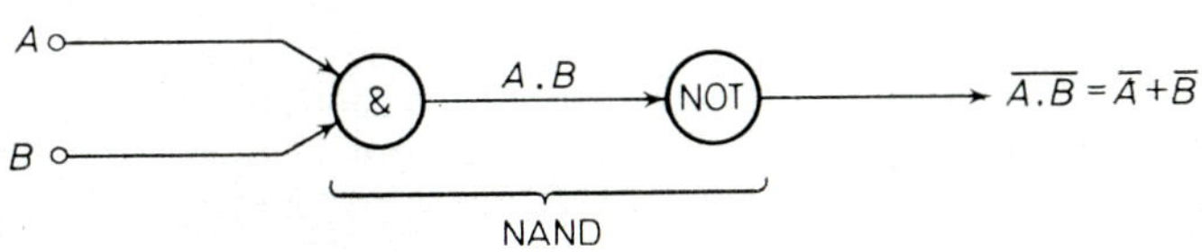

Figure 14.17. The action of a NAND gate

The NAND gate is derived from (NOT AND), i.e. NAND=$\overline{\text{AND}}$ (*Figure 14.17*) (Table 14.6).

Table 14.6

Inputs			*Outputs*
A	*B*	*A.B*	$\overline{A.B}$
0	0	0	1
0	1	0	1
1	0	0	1
1	1	1	0

De Morgan's theorem gives that $\overline{A+B}=\bar{A}.\bar{B}$, so that the output from a NAND gate can be considered as the OR function of the inputs to it. If only one input is used, then the output is $\bar{A}$, so that the NAND gate with a single *input* performs the NOT function (*Figure 14.18*). De Morgan's theorem gives $A+B=\bar{A}.\bar{B}$, so that an OR gate can be obtained from three NAND gates (*Figure 14.19*).

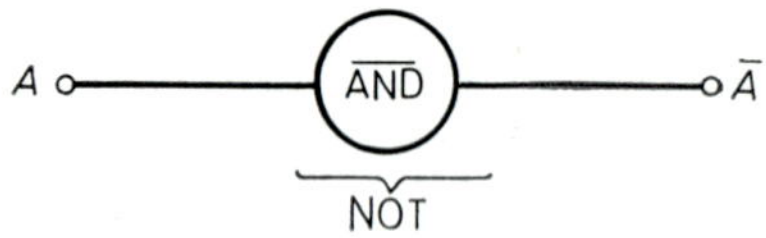

Figure 14.18. A NAND gate with a single input performing a NOT function

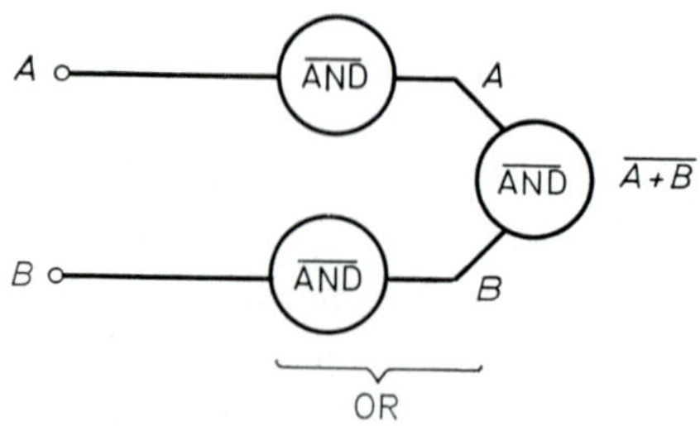

Figure 14.19. The use of three NAND gates to generate an OR function

Karnaugh (1953) describes a very useful 'mapping' method for the simplification of logical functions. Zissos and Copperwhite (1965) deal with the design of NOR/NAND circuits.

Logic Signal Levels

It is convenient to think in terms of a voltage near zero to represent logical '0' and a finite positive voltage to represent logical '1'. This is known as positive logic, since the more positive of the two levels represents logical '1'. In negative logic, a negative voltage is used to represent logical '1'.

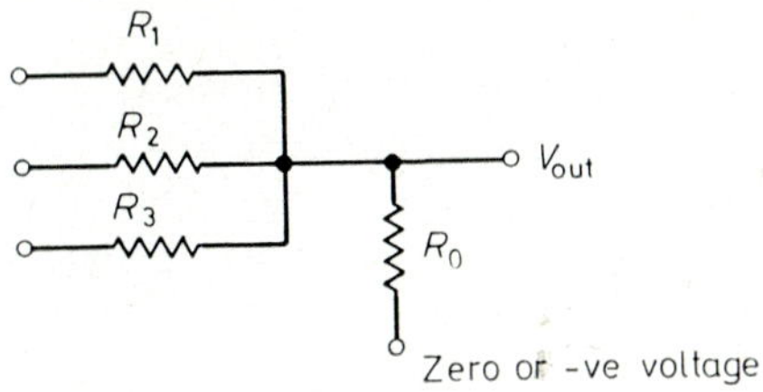

Figure 14.20. A positive logic resistor OR gate

Resistor Logic Gates

Figure 14.20 shows a positive logic resistor OR gate. The values of the input resistors R_1, R_2 and R_3 and the output resistor R_o are chosen so that if one or more of the input lines is at the logical '1' voltage level, the output voltage V_o rises above the minimum voltage level corresponding to logical '1'. When all the inputs are at logical '0', the output voltage falls below the minimum level for logical '1' and is then recognized as logical '0'. When there are X inputs to a logic gate, it is said to have a fan-in of X, and when there are X available outputs it is said to have a fan-out of X. By connecting R_o to a positive potential instead of to earth, the circuit is converted into an AND gate. The output voltage is arranged to stay below the logical '1' level when one or more of the input lines is at logical '0'. The output voltage rises to logical '1' only when all the inputs are at the logical '1' level.

Diode–Resistor Gates

With resistor logic gates, the inputs are always connected to the outputs via a conducting path. Thus the value of the output voltage

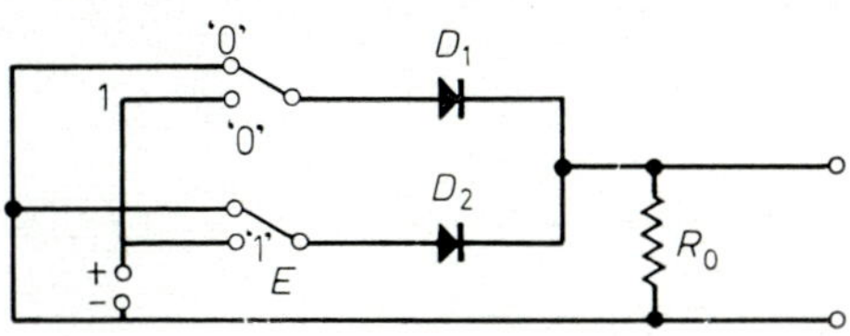

Figure 14.21. A positive logic diode–resistor OR gate

is dependent upon the number of input lines in use. Isolation can be achieved by the use of diodes as shown for a positive logic diode–

resistor OR gate (*Figure 14.21*). When both inputs are earthed, the output is also zero. If input 1 is connected to +E (logical '1'), diode 1 is forward biased and current flows through it and the output resistor R_0.

Since the voltage drop across the diode is now small, V_0 is almost equal to E, and diode 2 is reverse biased so that it is non-conducting. With resistor logic, the input lines at logical '0' reduce the value of the output voltage, but with diode–resistor logic these lines are isolated from the output.

A positive logic diode–resistor AND gate is illustrated in *Figure 14.22*. Connecting one or more of the input lines to the logical '0'

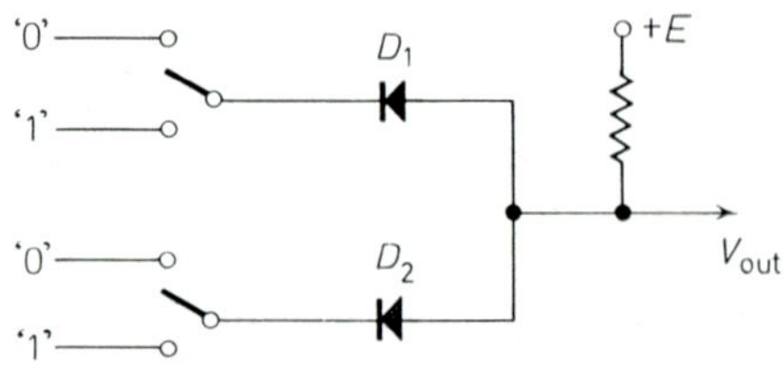

Figure 14.22. A positive logic diode–resistor AND gate

level makes the appropriate diodes conduct. A forward biased silicon junction has a voltage drop across it of about 0·7 V, so that this is the value of the output voltage. Only when both inputs are raised to the logical '1' level will the output voltage be able to attain the logical '1' level.

The truth table for the two gates is given in Table 14.7.

Table 14.7

Input A	*Input B*	*OR gate output*	*AND gate*
0	0	0	0
1	0	1	0
0	1	1	0
1	1	1	1

Resistor–Transistor Logic (*RTL*)

Figure 14.23 is the circuit of a positive logic resistor–transistor NOR gate with a fan-in of X and a fan-out of Y. The OR function is produced by the resistor network and logical inversion is provided by the transistor. The circuit works well provided that $V_{CE(sat)}$ is less than $V_{BE(sat)}$, so that the collector voltage when the transistor is ON is not sufficient to turn ON any transistor connected to it.

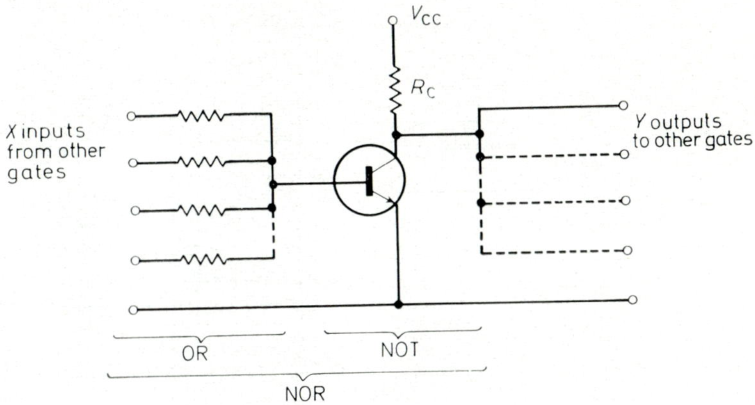

Figure 14.23. A positive logic resistor–transistor NOR gate

This fixes an upper temperature limit for the circuit operation. The most severe operating conditions arise when the transistor is OFF, since it then has to provide an adequate base current to all the connected transistors to maintain them in an ON condition.

Transistor–Transistor Logic (TTL)

The development of monolithic integrated circuits has led to attention being concentrated on TTL logic. This has been facilitated by the ability to lay down multiple emitter transistors on the chip. Referring to *Figure 14.24*, a TTL NAND gate is seen to consist of a multiple emitter transistor input, a phase splitter and a low output impedance totem pole output circuit.

In order to explain the action of the circuit, a simple two-diode model will be used as a substitute for each transistor (*Figure 14.25*). It will be assumed that the voltage drop across a conducting silicon *p–n* junction (diode) is about 0·75 V and that a saturated silicon transistor has an average collector–emitter voltage of 0·4 V. With either input at logical '0' level (0 to 0·8 V), the multiple emitter input transistor will be ON with its base at about 0·75+0·4=1·15 V. The chain of three diodes (*Figure 14.26*) comprising the base–collector diode of Q_1, the base–emitter diode of Q_2 and the base–emitter diode of Q_4 will have only 1·15 V across it, and will only be passing leakage current. To be forward conducting, a total of $3 \times 0{\cdot}75$ V= $2{\cdot}25$ V would be needed. Since an insignificant current flows into the base–emitter junction of Q_2, this transistor will be non-conducting

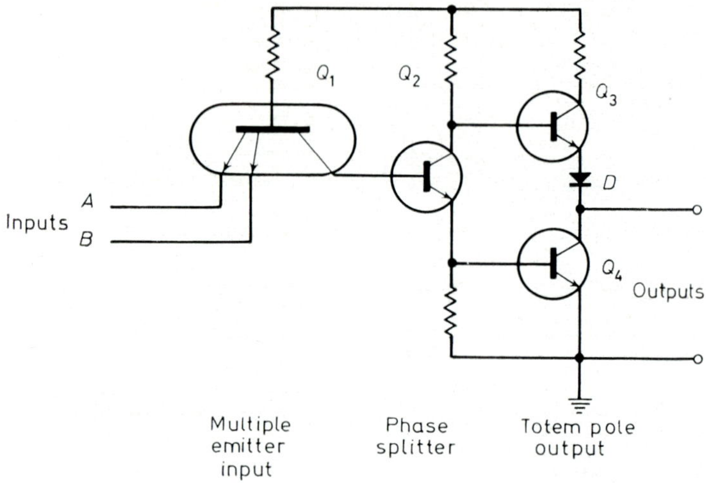

Figure 14.24. An integrated circuit transistor–transistor NAND gate

and its collector–emitter voltage will be high. Similarly for Q_4. Q_3 is now free to raise the output voltage to a high level. If both inputs are at logical '1' level, the diode chain will conduct and there will be a current path to earth through the collector load of Q_1 and the

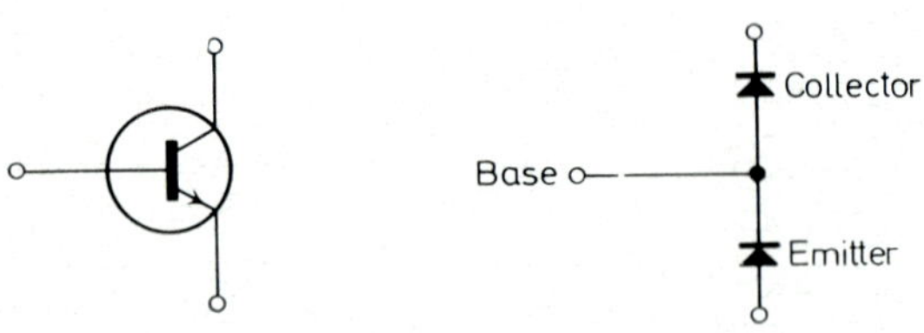

Figure 14.25. Two-diode model of a transistor

diode chain. Enough current flows in the base–emitter junctions of Q_2 and Q_4 to turn them ON. The action of the totem pole is such that when Q_2 is ON, Q_3 is OFF. The fact that Q_4 turns ON pulls the output voltage down to the logical '0' level (0 to 0·4 V). The collector voltage of Q_2 is low and Q_3 is turned OFF. The signal at the emitter of Q_2 switches Q_4, whilst that at its collector switches

Q_3. The use of the two transistors in the output circuit gives a low output impedance and a fast switching speed. Q_3 and Q_4 do not switch ON and OFF instantaneously, so that both will be ON during the change-over period. The addition of diode D improves the

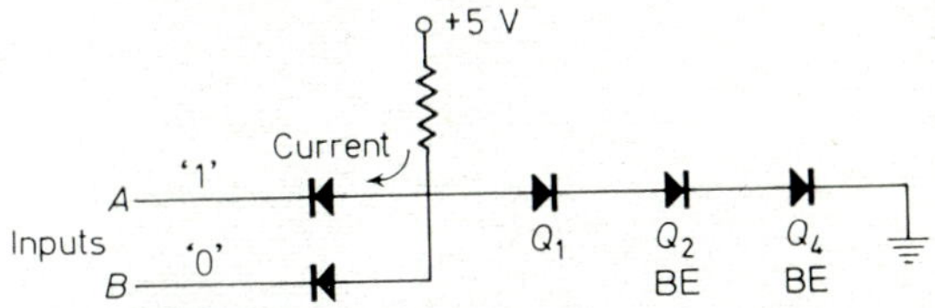

Figure 14.26. Diode equivalent circuit of the NAND gate of Figure 14.24

immunity of the circuit to noise, and its forward voltage drop helps to reduce the amplitude of the current transient produced during switching. When Q_4 is ON, the output impedance is low and approximately equal to the saturation resistance of Q_4. When Q_4 is OFF and Q_3 ON, the output impedance is again low, since now it is approximately equal to the sum of the forward resistance of D and the saturation resistance of Q_3.

Figure 14.27 shows the integrated circuit version of an AND/NOR gate based on the basic elements of a TTL NAND gate. The phase

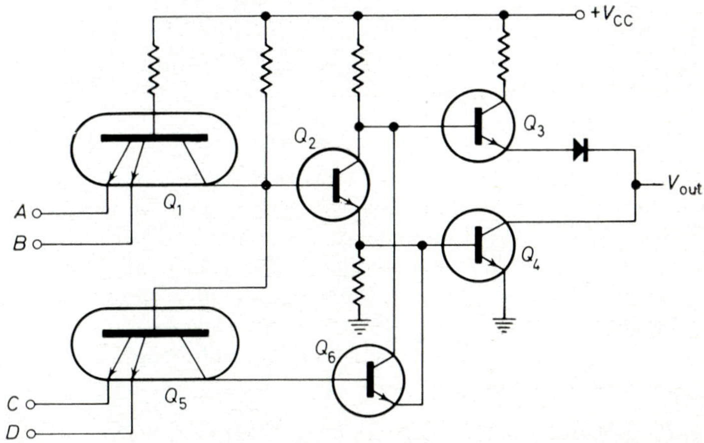

Figure 14.27. Circuit diagram of a positive logic integrated circuit AND/NOR gate

splitter Q_2 is now in parallel with an identical transistor Q_6. Q_6 is also controlled by a multiple emitter transistor. When either of the input pairs is at logical '1' level, the phase inverter acts to switch the output voltage level to logical '0'. With both inputs separate as shown in *Figure 14.28a*, the circuit functions as an AND gate, but if both

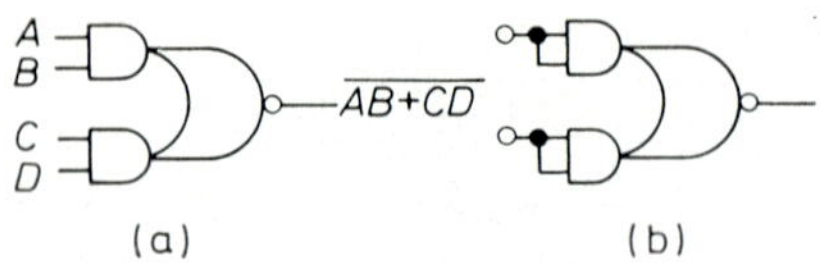

Figure 14.28. The use of the AND/NOR gate (a) as an AND gate and (b) as a NOR gate

AND inputs are connected together as in *Figure 14.28b*, the circuit performs as a NOR gate. *Figure 14.29* shows the voltage levels

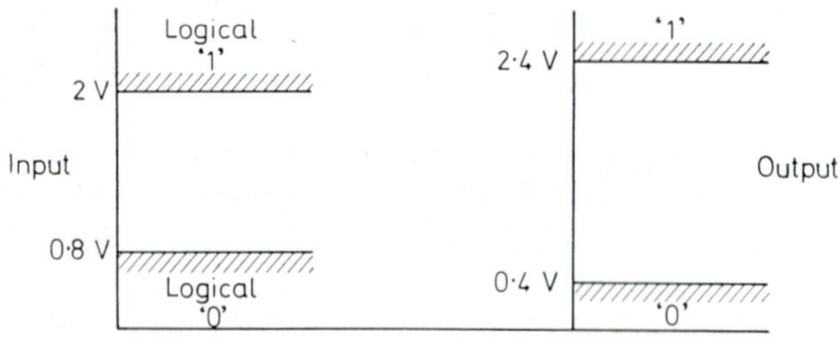

Figure 14.29. Logic circuit voltage levels
(By courtesy of Digital Equipment Corporation)

recommended by the Digital Equipment Corporation for use with their range of logic modules.

Packaging of TTL Logic Elements

Logic elements are commonly arranged in a dual in-line package approximately 19 mm ($\frac{3}{4}$ in) long by 6 mm ($\frac{1}{4}$ in) wide and 3 mm ($\frac{1}{8}$ in) deep. The connection leads enter the body from opposite sides, seven to a side. The spacing between each lead is usually 2·5 mm (0·1 in) and the leads are stiff enough to permit plugging directly into a printed circuit board. Each lead comes out horizontally from the body before being bent at right angles to allow a test probe to be clipped on.

FLIP-FLOPS

Logic gates are often used to steer pulses into counting and sequential networks. It is necessary to provide storage elements to hold, for example, the sum accumulated in a counter. Flip-flops or bistable circuits are often used for this. As has been mentioned in

Chapter 11, a flip-flop has two stable states. These are made to correspond with the logical '0' and '1' levels. It is a device which holds binary information in the form of a '0' or a '1'.

The simplest types of flip-flop take up the state of output A at '1' and output $\bar{A}$ at '0' when a pulse is applied to the set input (*Figure 14.30a*), and of output A at '0' and output $\bar{A}$ at '1' when a pulse is

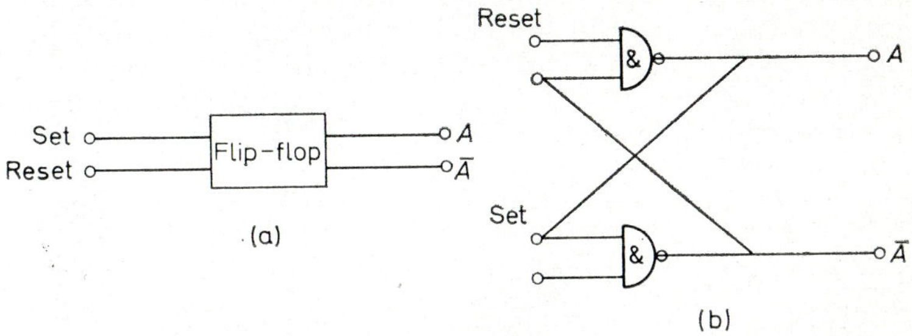

Figure 14.30. (a) Simple set–reset flip-flop. (b) Implementation of a set–reset flip-flop using a pair of NAND gates

applied to the reset input. The arrangement can be implemented by means of a pair of cross-coupled NAND or NOR gates (*Figure 14.30b*). Flip-flops are often connected in series, perhaps via intervening logic gates. This is known as asynchronous operation, since the input to a particular flip-flop in the chain is dependent upon the state of previous flip-flops. This is a ripple-through network. With this simple system there is a possibility, if the states of the flip-flops are read during a change-over, of recording a transient state of '0' '0'.

In synchronous operation, this possibility is avoided by designing the flip-flops so that they all change together on receipt of a common clock pulse.

One well-known form of clocked flip-flop is the J–K flip-flop. This device has the property that a clock pulse will not cause the flip-flop to change states if neither the J nor the K input is at the logical '1' level (enabled) during the presence of the clock pulse. On the other hand, if both the J and the K inputs are enabled during the clock pulse, the flip-flop will change states (complement). With the J–K flip-flop there is no indeterminate state. No change should be permitted in the J or K input when the clock pulse is on unless a change of state in the flip-flop is desired.

The J–K flip-flop consists of a master flip-flop and a slave flip-flop. The logical information present at the J and K inputs during the clock pulse will be passed to the master flip-flop. At the end of the clock pulse on its trailing edge, the information stored on the master flip-flop is transferred to the slave flip-flop. If the *J* input is at logical '1' and the *K* input at logical '0' during the clock pulse, the flip-flop will go to the '1' state on the trailing edge of the clock pulse. On the other hand, if the *J* input is at logical '0' and the *K* input at logical '1', the flip-flop will go to the '0' state on the trailing edge of the clock pulse. If both the *J* and the *K* inputs are at logical '1' before and during the clock pulse, the flip-flop will change states on the trailing edge. Finally, if both inputs are at logical '0', the flip-flop will remain in whatever condition existed prior to the clock pulse. The truth table is shown in Table 14.8.

Table 14.8

Input 1	*Input* 0	*Output* J	*Output* K	*Output after clock pulse* 1	*Output after clock pulse* 0
0	1	0	0	0	1
0	1	0	1	0	1
0	1	1	0	1	0
0	1	1	1	1	0
1	0	0	0	1	0
1	0	0	1	0	1
1	0	1	0	1	0
1	0	1	1	0	1

The logical action of the *J–K* flip-flop can be seen from *Figure 14.31*. The *J* inputs are applied to AND gate 1 and the *K* inputs to AND gate 2. When $J=K=0$, both AND gates are inhibited and the output of the flip-flop does not change. When $J=K=1$, the flip-flop output changes state on the end of each clock pulse. When $J=A=1$ and $K=\bar{A}=0$, both the AND gates are inhibited and there

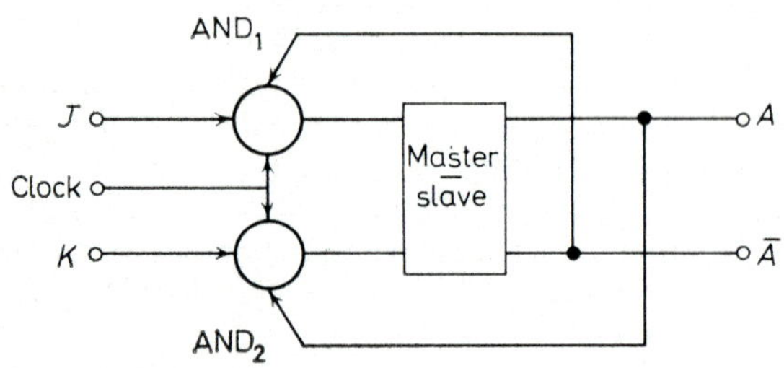

Figure 14.31. Logical action of a J–K flip-flop

is no output change. When $J = \bar{A}$, one of the AND gates is opened and the input conditions are transferred to the master–slave network. Binary coded decimal counters can be formed from a series of J–K flip-flops. Biwas (1966) discusses the design of counters using flip-flops.

REFERENCES

Biwas, N. N. (1966). 'The logic and input equations of flip-flops.' *Electron. Engng* **38,** 107.

Hartley, M. G. (1962). *An Introduction to Electronic Analogue Computers.* London: Methuen.

Kaye, D. (1968). *Boolean Systems.* London: Longmans Green.

Karnaugh, M. (1953). 'The map method for synthesis of combinational logic circuits.' *Communs Electron., Lond.* **9,** 539.

Macy, J. (1965). 'Analog–digital conversion systems.' In *Computers in Medical Research,* Vol. 2. Ed. by R. W. Stacy and B. Watson. New York: Academic Press.

Zissos, D. and Copperwhite, G. W. (1965). 'The design of minimal NOR/NAND logical circuits.' *Electron. Engng* **37,** 592.

Index